MW01165882

Disclaimer Notice:

Please note the information contained within this document is for educational and entertainment purposes only. All effort has been executed to present accurate, up to date, reliable, complete information. No warranties of any kind are declared or implied. Readers acknowledge that the author is not engaged in the rendering of legal, financial, medical, or professional advice. The content within this book has been derived from various sources. Please consult a licensed professional before attempting any techniques outlined in this book.

By reading this document, the reader agrees that under no circumstances is the author responsible for any losses, direct or indirect, that are incurred as a result of the use of the information contained within this document, including, but not limited to, errors, omissions, or inaccuracies.

CONTENTS

INTRODUCTION

The DASH diet focuses on long-term healthy eating habits. The diet doesn't force you to starve or battle constant cravings. Instead, it focuses on understanding food groups, controlling portion sizes, and making sure you get the optimal levels of potassium, calcium, magnesium, fiber, and protein.

The diet focuses certain food groups for specific reasons: Fruits and vegetables give you the magnesium and potassium your body needs, and low-fat dairy products provide calcium. Every food you eat should have a purpose, and that's the most important principle of the DASH diet: eat well so you feel well. Here are some additional points to remember when you're following the DASH principles:

Reduce your sodium intake. The diet recommends less than 2,300 mg of sodium per day. The National Heart, Lung and Blood Institute recommends lowering the sodium intake even further—to 1,500 mg—for people with high blood pressure, people with diabetes or chronic kidney disease, African Americans, and people aged 51 and over.

Eat fruits, vegetables, and low-fat dairy products

Focus on high-fiber foods

Eat more healthy fats, which are good for your heart, instead of saturated fats

Achieve and maintain a healthy body weight

Eat a lot of potassium and magnesium

Stay hydrated by drinking plenty of plain water

Avoid smoking

The DASH diet is more than just a diet—it's a lifestyle.

BREAKFAST

01. Shrimp Skillet

Preparation time: 10 minutes
Cooking time: 25 minutes
Servings: 5
Ingredients:
- 2 bell peppers
- 1 red onion
- 1-pound shrimps, peeled
- ½ teaspoon ground coriander
- ½ teaspoon white pepper
- ½ teaspoon paprika
- 1 tablespoon butter

Directions:
1. Remove the seeds from the bell peppers and cut the vegetable into the wedges.
2. Then place them in the skillet.
3. Add peeled shrimps, white pepper, paprika, and butter.
4. Peel and slice the red onion. Add it in the skillet too.
5. Preheat the oven to 365F.
6. Cover the skillet with foil and secure the edges.
7. Transfer it in the preheated oven and cook for 20 minutes.
8. When the time is over, discard the foil and cook the dish for 5 minutes more -use ventilation mode if you have.
Nutrition Values: calories 153, fat 4, fiber 1.3, carbs 7.3, protein 21.5

02. Coconut Yogurt with Chia Seeds

Preparation time: 2 hours
Cooking time: 10 minutes
Servings: 4
Ingredients:
- 1 probiotic capsule -yogurt capsule
- 1 cup of coconut milk
- 1 tablespoon coconut meat
- 4 tablespoons chia seeds

Directions:
1. Por coconut milk in the saucepan and preheat it till 108F.
2. Then add a probiotic capsule and stir well. Close the lid and leave the coconut milk for 40 minutes.
3. Meanwhile, shred coconut meat.
4. When the time is over, transfer the almond milk mixture into the cheesecloth and squeeze it. Leave it like this for 40 minutes more or untilof the liquid from yogurt is squeezed.
5. After this, transfer the yogurt into the serving glasses.
6. Add chia seeds and coconut meat in every glass and mix up well.

7. Let the cooked yogurt rest for 10 minutes before serving.
Nutrition Values: calories 177, fat 16.9, fiber 3.9, carbs 6.5, protein 2.6

03. Chia Pudding

Preparation time: 15 minutes
Cooking time: 3 minutes
Servings: 4
Ingredients:
- 2 cups almond milk
- 8 tablespoons chia seeds
- 1 oz blackberries
- 1 tablespoon Erythritol

Directions:
1. Preheat almond milk for 3 minutes, then remove it from the heat and add chia seeds.
2. Stir gently and add Erythritol. Mix it up.
3. In the bottom om serving glasses put blackberries.
4. Then pour almond milk mixture over berries. Let the pudding rest for at least 10 minutes before serving.
Nutrition Values: calories 331, fat 31.9, fiber 6.7, carbs 11.8, protein 4.6

04. Egg Fat Bombs

Preparation time: 10 minutes
Cooking time: 10 minutes
Servings: 4
Ingredients:
- 4 oz bacon, sliced
- 4 eggs, boiled
- 1 tablespoon butter, softened
- ½ teaspoon salt
- ½ teaspoon ground black pepper
- 1 tablespoonmayonnaise

Directions:
1. Line the tray with the baking paper. Place the bacon on the paper.
2. Preheat the oven to 365F and put the tray inside.
3. Cook the bacon for 10 minutes or until it is light brown.
4. Meanwhile, peeled and chop the boiled eggs and transfer them in the mixing bowl.
5. Add ground black pepper, mayonnaise, and salt.
6. When the bacon is cooked, chill it little and finely chop.
7. Add bacon in the egg mixture. Stir it well.
8. Add softened butter and mix up it again.
9. With the help of the scoop make medium size balls. Before serving, place them in the fridge for 10 minutes.
Nutrition Values: calories 255, fat 20.3, fiber 0.1, carbs 1.2, protein 16.1

05. Morning "Grits"

Preparation time: 10 minutes
Cooking time: 10 minutes
Servings: 4
Ingredients:
- 1 ½ cup almond milk
- 1 cup heavy cream, whipped
- 4 tablespoon chia seeds
- 3 oz Parmesan, grated
- ½ teaspoon chili flakes
- ½ teaspoon salt
- 1 tablespoon butter

Directions:
1. Pour almond milk in the saucepan and bring it to boil.
2. Meanwhile, grind the chia seeds with the help of the coffee grinder.
3. Remove the almond milk from the heat and add grinded chia seeds.
4. Add whipped cream, chili flakes, and salt. Stir it well and leave for 5 minutes.
5. After this, add butter and grated Parmesan. Stir well and preheat it over the low heat until the cheese is melted.
6. Stir it again and transfer in the serving bowls.

Nutrition Values: calories 439, fat 42.2, fiber 4.4, carbs 9.6, protein 10.7

06. Scotch Eggs

Preparation time: 15 minutes
Cooking time: 15 minutes
Servings: 4
Ingredients:
- 4 eggs, boiled
- 1 ½ cup ground beef
- 1 tablespoon onion, grated
- ½ teaspoon ground black pepper
- ½ teaspoon salt
- ½ teaspoon dried oregano
- ½ teaspoon dried basil
- 1 tablespoon butter
- ¾ cup of water

Directions:
1. In the mixing bowl, mix up together ground beef, grated onion, ground black pepper, salt, dried oregano, and basil.
2. Peel the boiled eggs.
3. Make 4 balls from the ground beef mixture.
4. Put peeled eggs inside every ground beef ball and press them gently to get the shape of eggs.
5. Spread the tray with the butter and place ground beef eggs on it.
6. Add water.
7. Preheat oven to 365F and transfer the tray inside.
8. Cook the dish for 15 minutes or until each side of Scotch eggs is light brown.

Nutrition Values: calories 188, fat 13.4, fiber 0.2, carbs 0.9, protein 15.4

07. Bacon Sandwich

Preparation time: 15 minutes
Cooking time: 20 minutes
Servings: 2
Ingredients:
- 1 oz bacon, sliced -4 slices
- 4 eggs, separated
- 2 teaspoons ricotta cheese
- ¾ teaspoon cream of tartar
- 1 teaspoon flax meal, ground
- 2 lettuce leaves

Directions:
1. Whisk the eggs yolks with 1 teaspoon of ricotta cheese until you get a soft and light fluffy mixture.
2. After this, whip together egg whites with remaining ricotta cheese, salt, and cream of tartar. When the mixture is fluffy, add ground flax meal and stir gently.
3. Preheat the oven to 310F.
4. Gently combine together egg yolk mixture and egg white mixture.
5. Line the tray with baking paper.
6. Make the 4 medium size clouds from the egg mixture using the spoon.
7. Transfer the tray in the oven and cook them for 20 minutes or until they are light brown.
8. Meanwhile, place bacon slices in the skillet and roast them for 1 minute from each side over the medium-high heat.
9. Chill the bacon little.
10. Transfer the cooked and chilled egg clouds on the plate.
11. Place bacon onto 2 clouds and then add lettuce leaves. Cover them with the remaining egg clouds.
12. Secure the sandwiches with toothpicks and transfer in the serving plate.

Nutrition Values: calories 218, fat 15.5, fiber 0.4, carbs 2.3, protein 17.2

08. Noatmeal

Preparation time: 10 minutes
Cooking time: 10 minutes
Servings: 3
Ingredients:
- 1 cup organic almond milk
- 2 tablespoons hemp seeds
- 1 tablespoon chia seeds, dried
- 1 tablespoon Erythritol
- 1 tablespoon almond flakes
- 2 tablespoons coconut flour
- 1 tablespoon flax meal
- 1 tablespoon walnuts, chopped
- ½ teaspoon vanilla extract
- ¼ teaspoon ground cinnamon

Directions:

1.   Put all the ingredients except vanilla extract in the saucepan and stir gently.
2.   Cook the mixture on the low heat for 10 minutes. Stir it constantly.
3.   When the mixture starts to be thick, add vanilla extract. Mix it up.
4.   Remove the noatmeal from the heat and let it rest little.
Nutrition Values: calories 350, fat 30.4, fiber 8.4, carbs 16.9, protein 9.1

09. Breakfast Bake with Meat

Preparation time: 10 minutes
Cooking time: 30 minutes
Servings: 4
Ingredients:
- 1 cup ground beef
- 1 cup cauliflower, shredded
- ½ cup coconut cream
- 1 onion, diced
- 1 teaspoon butter
- ½ teaspoon salt
- ½ teaspoon paprika
- ½ teaspoon garam masala
- 1 tablespoon fresh cilantro, chopped
- 1 oz celery root, grated
- 1 oz Cheddar cheese, grated

Directions:
1.   Mix up together garam masala mixture, celery root, paprika, salt, and ground beef.
2.   Mix up together shredded cauliflower and salt.
3.   Spread the casserole tray with butter.
4.   Make the layer of the ground beef mixture inside the casserole tray.
5.   Then place the layer of the cauliflower mixture and diced onion.
6.   Sprinkle it with grated cheese and fresh cilantro, Add coconut cream.
7.   Cover the surface of the casserole with the foil and secure the lids.
8.   Preheat the oven to 365F.
9.   Place the casserole tray in the oven and cook it for 30 minutes.
10.   When the time is over, transfer the casserole from the oven, remove the foil and let it chill for 15 minutes.
11.   Cut it into the serving and transfer in the serving bowls.
Nutrition Values: calories 192, fat 14.7, fiber 2.1, carbs 6.5, protein 10

10. Breakfast Bagel

Preparation time: 15 minutes
Cooking time: 30 minutes
Servings: 3
Ingredients:
- ½ cup almond flour
- 1 ½ teaspoon xanthan gum
- 1 egg, beaten
- 3 oz Parmesan, grated
- ½ teaspoon cumin seeds
- 1 teaspoon cream cheese
- 1 teaspoon butter, melted

Directions:
1.   In the mixing bowl, mix up together almond flour, xanthan gum, and egg.
2.   Stir it until homogenous.
3.   Put the cheese in the separate bowl, add cream cheese.
4.   Microwave the mixture until it is melted. Stir it well.
5.   Combine together cheese mixture and almond flour mixture and knead the dough.
6.   Roll the dough into the log.
7.   Cut the log into 3 pieces and make bagels.
8.   Line the tray with baking paper and place bagels on it.
9.   Brush the meal with melted butter and sprinkle with cumin seeds.
10.   Preheat the oven to 365F.
11.   Put the tray with bagels in the oven and cook 30 minutes.
12.   Check if the bagels are cooked with the help of the toothpicks.
13.   Cut the bagels and spread them with your favoritespread.
Nutrition Values: calories 262, fat 18.6, fiber 8.7, carbs 12, protein 15.1

11. Egg and Vegetable Hash

Preparation time: 8 minutes
Cooking time: 20 minutes
Servings: 6
Ingredients:
- 4 eggs
- 1 white onion, diced
- 6 oz turnip, chopped
- 2 bell peppers, chopped
- 1 garlic clove, peeled, diced
- 1 jalapeno pepper, sliced
- 5 oz Swiss cheese, grated
- 1 tablespoon lemon juice
- 1 tablespoon canola oil
- ½ teaspoon Taco seasoning

Directions:
1.   Beat the eggs in the bowl and whisk gently.
2.   Then pour canola oil in the pan and preheat it.
3.   Add chopped turnips and white onion. Mix up the vegetables and cook them for 5 minutes over the medium heat. Stir them from time to time.
4.   Then add diced garlic and chopped peppers.
5.   Sprinkle the vegetables with taco seasoning and mix up well.
6.   Add lemon juice and close the lid. Cook it for 5 minutes more.
7.   Then pour the whisked egg mixture over the vegetables. Sprinkle with the grated cheese.

8.   Close the lid and cook it on the low heat for 10 minutes.
9.   It is recommended to serve the dish hot.
Nutrition Values: calories 184, fat 12, fiber 1.5, carbs 8.7, protein 11

12. Cowboy Skillet

Preparation time: 5 minutes
Cooking time: 15 minutes
Servings: 4
Ingredients:
- 1 cup rutabaga, chopped
- 3 eggs, whisked
- ½ cup fresh cilantro, chopped
- 6 oz chorizo, chopped
- ½ teaspoon cayenne pepper
- 1 tablespoon olive oil
- ¾ cup heavy cream

Directions:
1.   Put rutabaga in the skillet. Add olive oil and chorizo.
2.   Mix the mixture up and close the lid. Cook it for 5 minutes over the medium heat.
3.   When rutabaga becomes tender, add whisked eggs and chopped cilantro.
4.   Add heavy cream and stir the meal with the help of a spatula.
5.   Close the lid and saute it for 10 minutes over the medium-low heat.
Nutrition Values: calories 362, fat 31.5, fiber 1, carbs 4.7, protein 15.4

13. Feta Quiche

Preparation time: 15 minutes
Cooking time: 25 minutes
Servings: 8
Ingredients:
- 8 oz Feta cheese, crumbled
- 5 eggs, whisked
- 1 cup spinach, chopped
- 1 garlic clove, diced
- 1 white onion, diced
- 1 teaspoon butter
- 5 oz Mozzarella, chopped
- ½ teaspoon chili flakes
- 1 teaspoon paprika
- ½ teaspoon white pepper
- ½ cup whipped cream

Directions:
1.   Toss butter in the skillet and preheat it.
2.   Add diced garlic and onion and cook it over the medium heat until the vegetables are soft.
3.   Transfer the cooked vegetables in the mixing bowl. Add crumbled cheese, whisked eggs, spinach, chopped Mozzarella, chili flakes, paprika, white pepper, and whipped cream.
4.   Mix the mixture well and transfer in the non-sticky mold. Flatten it gently with the spatula.
5.   Place the mold in the preheated to 365F oven and cook quiche for 25 minutes.

6.   Chill the quiche little and then cut into the servings.
Nutrition Values: calories 198, fat 14.7, fiber 0.5, carbs 4, protein 13

14. Bacon Pancakes

Preparation time: 10 minutes
Cooking time: 10 minutes
Servings: 2
Ingredients:
- 3 oz bacon, chopped
- ½ cup almond flour
- ¾ cup heavy cream
- ½ teaspoon baking powder
- ¼ teaspoon salt
- 1 egg, whisked

Directions:
1.   Place the chopped bacon in the skillet and cook it for 5-6 minutes over the medium-high heat. The cooked bacon should be a little bit crunchy.
2.   Meanwhile, mix up together almond flour, heavy cream, salt, baking powder, and whisked egg. When the mixture is smooth, the batter is cooked.
3.   Add the cooked bacon in the batter and stir it gently with the help of the spoon.
4.   Don't clean the skillet after t bacon. Ladle the bacon batter in the skillet and make the pancake.
5.   Cook it for 1 minute from one side and then flip onto another side.
6.   Cook it for 1.5 minutes more.
7.   Make the same steps with the remaining batter.
8.   Transfer the pancakes on the serving plate.
Nutrition Values: calories 458, fat 40.1, fiber 0.8, carbs 4.1, protein 20.9

15. Waffles

Preparation time: 10 minutes
Cooking time: 10 minutes
Servings: 4
Ingredients:
- 2 tablespoon butter, melted
- 4 eggs, whisked
- 1 teaspoon baking powder
- 1 teaspoon lemon juice
- 1 cup almond flour
- ½ teaspoon vanilla extract
- 1 tablespoon Erythritol
- ¾ cup organic almond milk

Directions:
1.   In the mixing bowl combine together all the ingredients.
2.   Whisk the smooth and homogenous batter.
3.   Preheat the waffle maker well.
4.   Pour enough of the batter in the waffle maker. Flatten it gently to get a waffle. Close it and cook until lightly golden.
5.   Repeat the same steps with all remaining batter.
6.   Serve the waffles warm.

Nutrition Values: calories 167, fat 13.7, fiber 1, carbs 3, protein 7.4

16. Chocolate Shake

Preparation time: 10 minutes
Servings: 4
Ingredients:
- 2 cups heavy cream, whipped
- 1 tablespoon cocoa powder
- 1 tablespoon peanut butter
- ½ cup of coconut milk
- 2 tablespoons Erythritol
- ½ teaspoon vanilla extract

Directions:
1. Mix up together coconut milk and whipped heavy cream.
2. Add cocoa powder and mix it with the help of the hand mixer.
3. When the liquid is homogenous, add peanut butter, vanilla extract, and Erythritol.
4. Whisk it well.
5. Pour the chocolate shake in the serving glasses.

Nutrition Values: calories 304, fat 31.5, fiber 1.3, carbs 4.9, protein 3.2

17. Rolled Omelette with Mushrooms

Preparation time: 10 minutes
Cooking time: 20 minutes
Servings: 3
Ingredients:
- 1 cup mushrooms, chopped
- ½ white onion, sliced
- ½ teaspoon tomato paste
- 2 tablespoons water
- ½ teaspoon salt
- ½ teaspoon cayenne pepper
- ¾ teaspoon chili flakes
- 3 eggs, beaten
- 1 tablespoon cream cheese
- 1 teaspoon butter
- 1 teaspoon avocado oil

Directions:
1. Pour olive oil in the skillet and preheat it.
2. Add chopped mushrooms and sliced onion.
3. Then add tomato paste and water. Stir the ingredients and saute them with the closed lid for 10 minutes.
4. Transfer the cooked vegetables in the mixing bowl.
5. Whisk together cream cheese, eggs, chili flakes, cayenne pepper, and salt.
6. Toss butter in the skillet and melt it.
7. Add egg mixture. Close the lid.
8. Cook it for 10 minutes over the medium-low heat.
9. Then spread the mushroom mixture over the cooked omelet and roll it.
10. Cut the cooked meal into 3 parts and transfer on the serving plates.

Nutrition Values: calories 102, fat 7.1, fiber 0.8, carbs 3.4, protein 6.8

18. Quiche Lorraine

Preparation time: 15 minutes
Cooking time: 18 minutes
Servings: 6
Ingredients:
- 1/3 cup butter, softened
- 1 cup almond flour
- ½ teaspoon salt
- 1 oz bacon, chopped
- 1 white onion, diced
- 1/3 cup heavy cream
- 5 oz Swiss cheese, grated
- 2 eggs, whisked
- ½ teaspoon ground black pepper
- 1 teaspoon olive oil

Directions:
1. Make the quiche crust: combine together softened butter, almond flour, and salt. Knead the dough. Roll it up.
2. Place it in the pie pan and flatten to get pie crust. Pin it with the help of the fork.
3. Preheat the oven to 360F and put the pan with pie crust inside. Cook it for 18 minutes.
4. Meanwhile, pour olive oil in the skillet.
5. Add diced onion and chopped bacon. Cook the ingredients for 5-6 minutes or until they are soft.
6. When the pie crust is cooked, remove it from the oven and chill little.
7. Spread it with the onion mixture and sprinkle with Swiss cheese.
8. Then combine together whisked eggs and heavy cream.
9. Pour the liquid over the cheese.
10. Transfer the pie in the oven and cook for 10 minutes at 355F.
11. Chill the cooked quiche well and cut into the servings.

Nutrition Values: calories 291, fat 25.8, fiber 0.9, carbs 4.5, protein 11.4

19. Shakshuka

Preparation time: 10 minutes
Cooking time: 20 minutes
Servings: 2
Ingredients:
- 1 tomato, diced
- 1 tablespoon tomato paste
- ¾ cup of water
- 1 teaspoon butter
- 1 white onion, diced
- 1 cup mushrooms, sliced
- 1 bell pepper, chopped
- ½ teaspoon salt
- ½ teaspoon sumac
- ½ teaspoon chili flakes

Directions:

1. Put butter in the pan and melt it.
2. Add diced onion and mushrooms. Saute the vegetables for 4 minutes.
3. Then add diced tomato, water, and tomato paste. Sprinkle the mixture with chopped pepper, salt, sumac, and chili flakes.
4. Mix it up and saute for 10 minutes.
5. Then beat eggs over the vegetables and close the lid. Cook the meal for 5 minutes over the medium heat.
6. Serve it immediately or leave the meal for 10 minutes with the closed lid.
Nutrition Values: calories 78, fat 2.3, fiber 3, carbs 13.5, protein 3

20. Breakfast Zucchini Bread

Preparation time: 15 minutes
Cooking time: 50 minutes
Servings: 8
Ingredients:
- ½ cup walnuts, chopped
- 1 teaspoon baking powder
- 1 tablespoon lemon juice
- 1 tablespoon flax meal
- 1 ½ cup almond flour
- 1 zucchini, grated
- 1 teaspoon xanthan gum
- 1 tablespoon butter, melted
- 3 eggs, beaten
- 1 teaspoon salt

Directions:
1. Preheat oven to 360F.
2. In the mixing bowl, combine all wet ingredients. Whisk the mixture well.
3. Then add baking powder, flax meal, almond flour, zucchini, xanthan gum, and salt.
4. Mix up the mixture. Add chopped walnuts and stir it well. You will get a liquid but thick dough. Check if you add all the ingredients.
5. Transfer the dough into the non-sticky loaf mold and flatten its surface with the spatula.
6. Place the bread in the oven and cook for 50 minutes.
7. Check if the bread cooked with the help of the toothpick -if it is clean – the bread is cooked.
8. Remove the zucchini bread from the oven and chill well, Then remove it from the mold and let it chill totally.
9. Slice it.
Nutrition Values: calories 123, fat 10.7, fiber 1.6, carbs 3.4, protein 5.6

21. Granola

Preparation time: 10 minutes
Cooking time: 25 minutes
Servings: 3
Ingredients:
- 4 tablespoons walnuts
- 3 tablespoons pecans
- 3 tablespoons hazelnuts
- 1 tablespoon chia seeds
- 2 tablespoons pumpkin seeds
- 2 tablespoons flax meal
- 1 tablespoon coconut shred
- 1 tablespoon Erythritol
- 2 tablespoons almond butter
- 1 tablespoon peanut butter

Directions:
1. Chop walnuts, pecans, hazelnuts, pumpkin seeds, and transfer in the mixing bowl.
2. Add chia seeds, flax meal coconut shred, Erythritol, almond butter, and peanut butter. Mix up the mixture. The mass should be sticky.
3. Preheat the oven to 300F.
4. Line the tray with parchment.
5. Transfer the nut mixture in the parchment and flatten it into the layer.
6. Place the tray in the oven and cook it for 25 minutes.
7. When the time is over, remove the tray from oven and chill granola.
8. Brake it into medium size pieces. Store granola in the glass jar with the closed lid.
Nutrition Values: calories 373, fat 34.5, fiber 7.4, carbs 11.7, protein 11.6

22. Cheddar Souffle

Preparation time: 10 minutes
Cooking time: 25 minutes
Servings: 2
Ingredients:
- 2 oz Cheddar cheese, grated
- ½ teaspoon ground black pepper
- ½ teaspoon salt
- ½ cup almond milk
- ½ onion
- 1 bay leaf
- ¼ teaspoon peppercorn
- 1 tablespoon coconut shred
- 2 teaspoon butter, melted
- 2 eggs
- 1 teaspoon coconut oil
- ½ teaspoon paprika

Directions:
1. Brush the ramekins with coconut oil and sprinkle with coconut shred.
2. Then pour almond milk in the saucepan. Add onion and peppercorns.
3. Bring it to boil.
4. Remove onion and peppercorns.
5. Toss butter in the pan and add the almond flour. Stir it well until smooth.
6. Add salt, ground black pepper, and paprika. Mix up well.
7. After this, separate egg yolk and egg whites.
8. Add egg yolks in the almond flour mixture. Stir it well.
9. Add almond milk and start to preheat it. Stir it all the time until the mixture is smooth.

10. After this, whisk the egg whites till the strong peaks.
11. Add grated Cheddar in the almond flour mixture. Mix it up.
12. Then chill the mixture little.
13. Add egg whites and mix up gently.
14. Preheat the oven to 365F.
15. Place the cheese mixture into the prepared ramekins and transfer on the tray.
16. Put the tray in the preheated oven and cook for 15 minutes.
17. When the souffle is cooked, it will have a light brown color.
Nutrition Values: calories 384, fat 34.3, fiber 2.4, carbs 7.6, protein 14.5

23. Mediterranean Omelette

Preparation time: 5 minutes
Cooking time: 10 minutes
Servings: 2
Ingredients:
- 3 eggs, beaten
- 1 tablespoon ricotta cheese
- 2 oz feta cheese, chopped
- 1 tomato, chopped
- 1 teaspoon butter
- ½ teaspoon salt
- 1 tablespoon scallions, chopped

Directions:
1. Mix up together ricotta cheese and eggs. Add salt and scallions.
2. Toss butter in the skillet and melt it.
3. Pour ½ part of whisked egg mixture in the skillet and cook it for 5-6 minutes or until it is solid - the omelet is cooked.
4. Then transfer omelet in the plate.
5. Make the second omelet with the remaining egg mixture.
6. Sprinkle each omelet with Feta and tomatoes. Roll them.
Nutrition Values: calories 203, fat 15.2, fiber 0.5, carbs 3.5, protein 13.6

24. Chicken Fritters

Preparation time: 10 minutes
Cooking time: 8 minutes
Servings: 4
Ingredients:
- 1-pound chicken fillet, finely chopped
- 2 tablespoons almond flour
- 1 egg, beaten
- 1 teaspoon dried dill
- 1 teaspoon dried oregano
- ½ teaspoon salt
- 1 teaspoon minced garlic
- 1 tablespoon olive oil

Directions:
1. Put finely chopped chicken fillet and almond flour in the mixing bowl.
2. Add beaten egg, dried dill, oregano, salt, and minced garlic. Mix it up.
3. Make the fritters.
4. Pour olive oil in the skillet and preheat it until hot.
5. Add fritters and cook them for 4 minutes from each side over the medium heat.
6. Dry the fritters with the help of the paper towel and transfer on the serving bowl.
Nutrition Values: calories 284, fat 14.8, fiber 0.6, carbs 1.4, protein 35.1

25. Eggs in Portobello Mushroom Hats

Preparation time: 10 minutes
Cooking time: 15 minutes
Servings: 2
Ingredients:
- 4 Portobello caps
- 4 quail eggs
- ½ teaspoon dried parsley
- ¾ teaspoon salt
- 1 teaspoon butter, melted

Directions:
1. Brush Portobello caps with melted butter from all sides.
2. Line the tray with baking paper.
3. Put Portobello caps on the tray.
4. Beat the quail eggs into the mushroom caps and sprinkle them with salt and dried parsley.
5. Transfer the tray in the preheated to the 355F oven. Cook the mushrooms for 15 minutes.
6. Chill the meal little and transfer on the serving plates.
Nutrition Values: calories 46, fat 3.9, fiber 0, carbs 0.2, protein 2.4

26. Matcha Fat Bombs

Preparation time: 15 minutes
Servings: 12
Ingredients:
- ½ cup cashew butter
- 1 cup coconut butter
- ¼ cup coconut cream
- 2 tablespoons matcha green tea
- ¼ teaspoon ground cinnamon
- ½ cup coconut shred

Directions:
1. Put the cashew butter, coconut butter, coconut cream, ½ tablespoon of matcha green tea, and ground cinnamon in the mixing bowl.
2. Blend the mixture with the hand blender until you get homogenous and fluffy mass.
3. In the separated bowl, combine together coconut shred and remaining matcha green tea.
4. Make the balls from the coconut butter mixture with the help of the scooper.
5. Then coat every ball in the coconut shred green mixture.
6. Transfer the meal on the plates and store them in the cold place -fridge.

Nutrition Values: calories 222, fat 20.7, fiber 4.1, carbs 9.2, protein 3.6

27. Smoothie Bowl

Preparation time: 7 minutes
Servings: 3
Ingredients:
- 1 teaspoon pumpkin seeds
- 1 teaspoon sunflower seeds
- ½ cup blackberries
- 1 cup almond milk
- ¼ cup coconut cream
- 2 tablespoons Erythritol
- 1 tablespoon Protein powder
- ½ teaspoon of cocoa powder

Directions:
1.   Blend together almond milk, coconut cream, blackberries, Erythritol, and protein powder.
2.   When the mixture is smooth, add cocoa powder and pulse it for 30 seconds more.
3.   Pour the liquid into the serving small bowls.
4.   Sprinkle the smoothie with pumpkin seeds and sunflower seeds.
Nutrition Values: calories 346, fat 11.5, fiber 3.4, carbs 11.5, protein 5.6

28. Salmon Omelet

Preparation Time: 15 minutes
Servings: 2
Ingredients
- 3 eggs
- 1 smoked salmon
- 3 links pork sausage
- ¼ cup onions
- ¼ cup provolone cheese

Directions:
1.   Whisk the eggs and pour them into a skillet.
2.   Follow the standard method for making an omelette.
3.   Add the onions, salmon and cheese before turning the omelet over.
4.   Sprinkle the omelet with cheese and serve with the sausages on the side.
5.   Serve!

29. Black's Bangin' Casserole

Preparation Time: 40 minutes
Servings: 4
Ingredients
- 5 eggs
- 3 tbsp chunky tomato sauce
- 2 tbsp heavy cream
- 2 tbsp grated parmesan cheese

Directions:
1.   Preheat your oven to 350°F/175°C.
2.   Combine the eggs and cream in a bowl.
3.   Mix in the tomato sauce and add the cheese.
4.   Spread into a glass baking dish and bake for 25-35 minutes.
5.   Top with extra cheese.

6.   Enjoy!

30. Hash Brown

Preparation Time: 20 minutes
Servings: 2
Ingredients
- 12 oz grated fresh cauliflower -about ½ a medium-sized head
- 4 slices bacon, chopped
- 3 oz onion, chopped
- 1 tbsp butter, softened

Directions:
1.   In a skillet, sauté the bacon and onion until brown.
2.   Add in the cauliflower and stir until tender and browned.
3.   Add the butter steadily as it cooks.
4.   Season to taste with salt and pepper.
5.   Enjoy!

31. Bacon Cups

Preparation Time: 40 minutes
Servings: 2
Ingredients
- 2 eggs
- 1 slice tomato
- 3 slices bacon
- 2 slices ham
- 2 tsp grated parmesan cheese

Directions:
1.   Preheat your oven to 375°F/190°C.
2.   Cook the bacon for half of the directed time.
3.   Slice the bacon strips in half and line 2 greased muffin tins with 3 half-strips of bacon
4.   Put one slice of ham and half slice of tomato in each muffin tin on top of the bacon
5.   Crack one egg on top of the tomato in each muffin tin and sprinkle each with half a teaspoon of grated parmesan cheese.
6.   Bake for 20 minutes.
7.   Remove and let cool.
8.   Serve!

32. Spinach Eggs and Cheese

Preparation Time: 40 minutes
Servings: 2
Ingredients
- 3 whole eggs
- 3 oz cottage cheese
- 3-4 oz chopped spinach
- ¼ cup parmesan cheese
- ¼ cup of milk

Directions:
1.   Preheat your oven to 375°F/190°C.
2.   In a large bowl, whisk the eggs, cottage cheese, the parmesan and the milk.
3.   Mix in the spinach.
4.   Transfer to a small, greased, oven dish.
5.   Sprinkle the cheese on top.
6.   Bake for 25-30 minutes.

7.   Let cool for 5 minutes and serve.

33. Fried Eggs

Preparation Time: 7 minutes
Servings: 2
Ingredients
- 2 eggs
- 3 slices bacon

Directions:
1.   Heat some oil in a deep fryer at 375°F/190°C.
2.   Fry the bacon.
3.   In a small bowl, add the 2 eggs.
4.   Quickly add the eggs into the center of the fryer.
5.   Using two spatulas, form the egg into a ball while frying.
6.   Fry for 2-3 minutes, until it stops bubbling.
7.   Place on a paper towel and allow to drain.
8.   Enjoy!

34. Scotch Eggs

Preparation Time: 40 minutes
Servings: 4
Ingredients
- 4 large eggs
- 1 package Jimmy Dean's Pork Sausage -12 oz
- 8 slices thick-cut bacon
- 4 toothpicks

Directions:
1.   Hard-boil the eggs, peel the shells and let them cool.
2.   Slice the sausage into four parts and place each part into a large circle.
3.   Put an egg into each circle and wrap it in the sausage.
4.   Place inside your refrigerator for 1 hour.
5.   Make a cross with two pieces of thick-cut bacon.
6.   Place a wrapped egg in the center, fold the bacon over top of the egg and secure with a toothpick.
7.   Cook inside your oven at 450°F/230°C for 25 minutes.
8.   Enjoy!

35. Toasties

Preparation Time: 30 minutes
Servings: 2
Ingredients
- ¼ cup milk or cream
- 2 sausages, boiled
- 3 eggs
- 1 slicebread, sliced lengthwise
- 4 tbsp. cheese, grated
- Sea salt to taste
- Chopped fresh herbs and steamed broccoli [optional]

Directions:

1.   Pre-heat your Air Fryer at 360°F and set the timer for 5 minutes.
2.   In the meantime, scramble the eggs in a bowl and add in the milk.
3.   Grease three muffin cups with a cooking spray. Divide the egg mixture in three and pour equal amounts into each cup.
4.   Slice the sausages and drop them, along with the slices ofbread, into the egg mixture. Add the cheese on top and a little salt as desired.
5.   Transfer the cups to the Fryer and cook for 15-20 minutes, depending on how firm you would like them. When ready, remove them from the fryer and serve with fresh herbs and steam broccoli if you prefer.

36. Egg Baked Omelet

Preparation Time: 15 minutes
Servings: 1
Ingredients
- tbsp. ricotta cheese
- 1 tbsp. chopped parsley
- 1 tsp. olive oil
- 3 eggs
- ¼ cup chopped spinach
- Salt and pepper to taste

Directions:
1.   Set your Air Fryer at 330°F and allow to warm with the olive oil inside.
2.   In a bowl, beat the eggs with a fork and sprinkle some salt and pepper as desired.
3.   Add in the ricotta, spinach, and parsley and then transfer to the Air Fryer. Cook for 10 minutes before serving.

37. Breakfast Omelet

Preparation Time: 30 minutes
Servings: 2
Ingredients
- 1 large onion, chopped
- 2 tbsp. cheddar cheese, grated
- 3 eggs
- ½ tsp. soy sauce
- Salt
- Pepper powder
- Cooking spray

Directions:
1.   In a bowl, mix the salt, pepper powder, soy sauce and eggs with a whisk.
2.   Take a small pan small enough to fit inside the Air Fryer and spritz with cooking spray. Spread the chopped onion across the bottom of the pan, then transfer the pan to the Fryer. Cook at 355°F for 6-7 minutes, ensuring the onions turn translucent.
3.   Add the egg mixture on top of the onions, coating everything well. Add the cheese on top, then resume cooking for another 5 or 6 minutes.
4.   Take care when taking the pan out of the fryer. Enjoy with some toastedbread.

38. Ranch Risotto

Preparation Time: 40 minutes
Servings: 2
Ingredients
- 1 onion, diced
- 2 cups chicken stock, boiling
- ½ cup parmesan OR cheddar cheese, grated
- 1 clove garlic, minced
- ¾ cup Arborio rice
- 1 tbsp. olive oil
- 1 tbsp. unsalted butter

Directions:
1. Set the Air Fryer at 390°F for 5 minutes to heat up.
2. With oil, grease a round baking tin, small enough to fit inside the fryer, and stir in the garlic, butter, and onion.
3. Transfer the tin to the Air Fryer and allow to cook for 4 minutes. Add in the rice and cook for a further 4 minutes, giving it a stir three times throughout the cooking time.
4. Turn the fryer down to 320°F and add in the chicken stock, before gently mixing it. Leave to cook for 22 minutes with the fryer uncovered. Before serving, throw in the cheese and give it one more stir. Enjoy!

39. Coffee Donuts

Preparation Time: 20 minutes
Servings: 6
Ingredients
- 1 cupalmond flour
- ¼ cup stevia
- ½ tsp. salt
- 1 tsp. baking powder
- 1 tbsp. aquafaba
- 1 tbsp. sunflower oil
- ¼ cup coffee

Directions:
1. In a large bowl, combine the stevia, salt, flour, and baking powder.
2. Add in the coffee, aquafaba, and sunflower oil and mix until a dough is formed. Leave the dough to rest in and the refrigerator.
3. Set your Air Fryer at 400°F to heat up.
4. Remove the dough from the fridge and divide up, kneading each section into a doughnut.
5. Put the doughnuts inside the Air Fryer, ensuring not to overlap any. Fry for 6 minutes. Do not shake the basket, to make sure the doughnuts hold their shape.

40. Taco Wraps

Preparation Time: 30 minutes
Servings: 4
Ingredients
- 1 tbsp. water
- 4 pc commercial vegan nuggets, chopped
- 1 small yellow onion, diced
- 1 small red bell pepper, chopped
- 2 cobs grilled corn kernels
- 4 large corn tortillas
- Mixed greens for garnish

Directions:
1. Pre-heat your Air Fryer at 400°F.
2. Over a medium heat, water-sauté the nuggets with the onions, corn kernels and bell peppers in a skillet, then remove from the heat.
3. Fill the tortillas with the nuggets and vegetables and fold them up. Transfer to the inside of the fryer and cook for 15 minutes. Once crispy, serve immediately, garnished with the mixed greens.

41. Bistro Wedges

Preparation Time: 20 minutes
Servings: 4
Ingredients
- 1 lb. fingerling potatoes, cut into wedges
- 1 tsp. extra virgin olive oil
- ½ tsp. garlic powder
- Salt and pepper to taste
- ½ cup raw cashews, soaked in water overnight
- ½ tsp. ground turmeric
- ½ tsp. paprika
- 1 tbsp. nutritional yeast
- 1 tsp. fresh lemon juice
- 2 tbsp. to ¼ cup water

Directions:
1. Pre-heat your Air Fryer at 400°F.
2. In a bowl, toss together the potato wedges, olive oil, garlic powder, and salt and pepper, making sure to coat the potatoes well.
3. Transfer the potatoes to the basket of your fryer and fry for 10 minutes.
4. In the meantime, prepare the cheese sauce. Pulse the cashews, turmeric, paprika, nutritional yeast, lemon juice, and water together in a food processor. Add more water to achieve your desired consistency.
5. When the potatoes are finished cooking, move them to a bowl that is small enough to fit inside the fryer and add the cheese sauce on top. Cook for an additional 3 minutes.

42. Spinach Balls

Preparation Time: 20 minutes
Servings: 4
Ingredients
- 1 carrot, peeled and grated
- 1 package fresh spinach, blanched and chopped
- ½ onion, chopped
- 1 egg, beaten
- ½ tsp. garlic powder
- 1 tsp. garlic, minced
- 1 tsp. salt
- ½ tsp. black pepper

- 1 tbsp. nutritional yeast
- 1 tbsp. almond flour
- 2 slices bread, toasted

Directions:

1. In a food processor, pulse the toasted bread to form breadcrumbs. Transfer into a shallow dish or bowl.
2. In a bowl, mix together all the other ingredients.
3. Use your hands to shape the mixture into small-sized balls. Roll the balls in the breadcrumbs, ensuring to cover them well.
4. Put in the Air Fryer and cook at 390°F for 10 minutes.

43. Cheese & Chicken Sandwich

Preparation Time: 15 minutes
Servings: 1
Ingredients

- ⅓ cup chicken, cooked and shredded
- 2 mozzarella slices
- 1 hamburger bun
- ¼ cup cabbage, shredded
- 1 tsp. mayonnaise
- 2 tsp. butter
- 1 tsp. olive oil
- ½ tsp. balsamic vinegar
- 1/4 tsp. smoked paprika
- ¼ tsp. black pepper
- ¼ tsp. garlic powder
- Pinch of salt

Directions:

1. Pre-heat your Air Fryer at 370°F.
2. Apply some butter to the outside of the hamburger bun with a brush.
3. In a bowl, coat the chicken with the garlic powder, salt, pepper, and paprika.
4. In a separate bowl, stir together the mayonnaise, olive oil, cabbage, and balsamic vinegar to make coleslaw.
5. Slice the bun in two. Start building the sandwich, starting with the chicken, followed by the mozzarella, the coleslaw, and finally the top bun.
6. Transfer the sandwich to the fryer and cook for 5 – 7 minutes.

44. Bacon & Horseradish Cream

Preparation Time: 1 hour 40 minutes
Servings: 4
Ingredients

- ½ lb. thick cut bacon, diced
- 2 tbsp. butter
- 2 shallots, sliced
- ½ cup milk
- 1 ½ lb. Brussels sprouts, halved
- 2 tbsp. almond flour
- 1 cup heavy cream
- 2 tbsp. prepared horseradish
- ½ tbsp. fresh thyme leaves

- 1/8 tsp. ground nutmeg
- 1 tbsp. olive oil
- ½ tsp. sea salt
- Ground black pepper to taste
- ½ cup water

Directions:

1. Pre-heat your Air Fryer at 400°F.
2. Coat the Brussels sprouts with olive oil and sprinkle some salt and pepper on top. Transfer to the fryer and cook for a half hour. At the halfway point, give them a good stir, then take them out of the fryer and set to the side.
3. Put the bacon in the basket of the fryer and pour the water into the drawer underneath to catch the fat. Cook for 10 minutes, stirring 2 or 3 times throughout the cooking time.
4. When 10 minutes are up, add in the shallots. Cook for a further 10 – 15 minutes, making sure the shallots soften up and the bacon turns brown. Add some more pepper and remove. Leave to drain on some paper towels.
5. Melt the butter over the stove or in the microwave, before adding in the flour and mixing with a whisk. Slowly add in the heavy cream and milk, and continue to whisk for another 3 – 5 minutes, making sure the mixture thickens.
6. Add the horseradish, thyme, salt, and nutmeg and stirring well once more.
7. Take a 9" x 13" baking dish and grease it with oil. Pre-heat your oven to 350°F.
8. Put the Brussels sprouts in the baking dish and spread them across the base. Pour over the cream sauce and then top with a layer of bacon and shallots.
9. Cook in the oven for a half hour and enjoy.

45. Vegetable Toast

Preparation Time: 25 minutes
Servings: 4
Ingredients

- 4 slices bread
- 1 red bell pepper, cut into strips
- 1 cup sliced button or cremini mushrooms
- 1 small yellow squash, sliced
- 2 green onions, sliced
- 1 tbsp. olive oil
- 2 tbsp. softened butter
- ½ cup soft goat cheese

Directions:

1. Drizzle the Air Fryer with the olive oil and pre-heat to 350°F.
2. Put the red pepper, green onions, mushrooms, and squash inside the fryer, give them a stir and cook for 7 minutes, shaking the basket once throughout the cooking time. Ensure the vegetables become tender.
3. Remove the vegetables and set them aside.
4. Spread some butter on the slices of bread and transfer to the Air Fryer, butter side-up. Brown for 2 to 4 minutes.

5.   Remove the toast from the fryer and top with goat cheese and vegetables. Serve warm.

46. Cinnamon Toasts

Preparation Time: 15 minutes
Servings: 4
Ingredients
- 10bread slices
- 1 pack salted butter
- 4 tbsp. stevia
- 2 tsp. ground cinnamon
- ½ tsp. vanilla extract

Directions:
1.   In a bowl, combine the butter, cinnamon, stevia, and vanilla extract. Spread onto the slices of bread.
2.   Set your Air Fryer to 380°F. When warmed up, put the bread inside the fryer and cook for 4 – 5 minutes.

47. Toasted Cheese

Preparation Time: 20 minutes
Servings: 2
Ingredients
- 2 slicesbread
- 4 oz cheese, grated

- Small amount of butter
- Directions:
- Grill thebread in the toaster.
- Butter the toast and top with the grated cheese.
- Set your Air Fryer to 350°F and allow to warm.
- Put the toast slices inside the fryer and cook for 4 - 6 minutes.
- Serve and enjoy!

48. Peanut Butter Bread

Preparation Time: 15 minutes
Servings: 3
Ingredients
- 1 tbsp. oil
- 2 tbsp. peanut butter
- 4 slicesbread
- 1 banana, sliced

Directions:
1.   Spread the peanut butter on top of each slice ofbread, then arrange the banana slices on top. Sandwich two slices together, then the other two.
2.   Oil the inside of the Air Fryer and cook the bread for 5 minutes at 300°F.

MAINS

49. Spinach Rolls

Preparation time: 10 minutes
Cooking time: 10 minutes
Servings: 4
Ingredients:
- 4 eggs, whisked
- 1/3 cup organic almond milk
- ½ teaspoon salt
- ½ teaspoon white pepper
- 1 teaspoon butter
- 9 oz chicken breast, boneless, skinless, cooked
- 2 cups spinach
- 2 tablespoon heavy cream

Directions:
1. Mix up together whisked eggs with almond milk and salt.
2. Preheat the skillet well and toss the butter in it.
3. Melt it.
4. Cook 4 crepes in the preheated skillet.
5. Meanwhile, chop the spinach and chicken breast.
6. Fill every egg crepe with chopped spinach, chicken breast, and heavy cream.
7. Roll the crepes and transfer on the serving plate.

Nutrition Values: calories 220, fat 14.5, fiber 0.8, carbs 2.4, protein 20.1

50. Goat Cheese Fold-Overs

Preparation time: 15 minutes
Cooking time: 8 minutes
Servings: 4
Ingredients:
- 8 oz goat cheese, crumbled
- 5 oz ham, sliced
- 1 cup almond flour
- ¼ cup of coconut milk
- 1 teaspoon olive oil
- ½ teaspoon dried dill
- 1 teaspoon Italian seasoning
- ½ teaspoon salt

Directions:
1. In the mixing bowl, mix up together almond flour, coconut milk, olive oil, and salt. You will get a smooth batter.
2. Preheat the non-stick skillet.
3. Separate batter into 4 parts. Pour 1st batter part in the preheated skillet and cook it for 1 minute from each side.
4. Repeat the same steps with all batter.
5. After this, mix up together crumbled goat cheese, dried dill, and Italian seasoning.
6. Spread every almond flour pancake with goat cheese mixture. Add sliced ham and fold them.

Nutrition Values: calories 402 fat 31.8, fiber 1.6, carbs 5.1, protein 25.1

51. Crepe Pie

Preparation time: 10 minutes
Cooking time: 15 minutes
Servings: 8
Ingredients:
- 1 cup almond flour
- 1 cup coconut flour
- ½ cup heavy cream
- 1 teaspoon baking powder
- ½ teaspoon salt
- 10 oz ham, sliced
- ½ cup cream cheese
- 1 teaspoon chili flakes
- 1 tablespoon fresh cilantro, chopped
- 4 oz Cheddar cheese, shredded

Directions:
1. Make crepes: in the mixing bowl, mix up together almond flour, coconut flour, heavy cream, salt, and baking powder. Whisk the mixture.
2. Preheat the non-sticky skillet well and ladle 1 ladle of the crepe batter in it.
3. Make the crepes: cook them for 1 minute from each side over the medium heat.
4. Mix up together cream cheese, chili flakes, cilantro, and shredded Cheddar cheese.
5. After this, transfer 1st crepe in the plate. Spread it with cream cheese mixture. Add ham.
6. Repeat the steps until you use all the ingredients.
7. Bake the crepe pie for 5 minutes in the preheated to the 365F oven.
8. Cut it into the serving and serve hot.

Nutrition Values: calories 272, fat 18.8, fiber 6.9, carbs 13.2, protein 13.4

52. Coconut Soup

Preparation time: 15 minutes
Cooking time: 25 minutes
Servings: 4
Ingredients:
- 1 cup of coconut milk
- 2 cups of water
- 1 teaspoon curry paste
- 4 chicken thighs
- ½ teaspoon fresh ginger, grated
- 1 garlic clove, diced
- 1 teaspoon butter
- 1 teaspoon chili flakes
- 1 tablespoon lemon juice

Directions:
1. Toss the butter in the skillet and melt it.
2. Add diced garlic and grated ginger. Cook the ingredients for 1 minute. Stir them constantly.

3. Pour water in the saucepan. Add coconut milk and curry paste. Mix up the liquid until homogenous.
4. Add chicken thighs, chili flakes, and cooked ginger mixture.
5. Close the lid and cook soup for 15 minutes.
6. Then start to whisk soup with the hand whisker and add lemon juice.
7. When all lemon juice is added, stop to whisk it.
8. Close the lid and cook soup for 5 minutes more over the medium heat.
9. Then remove soup from the heat and let it rest for 15 minutes.
Nutrition Values: calories 318, fat 26, fiber 1.4, carbs 4.2, protein 20.6

53. Fish Tacos

Preparation time: 10 minutes
Cooking time: 5 minutes
Servings: 4
Ingredients:
- 4 lettuce leaves
- ½ red onion, diced
- ½ jalapeno pepper, minced
- 1 tablespoon olive oil
- 1-pound cod fillet
- 1 tablespoon lemon juice
- ¼ teaspoon ground coriander

Directions:
1. Sprinkle cod fillet with a ½ tablespoon of olive oil and ground coriander.
2. Preheat the grill well.
3. Grill the fish for 2 minutes from each side. The cooked fish has a light brown color.
4. After this, mix up together diced red onion, minced jalapeno pepper, remaining olive oil, and lemon juice.
5. Cut the grilled cod fillet into 4 pieces.
6. Place the fish in the lettuce leaves. Add mixed red onion mixture over the fish and transfer the tacos on the serving plates.
Nutrition Values: calories 157, fat 4.5, fiber 0.4, carbs 1.6, protein 26.1

54. Cobb Salad

Preparation time: 10 minutes
Cooking time: 5 minutes
Servings: 2
Ingredients:
- 2 oz bacon, sliced
- 1 egg, boiled, peeled
- ½ tomato, chopped
- 1 oz Blue cheese
- 1 teaspoon chives
- 1/3 cup lettuce, chopped
- 1 tablespoon mayonnaise
- 1 tablespoon lemon juice

Directions:

1. Place the bacon in the preheated skillet and roast it 1.5 minutes from each side.
2. When the bacon is cooked, chop it roughly and transfer in the salad bowl.
3. Chop the eggs roughly and add them in the salad bowl too.
4. After this, add chopped tomato, chives, and lettuce.
5. Chop Blue cheese and add it in the salad.
6. Then make seasoning: whisk together mayonnaise with lemon juice.
7. Pour the mixture over the salad and shake little.
Nutrition Values: calories 270, fat 20.7, fiber 0.3, carbs 3.7, protein 16.6

55. Cheese Soup

Preparation time: 10 minutes
Cooking time:15 minutes
Servings: 3
Ingredients:
- 2 white onion, peeled, diced
- 1 cup Cheddar cheese, shredded
- ½ cup heavy cream
- ½ cup of water
- 1 teaspoon ground black pepper
- 1 tablespoon butter
- ½ teaspoon salt

Directions:
1. Pour water and heavy cream in the saucepan.
2. Bring it to boil.
3. Meanwhile, toss the butter in the pan, add diced onions and saute them.
4. When the onions are translucent, transfer them in the boiling liquid.
5. Add ground black pepper, salt, and cheese. Cook the soup for 5 minutes.
6. Then let it chill little and ladle it into the bowls.
Nutrition Values: calories 286, fat 23.8, fiber 1.8, carbs 8.3, protein 10.7

56. Tuna Tartare

Preparation time: 10 minutes
Servings: 4
Ingredients:
- 1-pound tuna steak
- 1 tablespoon mayonnaise
- 3 oz avocado, chopped
- 1 cucumber, chopped
- 1 tablespoon lemon juice
- 1 teaspoon cayenne pepper
- 1 teaspoon soy sauce
- 1 teaspoon chives
- ½ teaspoon cumin seeds
- 1 teaspoon canola oil

Directions:
1. Chop tuna steak and place it in the big bowl.
2. Add avocado, cucumber, and chives.

3.   Mix up together lemon juice, cayenne pepper, soy sauce, cumin seeds, and canola oil.
4.   Add mixed liquid in the tuna mixture and mix up well.
5.   Place tuna tartare in the serving plates.
Nutrition Values: calories 292, fat 13.9, fiber 2, carbs 6, protein 35.1

57. Clam Chowder

Preparation time: 5 minutes
Cooking time: 15 minutes
Servings: 3
Ingredients:
- 1 cup of coconut milk
- 1 cup of water
- 6 oz clam, chopped
- 1 teaspoon chives
- ½ teaspoon white pepper
- ¾ teaspoon chili flakes
- ½ teaspoon salt
- 1 cup broccoli florets, chopped

Directions:
1.   Pour coconut milk and water in the saucepan.
2.   Add chopped clams, chives, white pepper, chili flakes, salt, and broccoli florets.
3.   Close the lid and cook chowder over the medium-low heat for 15 minutes or until all the ingredients are soft.
4.   It is recommended to serve the soup hot.
Nutrition Values: calories 139, fat 9.8, fiber 1.1, carbs 10.8, protein 2.4

58. Asian Beef Salad

Preparation time: 10 minutes
Cooking time: 25 minutes
Servings: 4
Ingredients:
- 14 oz beef brisket
- 1 teaspoon sesame seeds
- ½ teaspoon cumin seeds
- 1 tablespoon apple cider vinegar
- 1 tablespoon avocado oil
- 1 red bell pepper, sliced
- 1 white onion, sliced
- 1 teaspoon butter
- 1 teaspoon ground black pepper
- 1 teaspoon soy sauce
- 1 garlic clove, sliced
- 1 cup water, for cooking

Directions:
1.   Slice beef brisket and place it in the pan. Add water and close the lid.
2.   Cook the beef for 25 minutes.
3.   Then drain water and transfer beef brisket in the pan.
4.   Add butter and roast it for 5 minutes.
5.   Put the cooked beef brisket in the salad bowl.

6.   Add sesame seeds, cumin seeds, apple cider vinegar, avocado oil, sliced bell pepper, onion, ground black pepper, and soy sauce.
7.   Sprinkle the salad with garlic and mix it up.
Nutrition Values: calories 227, fat 8.1, fiber 1.4, carbs 6, protein 31.1

59. Carbonara

Preparation time: 10 minutes
Cooking time: 25 minutes
Servings: 6
Ingredients:
- 3 zucchini, trimmed
- 1 cup heavy cream
- 5 oz bacon, chopped
- 2 egg yolks
- 4 oz Cheddar cheese, grated
- 1 tablespoon butter
- 1 teaspoon chili flakes
- 1 teaspoon salt
- ½ cup water, for cooking

Directions:
1.   Make the zucchini noodles with the help of the spiralizer.
2.   Toss bacon in the skillet and roast it for 5 minutes on the medium heat. Stir it from time to time.
3.   Meanwhile, in the saucepan, mix up together heavy cream, butter, salt, and chili flakes.
4.   Add egg yolk and whisk the mixture until smooth.
5.   Start to preheat the liquid, stir it constantly.
6.   When the liquid starts to boil, add grated cheese and fried bacon. Mix it up and close the lid. Saute it on the low heat for 5 minutes.
7.   Meanwhile, place the zucchini noodles in the skillet where bacon was and roast it for 3 minutes.
8.   Then pour heavy cream mixture over zucchini and mix up well. Cook it for 1 minute more and transfer on the serving plates.
Nutrition Values: calories 324, fat 27.1, fiber 1.1, carbs 4.6, protein 16

60. Cauliflower Soup with Seeds

Preparation time: 10 minutes
Cooking time: 20 minutes
Servings: 4
Ingredients:
- 2 cups cauliflower
- 1 tablespoon pumpkin seeds
- 1 tablespoon chia seeds
- ½ teaspoon salt
- 1 teaspoon butter
- ¼ white onion, diced
- ½ cup coconut cream
- 1 cup of water
- 4 oz Parmesan, grated
- 1 teaspoon paprika
- 1 tablespoon dried cilantro

Directions:
1. Chop cauliflower and put in the saucepan.
2. Add salt, butter, diced onion, paprika, and dried cilantro.
3. Cook the cauliflower over the medium heat for 5 minutes.
4. Then add coconut cream and water.
5. Close the lid and boil soup for 15 minutes.
6. Then blend the soup with the help of hand blender.
7. Dring to boil it again.
8. Add grated cheese and mix up well.
9. Ladle the soup into the serving bowls and top every bowl with pumpkin seeds and chia seeds.
Nutrition Values: calories 214, fat 16.4, fiber 3.6, carbs 8.1, protein 12.1

61. Prosciutto-Wrapped Asparagus

Preparation time: 15 minutes
Cooking time: 20 minutes
Servings: 6
Ingredients:
- 2-pound asparagus
- 8 oz prosciutto, sliced
- 1 tablespoon butter, melted
- ½ teaspoon ground black pepper
- 4 tablespoon heavy cream
- 1 tablespoon lemon juice

Directions:
1. Slice prousciutto slices into strips.
2. Wrap asparagus into prosciutto strips and place on the tray.
3. Sprinkle the vegetables with ground black pepper, heavy cream, and lemon juice. Add butter.
4. Preheat the oven to 365F.
5. Place the tray with asparagus in the oven and cook for 20 minutes.
6. Serve the cooked meal only hot.
Nutrition Values: calories 138, fat 7.9, fiber 3.2, carbs 6.9, protein 11.5

62. Stuffed Bell Peppers

Preparation time: 10 minutes
Cooking time: 25 minutes
Servings: 4
Ingredients:
- 4 bell peppers
- 1 ½ cup ground beef
- 1 zucchini, grated
- 1 white onion, diced
- ½ teaspoon ground nutmeg
- 1 tablespoon olive oil
- 1 teaspoon ground black pepper
- ½ teaspoon salt
- 3 oz Parmesan, grated

1. Directions:
2. Cut the bell peppers into halves and remove seeds.
3. Place ground beef in the skillet.

4. Add grated zucchini, diced onion, ground nutmeg, olive oil, ground black pepper, and salt.
5. Roast the mixture for 5 minutes.
6. Place bell pepper halves in the tray.
7. Fill every pepper half with ground beef mixture and top with grated Parmesan.
8. Cover the tray with foil and secure the edges.
9. Cook the stuffed bell peppers for 20 minutes at 360F.
Nutrition Values: calories 241, fat 14.6, fiber 3.4, carbs 11, protein 18.6

63. Stuffed Eggplants with Goat Cheese

Preparation time: 15 minutes
Cooking time: 25 minutes
Servings: 4
Ingredients:
- 1 large eggplant, trimmed
- 1 tomato, crushed
- 1 garlic clove, diced
- ½ teaspoon ground black pepper
- ½ teaspoon smoked paprika
- 1 cup spinach, chopped
- 4 oz goat cheese, crumbled
- 1 teaspoon butter
- 2 oz Cheddar cheese, shredded

Directions:
1. Cut the eggplants into halves and then cut every half into 2 parts.
2. Remove the flesh from the eggplants to get eggplant boards.
3. Mix up together crushed tomato, diced garlic, ground black pepper, smoked paprika, chopped spinach, crumbled goat cheese, and butter.
4. Fill the eggplants with this mixture.
5. Top every eggplant board with shredded Cheddar cheese.
6. Put the eggplants in the tray.
7. Preheat the oven to 365F.
8. Place the tray with eggplants in the oven and cook for 25 minutes.
Nutrition Values: calories 229, fat 16.1, fiber 4.6, carbs 9, protein 13.8

64. Korma Curry

Preparation time: 10 minutes
Cooking time: 25 minutes
Servings: 6
Ingredients:
- 3-pound chicken breast, skinless, boneless
- 1 teaspoon garam masala
- 1 teaspoon curry powder
- 1 tablespoon apple cider vinegar
- ½ coconut cream
- 1 cup organic almond milk
- 1 teaspoon ground coriander
- ¾ teaspoon ground cardamom
- ½ teaspoon ginger powder

- ¼ teaspoon cayenne pepper
- ¾ teaspoon ground cinnamon
- 1 tomato, diced
- 1 teaspoon avocado oil
- ½ cup of water

Directions:
1. Chop the chicken breast and put it in the saucepan.
2. Add avocado oil and start to cook it over the medium heat.
3. Sprinkle the chicken with garam masala, curry powder, apple cider vinegar, ground coriander, cardamom, ginger powder, cayenne pepper, ground cinnamon, and diced tomato. Mix up the ingredients carefully. Cook them for 10 minutes.
4. Add water, coconut cream, and almond milk. Saute the meal for 10 minutes more.

Nutrition Values: calories 411, fat 19.3, fiber 0.9, carbs 6, protein 49.9

65. Zucchini Bars

Preparation time: 10 minutes
Cooking time: 15 minutes
Servings: 8
Ingredients:
- 3 zucchini, grated
- ½ white onion, diced
- 2 teaspoons butter
- 3 eggs, whisked
- 4 tablespoons coconut flour
- 1 teaspoon salt
- ½ teaspoon ground black pepper
- 5 oz goat cheese, crumbled
- 4 oz Swiss cheese, shredded
- ½ cup spinach, chopped
- 1 teaspoon baking powder
- ½ teaspoon lemon juice

Directions:
1. In the mixing bowl, mix up together grated zucchini, diced onion, eggs, coconut flour, salt, ground black pepper, crumbled cheese, chopped spinach, baking powder, and lemon juice.
2. Add butter and churn the mixture until homogenous.
3. Line the baking dish with baking paper.
4. Transfer the zucchini mixture in the baking dish and flatten it.
5. Preheat the oven to 365F and put the dish inside.
6. Cook it for 15 minutes. Then chill the meal well.
7. Cut it into bars.

Nutrition Values: calories 199, fat 1316, fiber 215, carbs 7.1, protein 13.1

66. Mushroom Soup

Preparation time: 10 minutes
Cooking time: 25 minutes
Servings: 4
Ingredients:

- 1 cup of water
- 1 cup of coconut milk
- 1 cup white mushrooms, chopped
- ½ carrot, chopped
- ¼ white onion, diced
- 1 tablespoon butter
- 2 oz turnip, chopped
- 1 teaspoon dried dill
- ½ teaspoon ground black pepper
- ¾ teaspoon smoked paprika
- 1 oz celery stalk, chopped

Directions:
1. Pour water and coconut milk in the saucepan. Bring the liquid to boil.
2. Add chopped mushrooms, carrot, and turnip. Close the lid and boil for 10 minutes.
3. Meanwhile, put butter in the skillet. Add diced onion. Sprinkle it with dill, ground black pepper, and smoked paprika. Roast the onion for 3 minutes.
4. Add the roasted onion in the soup mixture.
5. Then add chopped celery stalk. Close the lid.
6. Cook soup for 10 minutes.
7. Then ladle it into the serving bowls.

Nutrition Values: calories 181, fat 17.3, fiber 2.5, carbs 6.9, protein 2.4

67. Stuffed Portobello Mushrooms

Preparation time: 10 minutes
Cooking time: 10 minutes
Servings: 4
Ingredients:
- 2 portobello mushrooms
- 1 cup spinach, chopped, steamed
- 2 oz artichoke hearts, drained, chopped
- 1 tablespoon coconut cream
- 1 tablespoon cream cheese
- 1 teaspoon minced garlic
- 1 tablespoon fresh cilantro, chopped
- 3 oz Cheddar cheese, grated
- ½ teaspoon ground black pepper
- 2 tablespoons olive oil
- ½ teaspoon salt

Directions:
1. Sprinkle mushrooms with olive oil and place in the tray.
2. Transfer the tray in the preheated to 360F oven and broil them for 5 minutes.
3. Meanwhile, blend together artichoke hearts, coconut cream, cream cheese, minced garlic, and chopped cilantro.
4. Add grated cheese in the mixture and sprinkle with ground black pepper and salt.
5. Fill the broiled mushrooms with the cheese mixture and cook them for 5 minutes more. Serve the mushrooms only hot.

Nutrition Values: calories 183, fat 16.3, fiber 1.9, carbs 3, protein 7.7

68. Lettuce Salad

Preparation time: 10 minutes
Servings: 1
Ingredients:
- 1 cup Romaine lettuce, roughly chopped
- 3 oz seitan, chopped
- 1 tablespoon avocado oil
- 1 teaspoon sunflower seeds
- 1 teaspoon lemon juice
- 1 egg, boiled, peeled
- 2 oz Cheddar cheese, shredded

Directions:
1.　　Place lettuce in the salad bowl. Add chopped seitan and shredded cheese.
2.　　Then chop the egg roughly and add in the salad bowl too.
3.　　Mix up together lemon juice with the avocado oil.
4.　　Sprinkle the salad with the oil mixture and sunflower seeds. Don't stir the salad before serving.
Nutrition Values: calories 663, fat 29.5, fiber 4.7, carbs 3.8, protein 84.2

69. Onion Soup

Preparation time: 10 minutes
Cooking time: 25 minutes
Servings: 6
Ingredients:
- 2 cups white onion, diced
- 4 tablespoon butter
- ½ cup white mushrooms, chopped
- 3 cups of water
- 1 cup heavy cream
- 1 teaspoon salt
- 1 teaspoon chili flakes
- 1 teaspoon garlic powder

Directions:
1.　　Put butter in the saucepan and melt it.
2.　　Add diced white onion, chili flakes, and garlic powder. Mix it up and saute for 10 minutes over the medium-low heat.
3.　　Then add water, heavy cream, and chopped mushrooms. Close the lid.
4.　　Cook the soup for 15 minutes more.
5.　　Then blend the soup until you get the creamy texture. Ladle it in the bowls.
Nutrition Values: calories 155, fat 15.1, fiber 0.9, carbs 4.7, protein 1.2

70. Asparagus Salad

Preparation time: 10 minutes
Cooking time: 15 minutes
Servings: 3
Ingredients:
- 10 oz asparagus
- 1 tablespoon olive oil
- ½ teaspoon white pepper
- 4 oz Feta cheese, crumbled
- 1 cup lettuce, chopped
- 1 tablespoon canola oil
- 1 teaspoon apple cider vinegar
- 1 tomato, diced

Directions:
1.　　Preheat the oven to 365F.
2.　　Place asparagus in the tray, sprinkle with olive oil and white pepper and transfer in the preheated oven. Cook it for 15 minutes.
3.　　Meanwhile, put crumbled Feta in the salad bowl.
4.　　Add chopped lettuce and diced tomato.
5.　　Sprinkle the ingredients with apple cider vinegar.
6.　　Chill the cooked asparagus to the room temperature and add in the salad.
7.　　Shake the salad gently before serving.
Nutrition Values: calories 207, fat 17.6, fiber 2.4, carbs 6.8, protein 7.8

71. Cauliflower Tabbouleh

Preparation time: 10 minutes
Cooking time: 4 minutes
Servings: 4
Ingredients:
- 1-pound cauliflower head
- 1 cucumber, chopped
- 2 tablespoons lemon juice
- 2 tablespoons olive oil
- ½ cup fresh parsley
- 1 garlic clove, diced
- 1 oz scallions, chopped
- 1 teaspoon mint

Directions:
1.　　Trim and chop cauliflower head. Transfer it in the food processor and pulse until you get cauliflower rice.
2.　　Transfer the cauliflower rice in the glass mixing bowl. Add lemon juice and chopped scallions. Mix up the mixture.
3.　　Microwave it for 4 minutes.
4.　　Meanwhile, blend together olive oil, parsley, and diced garlic.
5.　　Mix up together cooked cauliflower rice with parsley mixture. Add mint and chopped cucumbers.
6.　　Mix it up and transfer on the serving plates.
Nutrition Values: calories 108, fat 7.3, fiber 3.7, carbs 10.2, protein 3.2

72. Stuffed Artichoke

Preparation time: 10 minutes
Cooking time: 15 minutes
Servings: 4
Ingredients:
- 2 artichokes
- 4 tablespoon Parmesan, grated
- 2 teaspoon almond flour
- 1 teaspoon minced garlic
- 3 tablespoons sour cream
- 1 teaspoon avocado oil

- 1 cup water, for cooking

Directions:

1. Pour water in the saucepan and bring it to boil.
2. When the water is boiling, add artichokes and boil them for 5 minutes.
3. Drain water from artichokes and trim them.
4. Remove the artichoke hearts.
5. Preheat the oven to 365F.
6. Mix up together almond flour, grated Parmesan, minced garlic, sour cream, and avocado oil.
7. Fill the artichokes with cheese mixture and place on the baking tray.
8. Cook the vegetables for 10 minutes.
9. Then cut every artichoke into halves and transfer on the serving plates.

Nutrition Values: calories 162, fat 10.7, fiber 5.9, carbs 12.4, protein 8.2

73. Beef Salpicao

Preparation time: 10 minutes
Cooking time: 18 minutes
Servings: 2
Ingredients:

- 1-pound rib eye, boneless
- 2 garlic cloves, peeled, diced
- 2 tablespoons butter
- 1 tablespoon sour cream
- ½ teaspoon salt
- ½ teaspoon chili pepper
- 1 tablespoon lime juice

Directions:

1. Cut rib eye into the strips.
2. Sprinkle the meat with salt, chili pepper, and lime juice.
3. Toss butter in the skillet. Add diced garlic and roast it for 2 minutes over the medium heat.
4. Then add meat strips and roast them over the high heat for 2 minutes from each side.
5. Add sour cream and close the lid. Cook the meal for 10 minutes more over the medium heat. Stir it from time to time.
6. Transfer cooked beef salpicao on the serving plates.

Nutrition Values: calories 641, fat 52.8, fiber 0.1, carbs 1.9, protein 42.5

SIDES

74. Tomatoes Side Salad

Preparation time: 10 minutes
Cooking time: 0 minutes
Servings: 4
Ingredients:
- ½ bunch mint, chopped
- 8 plum tomatoes, sliced
- 1 teaspoon mustard
- 1 tablespoon rosemary vinegar
- A pinch of black pepper

Directions:
1. In a bowl, mix vinegar with mustard and pepper and whisk.
2. In another bowl, combine the tomatoes with the mint and the vinaigrette, toss, divide between plates and serve as a side dish.
3. Enjoy!
Nutrition Values: calories 70, fat 2, fiber 2, carbs 6, protein 4

75. Squash Salsa

Preparation time: 10 minutes
Cooking time: 13 minutes
Servings: 6
Ingredients:
- 3 tablespoons olive oil
- 5 medium squash, peeled and sliced
- 1 cup pepitas, toasted
- 7 tomatillos
- A pinch of black pepper
- 1 small onion, chopped
- 2 tablespoons fresh lime juice
- 2 tablespoons cilantro, chopped

Directions:
1. Heat up a pan over medium heat, add tomatillos, onion and black pepper, stir, cook for 3 minutes, transfer to your food processor and pulse.
2. Add lime juice and cilantro, pulse again and transfer to a bowl.
3. Heat up your kitchen grill over high heat, drizzle the oil over squash slices, grill them for 10 minutes, divide them between plates, add pepitas and tomatillos mix on top and serve as a side dish.
4. Enjoy!
Nutrition Values: calories 120, fat 2, fiber 1, carbs 7, protein 1

76. Apples And Fennel Mix

Preparation time: 10 minutes
Cooking time: 0 minutes
Servings: 3
Ingredients:
- 3 big apples, cored and sliced
- 1 and ½ cup fennel, shredded
- 1/3 cup coconut cream
- 3 tablespoons apple vinegar
- ½ teaspoon caraway seeds
- Black pepper to the taste

Directions:
1. In a bowl, mix fennel with apples and toss.
2. In another bowl, mix coconut cream with vinegar, black pepper and caraway seeds, whisk well, add over the fennel mix, toss, divide between plates and serve as a side dish.
3. Enjoy!
Nutrition Values: calories 130, fat 3, fiber 6, carbs 10, protein 3

77. Simple Roasted Celery Mix

Preparation time: 10 minutes
Cooking time: 25 minutes
Servings: 3
Ingredients:
- 3 celery roots, cubed
- 2 tablespoons olive oil
- A pinch of black pepper
- 2 cups natural and unsweetened apple juice
- ¼ cup parsley, chopped
- ¼ cup walnuts, chopped

Directions:
1. In a baking dish, combine the celery with the oil, pepper, parsley, walnuts and apple juice, toss to coat, introduce in the oven at 450 degrees F, bake for 25 minutes, divide between plates and serve as a side dish.
2. Enjoy!
Nutrition Values: calories 140, fat 2, fiber 2, carbs 7, protein 7

78. Thyme Spring Onions

Preparation time: 10 minutes
Cooking time: 40 minutes
Servings: 8
Ingredients:
- 15 spring onions
- A pinch of black pepper
- 1 teaspoon thyme, chopped
- 1 tablespoon olive oil

Directions:
1. Put onions in a baking dish, add thyme, black pepper and oil, toss, bake in the oven at 350 degrees F for 40 minutes, divide between plates and serve as a side dish.
2. Enjoy!
Nutrition Values: calories 120, fat 2, fiber 2, carbs 7, protein 2

79. Carrot Slaw

Preparation time: 10 minutes
Cooking time: 10 minutes
Servings: 4
Ingredients:
- ¼ yellow onion, chopped
- 5 carrots, cut into thin matchsticks
- 1 tablespoon olive oil

- 1 garlic clove, minced
- 1 tablespoon Dijon mustard
- 1 tablespoon red vinegar
- A pinch of black pepper
- 1 tablespoon lemon juice

Directions:

1. In a bowl, mix vinegar with black pepper, mustard and lemon juice and whisk.
2. Heat up a pan with the oil over medium heat, add onion, stir and cook for 5 minutes.
3. Add garlic and carrots, stir, cook for 5 minutes more, transfer to a salad bowl, cool down, add the vinaigrette, toss, divide between plates and serve as a side dish.
4. Enjoy!

Nutrition Values: calories 120, fat 3, fiber 3, carbs 7, protein 5

80. Watermelon Tomato Salsa

Preparation time: 10 minutes
Cooking time: 0 minutes
Servings: 16
Ingredients:
- 4 yellow tomatoes, seedless and chopped
- A pinch of black pepper
- 1 cup watermelon, seedless and chopped
- 1/3 cup red onion, chopped
- 2 jalapeno peppers, chopped
- ¼ cup cilantro, chopped
- 3 tablespoons lime juice

Directions:

1. In a bowl, mix tomatoes with watermelon, onion and jalapeno.
2. Add cilantro, lime juice and pepper, toss, divide between plates and serve as a side dish.
3. Enjoy!

Nutrition Values: calories 87, fat 1, fiber 2, carbs 4, protein 7

81. Sprouts Side Salad

Preparation time: 10 minutes
Cooking time: 0 minutes
Servings: 4
Ingredients:
- 2 zucchinis, cut with a spiralizer
- 2 cups bean sprouts
- 4 green onions, chopped
- 1 red bell pepper, chopped
- Juice of 1 lime
- 1 tablespoon olive oil
- ½ cup cilantro, chopped
- ¾ cup almonds, chopped
- Black pepper to the taste

Directions:

1. In a salad bowl, mix zucchinis with bean sprouts, onions and bell pepper.
2. Add black pepper, lime juice, almonds, cilantro and olive oil, toss everything, divide between plates and serve as a side dish.

3. Enjoy!

Nutrition Values: calories 120, fat 4, fiber 2, carbs 7, protein 12

82. Cabbage Slaw

Preparation time: 10 minutes
Cooking time: 0 minutes
Servings: 4
Ingredients:
- 1 green cabbage head, shredded
- 1/3 cup coconut, shredded
- ¼ cup olive oil
- 2 tablespoons lemon juice
- ¼ cup coconut aminos
- 3 tablespoons sesame seeds
- ½ teaspoon curry powder
- 1/3 teaspoon turmeric powder
- ½ teaspoon cumin, ground

Directions:

1. In a bowl, mix cabbage with coconut and lemon juice and stir.
2. Add oil, aminos, sesame seeds, curry powder, turmeric and cumin, toss to coat and serve as a side dish.
3. Enjoy!

Nutrition Values: calories 130, fat 4, fiber 5, carbs 8, protein 6

83. Edamame Side Salad

Preparation time: 10 minutes
Cooking time: 0 minutes
Servings: 4
Ingredients:
- 1 tablespoon ginger, grated
- 2 green onions, chopped
- 3 cups edamame, blanched
- 2 tablespoons rice vinegar
- 1 tablespoon sesame seeds

Directions :

1. In a bowl, combine the ginger with the onions, edamame, vinegar and sesame seeds, toss, divide between plates and serve as a side dish.
2. Enjoy!

Nutrition Values: calories 120, fat 3, fiber 2, carbs 5, protein 9

84. Flavored Beets Side Salad

Preparation time: 10 minutes
Cooking time: 0 minutes
Servings: 4
Ingredients:
- 4 carrots, sliced
- 12 radishes, sliced
- 1 beet, peeled and grated
- 2 tablespoons raisins
- Juice of 2 lemons
- 1 sugar beet, peeled and chopped
- 1 tablespoon chives, chopped
- 1 tablespoon parsley, chopped

- 1 tablespoon lemon thyme, chopped
- 1 tablespoon white sesame seeds
- 4 handfuls spinach leaves
- 4 tablespoons olive oil
- Black pepper to the taste

Directions:
1. In a salad bowl, mix carrots, radishes, beets, sugar beet, raisins, chives, parsley, spinach, thyme and sesame seeds.
2. Add lemon juice, oil and black pepper, toss well and serve as a side dish.
3. Enjoy!
Nutrition Values: calories 110, fat 2, fiber 2, carbs 4, protein 7

85. Tomato And Avocado Salad

Preparation time: 10 minutes
Cooking time: 0 minutes
Servings: 4
Ingredients:
- 1 cucumber, chopped
- 1 pound tomatoes, chopped
- 2 avocados, pitted, peeled and chopped
- 1 small red onion, sliced
- 2 tablespoons olive oil
- 2 tablespoons lemon juice
- ¼ cup cilantro, chopped
- Black pepper to the taste

Directions:
1. In a salad bowl, mix tomatoes with onion, avocado, cucumber and cilantro.
2. In a small bowl, mix oil with lemon juice and black pepper, whisk well, pour this over the salad, toss and serve as a side dish.
3. Enjoy!
Nutrition Values: calories 120, fat 2, fiber 2, carbs 3, protein 4

86. Greek Side Salad

Preparation time: 10 minutes
Cooking time: 0 minutes
Servings: 4
Ingredients:
- 4 pounds heirloom tomatoes, sliced
- 1 yellow bell pepper, thinly sliced
- 1 green bell pepper, thinly sliced
- 1 red onion, thinly sliced
- Black pepper to the taste
- ½ teaspoon oregano, dried
- 2 tablespoons mint leaves, chopped
- A drizzle of olive oil

Directions:
1. In a salad bowl, mix tomatoes with yellow and green peppers, onion, salt and pepper, toss to coat and leave aside for 10 minutes.
2. Add oregano, mint and olive oil, toss to coat and serve as a side salad.
3. Enjoy!

Nutrition Values: calories 100, fat 2, fiber 2, carbs 3, protein 6

87. Cucumber Salad

Preparation time: 10 minutes
Cooking time: 0 minutes
Servings: 4
Ingredients:
- 2 English cucumbers, chopped
- 8 dates, pitted and sliced
- ¾ cup fennel, sliced
- 2 tablespoons chives, chopped
- ½ cup walnuts, chopped
- 2 tablespoons lemon juice
- 4 tablespoons olive oil
- Black pepper to the taste

Directions:
1. In a salad bowl, combine the cucumbers with dates, fennel, chives, walnuts, lemon juice, oil and black pepper, toss, divide between plates and serve as a side dish.
2. Enjoy!
Nutrition Values: calories 100, fat 1, fiber 1, carbs 7, protein 6

88. Black Beans And Veggies Side Salad

Preparation time: 10 minutes
Cooking time: 0 minutes
Servings: 4
Ingredients:
- 1 big cucumber, cut into chunks
- 15 ounces canned black beans, no-salt-added, drained and rinsed
- 1 cup corn
- 1 cup cherry tomatoes, halved
- 1 small red onion, chopped
- 3 tablespoons olive oil
- 4 and ½ teaspoons orange marmalade
- Black pepper to the taste
- ½ teaspoon cumin, ground
- 1 tablespoon lemon juice

Directions:
1. In a bowl, mix beans with cucumber, corn, onion and tomatoes.
2. In another bowl, mix marmalade with oil, lemon juice, black pepper to the taste and cumin, whisk, pour over the salad, toss and serve as a side dish.
3. Enjoy!
Nutrition Values: calories 110, fat 0, fiber 3, carbs 6, protein 8

89. Endives And Escarole Side Salad

Preparation time: 10 minutes
Cooking time: 0 minutes
Servings: 4
Ingredients:
- 1 teaspoon shallot, minced
- ¼ cup apple cider vinegar
- 1 teaspoon Dijon mustard

- 3 Belgian endives, roughly chopped
- ¾ cup olive oil
- 1 cup escarole leaves, torn

Directions:
1. In a bowl, mix escarole leaves with endives, shallot, vinegar, mustard and oil, toss, divide between plates and serve as a side salad.
2. Enjoy!

Nutrition Values: calories 100, fat 1, fiber 3, carbs 6, protein 7

90. Radicchio And Lettuce Side Salad

Preparation time: 10 minutes
Cooking time: 0 minutes
Servings: 4

Ingredients:
- ½ cup olive oil
- Black pepper to the taste
- 2 tablespoons shallot, chopped
- ¼ cup mustard
- Juice of 2 lemons
- ½ cup basil, chopped
- 5 baby romaine lettuce heads, chopped
- 3 radicchios, sliced
- 3 endives, roughly chopped

Directions:
1. In a salad bowl, mix romaine lettuce with radicchios and endives.
2. In another bowl, mix oil with the pepper, shallot, mustard, lemon juice and basil, whisk, add to the salad, toss and serve as a side salad.
3. Enjoy!

Nutrition Values: calories 120, fat 2, fiber 1, carbs 8, protein 2

91. Jicama Side Salad

Preparation time: 10 minutes
Cooking time: 0 minutes
Servings: 4

Ingredients:
- 1 romaine lettuce head, leaves torn
- 1 Jicama, peeled and grated
- 1 cup cherry tomatoes, halved
- 1 yellow bell pepper, chopped
- 1 cup carrot, shredded
- 3 ounces low-fat cheese, crumbled
- 3 tablespoons red wine vinegar
- 5 tablespoons non-fat yogurt
- 1 and ½ tablespoons olive oil
- 1 teaspoon parsley, chopped
- 1 teaspoon dill, chopped
- Black pepper to the taste

Directions:
1. In a salad bowl, mix lettuce leaves with Jicama, tomatoes, bell pepper and carrot and toss.
2. In another bowl, combine the cheese with vinegar, yogurt, oil, pepper, dill and parsley, whisk, add to the salad, toss to coat, divide between plates and serve as a side dish.

3. Enjoy!

Nutrition Values: calories 170, fat 4, fiber 8, carbs 14, protein 11

92. Cauliflower Risotto

Preparation time: 10 minutes
Cooking time: 7 minutes
Servings: 4

Ingredients:
- 2 tablespoons olive oil
- 2 garlic cloves, minced
- 12 ounces cauliflower rice
- 2 tablespoons thyme, chopped
- 1 tablespoon lemon juice
- Zest of ½ lemon, grated
- A pinch of black pepper

Directions:
1. Heat up a pan with the oil over medium-high heat, add cauliflower rice and garlic, stir and cook for 5 minutes.
2. Add lemon juice, lemon zest, thyme, salt and pepper, stir, cook for 2 minutes more, divide between plates and serve as a side dish.
3. Enjoy!

Nutrition Values: calories 130, fat 2, fiber 2, carbs 6, protein 8

93. Cranberry And Broccoli Mix

Preparation time: 10 minutes
Cooking time: 0 minutes
Servings: 4

Ingredients:
- ½ cup avocado mayonnaise
- 1 tablespoon apple cider vinegar
- 1 tablespoon lemon juice
- 1 tablespoon coconut sugar
- ¼ cup cranberries
- ½ cup almonds, sliced
- 9 ounces broccoli florets, separated

Directions:
1. In a bowl, mix broccoli with cranberries and almond slices and toss.
2. In another bowl, mix coconut sugar with vinegar, mayo and lemon juice, whisk well, add to the broccoli mix, toss, divide between plates and serve as a side dish.
3. Enjoy!

Nutrition Values: calories 120, fat 1, fiber 3, carbs 7, protein 8

94. Three Beans Mix

Preparation time: 10 minutes
Cooking time: 0 minutes
Servings: 4

Ingredients:
- 15 ounces canned kidney beans, no-salt-added, drained and rinsed
- 15 ounces canned garbanzo beans, no-salt-added and drained

- 15 ounces canned pinto beans, no-salt-added and drained
- 3 tablespoons balsamic vinegar
- 2 tablespoons olive oil
- 2 teaspoon Italian seasoning
- 2 teaspoons garlic powder
- 1 teaspoon onion powder

Directions:
1. In a large salad bowl, combine the beans with vinegar, oil, seasoning, garlic powder and onion powder, toss, divide between plates and serve as a side dish.
2. Enjoy!

Nutrition Values: calories 140, fat 1, fiber 10, carbs 10, protein 7

95. Creamy Cucumber Mix

Preparation time: 10 minutes
Cooking time: 0 minutes
Servings: 2
Ingredients:
- 1 big cucumber, peeled and chopped
- 1 small red onion, chopped
- 4 tablespoons non-fat yogurt
- 1 teaspoon balsamic vinegar

Directions:
1. In a bowl, mix onion with cucumber, yogurt and vinegar, toss, divide between plates and serve as a side dish.
2. Enjoy!

Nutrition Values: calories 90, fat 1, fiber 3, carbs 7, protein 2

96. Bell Peppers Mix

Preparation time: 10 minutes
Cooking time: 10 minutes
Servings: 2
Ingredients:
- 1 tablespoon olive oil
- 2 teaspoons garlic powder
- 2 red bell peppers, chopped
- 2 yellow bell peppers, chopped
- 2 orange bell peppers, chopped
- Black pepper to the taste

Directions:
1. Heat up a pan with the oil over medium-high heat, add all the bell peppers, stir and cook for 5 minutes.
2. Add garlic powder and black pepper, stir, cook for 5 minutes, divide between plates and serve as a side dish.
3. Enjoy!

Nutrition Values: calories 145, fat 3, fiber 5, carbs 5, protein 8

97. Sweet Potato Mash

Preparation time: 10 minutes
Cooking time: 1 hour
Servings: 6
Ingredients:

- ¼ cup olive oil
- 3 pounds sweet potatoes
- Black pepper to the taste

Directions:
1. Arrange the sweet potatoes on a lined baking sheet, introduce in the oven, bake at 375 degrees F for 1 hour, cool them down, peel, mash them and put them in a bowl.
2. Add black pepper and the oil, whisk well, divide between plates and serve as a side dish.
3. Enjoy!

Nutrition Values: calories 140, fat 1, fiber 4, carbs 6, protein 4

98. Bok Choy Mix

Preparation time: 10 minutes
Cooking time: 15 minutes
Servings: 4
Ingredients:
- 2 tablespoons olive oil
- 3 tablespoons coconut aminos
- 1-inch ginger, grated
- A pinch of red pepper flakes
- 4 bok choy heads, cut into quarters
- 2 garlic cloves, minced
- 1 tablespoon sesame seeds, toasted

Directions:
1. Heat up a pan with the olive oil over medium heat, add coconut aminos, garlic, pepper flakes and ginger, stir and cook for 3-4 minutes.
2. Add the bok choy and the sesame seeds, toss, cook for 5 minutes more, divide between plates and serve as a side dish.
3. Enjoy!

Nutrition Values: calories 140, fat 2, fiber 2, carbs 4, protein 6

99. Flavored Turnips Mix

Preparation time: 10 minutes
Cooking time: 15 minutes
Servings: 4
Ingredients:
- 1 tablespoon lemon juice
- Zest of 2 oranges, grated
- 16 ounces turnips, sliced
- 3 tablespoons olive oil
- 1 tablespoon rosemary, chopped
- Black pepper to the taste

Directions:
1. Heat up a pan with the oil over medium-high heat, add turnips, stir and cook for 5 minutes.
2. Add lemon juice, black pepper, orange zest and rosemary, stir, cook for 10 minutes more, divide between plates and serve as a side dish.
3. Enjoy!

Nutrition Values: calories 130, fat 1, fiber 2, carbs 8, protein 4

100. Lemony Fennel Mix

Preparation time: 10 minutes

Cooking time: 0 minutes
Servings: 4
Ingredients:
- 3 tablespoons lemon juice
- 1 pound fennel, chopped
- 2 tablespoons olive oil
- A pinch of black pepper

Directions:
1. In a salad bowl, mix fennel with and black pepper, oil and lemon juice, toss well, divide between plates and serve as a side dish.
2. Enjoy!

Nutrition Values: calories 130, fat 1, fiber 1, carbs 7, protein 7

101. Simple Cauliflower Mix

Preparation time: 10 minutes
Cooking time: 35 minutes
Servings: 4
Ingredients:
- 6 cups cauliflower florets
- 2 teaspoons sweet paprika
- 2 cups chicken stock
- ¼ cup avocado oil
- Black pepper to the taste

Directions:
1. In a baking dish, combine the cauliflower with stock, oil, black pepper and paprika, toss, introduce in the oven and bake at 375 degrees F for 35 minutes.
2. Divide between plates and serve as a side dish.
3. Enjoy!

Nutrition Values: calories 180, fat 3, fiber 2, carbs 46, protein 6

102. Broccoli Mix

Preparation time: 10 minutes
Cooking time: 3 hours
Servings: 10
Ingredients:
- 6 cups broccoli florets
- 10 ounces tomato sauce, sodium-free
- 1 and ½ cups low-fat cheddar cheese, shredded
- ½ teaspoon cider vinegar
- ¼ cup yellow onion, chopped
- A pinch of black pepper
- 2 tablespoons olive oil

Directions:
1. Grease your slow cooker with the oil, add broccoli, tomato sauce, cider vinegar, onion and black pepper, cover and cook on High for 2 hours and 30 minutes.
2. Sprinkle the cheese all over, cover, cook on High for 30 minutes more, divide between plates and serve as a side dish.
3. Enjoy!

Nutrition Values: calories 160, fat 6, fiber 4, carbs 11, protein 6

103. Tasty Bean Side Dish

Preparation time: 10 minutes
Cooking time: 5 hours
Servings: 10
Ingredients:
- 1 and ½ cups tomato sauce, salt-free
- 1 yellow onion, chopped
- 2 celery ribs, chopped
- 1 sweet red pepper, chopped
- 1 green bell pepper, chopped
- ½ cup water
- 2 bay leaves
- 1 teaspoon ground mustard
- 1 tablespoon cider vinegar
- 16 ounces canned kidney beans, no-salt-added, drained and rinsed
- 16 ounces canned black-eyed peas, no-salt-added, drained and rinsed
- 15 ounces corn
- 15 ounces canned lima beans, no-salt-added, drained and rinsed
- 15 ounces canned black beans, no-salt-added, drained and rinsed

Directions:
1. In your slow cooker, mix the tomato sauce with the onion, celery, red pepper, green bell pepper, water, bay leaves, mustard, vinegar, kidney beans, black-eyed peas, corn, lima beans and black beans, cover and cook on Low for 5 hours.
2. Discard bay leaves, divide the whole mix between plates and serve.
3. Enjoy!

Nutrition Values: calories 211, fat 4, fiber 8, carbs 20, protein 7

104. Easy Green Beans

Preparation time: 10 minutes
Cooking time: 2 hours
Servings: 12
Ingredients:
- 16 ounces green beans
- 3 tablespoons olive oil
- ½ cup coconut sugar
- 1 teaspoon low-sodium soy sauce
- ½ teaspoon garlic powder

Directions:
1. In your slow cooker, mix the green beans with the oil, sugar, soy sauce and garlic powder, cover and cook on Low for 2 hours.
2. Toss the beans, divide them between plates and serve as a side dish.
3. Enjoy!

Nutrition Values: calories 142, fat 7, fiber 4, carbs 15, protein 3

105. Creamy Corn

Preparation time: 10 minutes
Cooking time: 4 hours
Servings: 12

Ingredients:
- 10 cups corn
- 20 ounces fat-free cream cheese
- ½ cup fat-free milk
- ½ cup low-fat butter
- A pinch of black pepper
- 2 tablespoons green onions, chopped

Directions:
1. In your slow cooker, mix the corn with cream cheese, milk, butter, black pepper and onions, toss, cover and cook on Low for 4 hours.
2. Toss one more time, divide between plates and serve as a side dish.
3. Enjoy!

Nutrition Values: calories 256, fat 11, fiber 2, carbs 17, protein 5

106. Classic Peas and Carrots

Preparation time: 10 minutes
Cooking time: 5 hours
Servings: 12

Ingredients:
- 1 pound carrots, sliced
- ¼ cup water
- 1 yellow onion, chopped
- 2 tablespoons olive oil
- 2 tablespoons stevia
- 4 garlic cloves, minced
- 1 teaspoon marjoram, dried
- A pinch of white pepper
- 16 ounces peas

Directions:
1. In your slow cooker, mix the carrots with water, onion, oil, stevia, garlic, marjoram, white pepper and peas, toss, cover and cook on High for 5 hours.
2. Divide between plates and serve as a side dish.
3. Enjoy!

Nutrition Values: calories 107, fat 3, fiber 3, carbs 14, protein 4

107. Mushroom Pilaf

Preparation time: 10 minutes
Cooking time: 3 hours
Servings: 6

Ingredients:
- 1 cup wild rice
- 2 garlic cloves, minced
- 6 green onions, chopped
- 2 tablespoons olive oil
- ½ pound baby Bella mushrooms
- 2 cups water

Directions:
1. In your slow cooker, mix the rice with garlic, onions, oil, mushrooms and water, toss, cover and cook on Low for 3 hours.
2. Stir the pilaf one more time, divide between plates and serve.

3. Enjoy!

Nutrition Values: calories 210, fat 7, fiber 1, carbs 16, protein 4

108. Butternut Mix

Preparation time: 10 minutes
Cooking time: 4 hours
Servings: 8

Ingredients:
- 1 cup carrots, chopped
- 1 tablespoon olive oil
- 1 yellow onion, chopped
- ½ teaspoon stevia
- 1 garlic clove, minced
- ½ teaspoon curry powder
- ½ teaspoon cinnamon powder
- ¼ teaspoon ginger, grated
- 1 butternut squash, cubed
- 2 and ½ cups low-sodium veggie stock
- ½ cup basmati rice
- ¾ cup coconut milk

Directions:
1. Heat up a pan with the oil over medium-highheat, add the oil, onion, garlic, stevia, carrots, curry powder, cinnamon and ginger, stir, cook for 5 minutes and transfer to your slow cooker.
2. Add squash, stock and coconut milk, stir, cover and cook on Low for 4 hours.
3. Divide the butternut mix between plates and serve as a side dish.
4. Enjoy!

Nutrition Values: calories 200, fat 4, fiber 4, carbs 17, protein 3

109. Sausage Side Dish

Preparation time: 10 minutes
Cooking time: 2 hours
Servings: 12

Ingredients:
- 1 pound no-sugar, beef sausage, chopped
- 2 tablespoons olive oil
- ½ pound mushrooms, chopped
- 6 celery ribs, chopped
- 2 yellow onions, chopped
- 2 garlic cloves, minced
- 1 tablespoon sage, dried
- 1 cup low-sodium veggie stock
- 1 cup cranberries, dried
- ½ cup sunflower seeds, peeled
- 1 whole wheat bread loaf, cubed

Directions:
1. Heat up a pan with the oil over medium-high heat, add beef, stir and brown for a few minutes.
2. Add mushrooms, onion, celery, garlic and sage, stir, cook for a few more minutes and transfer to your slow cooker.
3. Add stock, cranberries, sunflower seeds and the bread cubes, cover and cook on High for 2 hours.

4.   Stir the whole mix, divide between plates and serve as a side dish.
5.   Enjoy!
Nutrition Values: calories 200, fat 3, fiber 6, carbs 13, protein 4

110. Easy Potatoes Mix

Preparation time: 10 minutes
Cooking time: 6 hours
Servings: 8
Ingredients:
- 16 baby red potatoes, halved
- 1 carrot, sliced
- 1 celery rib, chopped
- ¼ cup yellow onion, chopped
- 2 cups low-sodium chicken stock
- 1 tablespoon parsley, chopped
- A pinch of black pepper
- 1 garlic clove minced
- 2 tablespoons olive oil

Directions:
1.   In your slow cooker, mix the potatoes with the carrot, celery, onion, stock, parsley, garlic, oil and black pepper, toss, cover and cook on Low for 6 hours.
2.   Divide between plates and serve as a side dish.
3.   Enjoy!
Nutrition Values: calories 114, fat 3, fiber 3, carbs 18, protein 4

111. Black-Eyed Peas Mix

Preparation time: 10 minutes
Cooking time: 5 hours
Servings: 12
Ingredients:
- 17 ounces black-eyed peas
- ½ cup sausage, chopped
- 1 yellow onion, chopped
- 1 sweet red pepper, chopped
- 1 jalapeno, chopped
- 2 garlic cloves minced
- ½ teaspoon cumin, ground
- A pinch of black pepper
- 6 cups water
- 2 tablespoons cilantro, chopped

Directions:
1.   In your slow cooker, mix the peas with the sausage, onion, red pepper, jalapeno, garlic, cumin, black pepper, water and cilantro, cover and cook on Low for 5 hours.
2.   Divide between plates and serve as a side dish.
3.   Enjoy!
Nutrition Values: calories 170, fat 3, fiber 7, carbs 20, protein 13

112. Green Beans and Corn Mix

Preparation time: 10 minutes
Cooking time: 4 hours

Servings: 8
Ingredients:
- 15 ounces green beans
- 14 ounces corn
- 11 ounces cream of mushroom soup, low-fat and sodium-free
- 4 ounces mushrooms, sliced
- ½ cup almonds, chopped
- ½ cup low-fat cheddar cheese, shredded
- ½ cup low-fat sour cream

Directions:
1.   In your slow cooker, mix the green beans with the corn, mushrooms soup, mushrooms, almonds, cheese and sour cream, toss, cover and cook on Low for 4 hours.
2.   Stir one more time, divide between plates and serve as a side dish.
3.   Enjoy!
Nutrition Values: calories 211, fat 8, fiber 3, carbs 16, protein 4

113. Spiced Carrots

Preparation time: 10 minutes
Cooking time: 6 hours
Servings: 6
Ingredients:
- 2 pounds small carrots, peeled
- ½ cup low-fat butter, melted
- ½ cup canned peach, unsweetened
- 3 tablespoons stevia
- ½ teaspoon cinnamon powder
- 1 teaspoon vanilla extract
- A pinch of nutmeg, ground
- 2 tablespoons water
- 2 tablespoons cornstarch

Directions:
1.   In your slow cooker, mix the carrots with the butter, peach, stevia, cinnamon, vanilla, nutmeg and cornstarch mixed with water, toss, cover and cook on Low for 6 hours.
2.   Toss the carrots one more time, divide between plates and serve as a side dish.
3.   Enjoy!
Nutrition Values: calories 200, fat 12, fiber 4, carbs 20, protein 3

114. Squash and Grains Mix

Preparation time: 10 minutes
Cooking time: 4 hours
Servings: 12
Ingredients:
- 1 butternut squash, peeled and cubed
- 1 cup whole grain blend, uncooked
- 1 yellow onion, chopped
- 3 garlic cloves, minced
- ½ cup water
- 2 teaspoons thyme, chopped
- A pinch of black pepper
- 12 ounces low-sodium veggie stock

- 6 ounces baby spinach

Directions:
1.   In your slow cooker, mix the squash with whole grain, onion, garlic, water, thyme, black pepper, stock and spinach, cover and cook on Low for 4 hours.
2.   Divide between plates and serve as a side dish.
3.   Enjoy!
Nutrition Values: calories 100, fat 1, fiber 4, carbs 22, protein 3

115. Mushroom Mix

Preparation time: 10 minutes
Cooking time: 4 hours
Servings: 6
Ingredients:
- 1 pound mushrooms, halved
- 3 tablespoons olive oil
- 1 yellow onion, chopped
- 1 teaspoon Italian seasoning
- 1 cup tomato sauce, no-salt-added

Directions:
1.   In your slow cooker, mix the mushrooms with the oil, onion, Italian seasoning and tomato sauce, toss, cover and cook on Low for 4 hours.
2.   Divide between plates and serve as a side dish.
3.   Enjoy!
Nutrition Values: calories 100, fat 5, fiber 2, carbs 9, protein 4

116. Spinach and Rice

Preparation time: 10 minutes
Cooking time: 4 hours
Servings: 8
Ingredients:
- 2 tablespoons olive oil
- 1 yellow onion, chopped
- ¼ teaspoon thyme, dried
- 2 garlic cloves, minced
- 4 cups low-sodium chicken stock
- 20 ounces spinach, chopped
- 8 ounces fat-free cream cheese
- 2 cups wild rice
- 2 cups low-fat cheddar cheese, shredded
- ½ cup whole wheat bread, crumbled

Directions:
1.   In your slow cooker, mix the oil with the onion, thyme, garlic, stock, spinach, cream cheese and rice, toss, cover and cook on Low for 4 hours.
2.   Add the cheese and the breadcrumbs, cover the pot, leave it aside for a few minutes, divide between plates and serve as a side dish.
3.   Enjoy!
Nutrition Values: calories 199, fat 2, fiber 6, carbs 9, protein 6

117. Creamy Mushrooms Mix

Preparation time: 10 minutes
Cooking time: 8 hours

Servings: 8
Ingredients:
- 1 and ½ pounds cremini mushrooms, halved
- 2 garlic cloves, minced
- 1 shallot, chopped
- ¼ cup low sodium chicken stock
- 2 tablespoons parsley, chopped
- ½ cup coconut cream
- 1 teaspoon cornstarch

Directions:
1.   In your slow cooker, mix the mushrooms with garlic, shallot, stock and parsley, cover and cook on Low for 7 hours.
2.   Add coconut cream mixed with the cornstarch, cover, cook on Low for 1 more hour, divide between plates and serve as a side dish.
3.   Enjoy!
Nutrition Values: calories 188, fat 3, fiber 8, carbs 17, protein 4

118. Ginger Beets

Preparation time: 10 minutes
Cooking time: 6 hours
Servings: 8
Ingredients:
- 6 beets, peeled and sliced
- 1 teaspoon orange peel, grated
- 2 tablespoons stevia
- 1/3 cup orange juice
- 2 tablespoons white vinegar
- 2 tablespoons olive oil
- 1 tablespoon ginger, grated
- A pinch of black pepper

Directions:
1.   In your slow cooker, mix the beets with the orange peel, orange juice, stevia, vinegar, oil, ginger and black pepper, toss, cover and cook on Low for 6 hours.
2.   Divide between plates and serve as a side dish.
3.   Enjoy!
Nutrition Values: calories 177, fat 2, fiber 7, carbs 11, protein 3

119. Artichokes Mix

Preparation time: 10 minutes
Cooking time: 5 hours
Servings: 8
Ingredients:
- 4 artichokes, trimmed and halved
- 2 cups whole wheat breadcrumbs
- 1 tablespoon olive oil
- Juice of 1 lemon
- 3 garlic cloves, minced
- 1/3 cup low-fat parmesan, grated
- 1 tablespoon lemon zest, grated
- 2 tablespoons parsley, chopped
- Black pepper to the taste

- 1 cup low-sodium vegetable stock
- 1 tablespoon shallot, minced
- 1 teaspoon oregano, chopped

Directions:
1. Rub artichokes with the lemon juice and the oil and put them in your slow cooker.
2. Add breadcrumbs, garlic, parsley, parmesan, lemon zest, black pepper, shallot, oregano and stock, cover and cook on Low for 5 hours.
3. Divide the whole mix between plates, sprinkle parsley on top and serve as a side dish.
4. Enjoy!

Nutrition Values: calories 200, fat 4, fiber 4, carbs 10, protein 6

120. Asparagus Mix

Preparation time: 10 minutes
Cooking time: 2 hours
Servings: 4
Ingredients:
- 1 pound asparagus, trimmed and halved
- 1 tablespoon parsley, chopped
- ½ cup low-sodium veggie stock
- 1 garlic clove, minced
- ¼ teaspoon lemon zest, grated
- 2 teaspoons lemon juice

Directions:
1. In your slow cooker, mix the asparagus with the parsley, stock, garlic, lemon zest and lemon juice, toss a bit, cover and cook on High for 2 hours.
2. Divide the asparagus between plates and serve as a side dish.
3. Enjoy!

Nutrition Values: calories 130, fat 3, fiber 2, carbs 10, protein 4

121. Black Bean and Corn Mix

Preparation time: 10 minutes
Cooking time: 6 hours
Servings: 6
Ingredients:
- 4 tomatoes, chopped
- 1 cup corn kernels
- 16 ounces canned black beans, drained
- 2 garlic cloves, minced
- ½ cup parsley, chopped
- 1 small red onion, chopped
- 1 red bell pepper, chopped
- Juice of 1 lemon
- 2 tablespoons stevia

Directions:
1. In your slow cooker, mix the tomatoes with corn, black beans, garlic, parsley, lemon juice, bell pepper, onion and stevia, toss, cook on Low for 6 hours, divide between plates and serve as a side dish.
2. Enjoy!

Nutrition Values: calories 210, fat 1, fiber 5, carbs 15, protein 7

122. Celery Mix

Preparation time: 10 minutes
Cooking time: 3 hours
Servings: 3
Ingredients:
- 2 celery roots, cut into medium wedges
- 1 cup low-sodium veggie stock
- 1 teaspoon mustard
- ¼ cup low-fat sour cream
- Black pepper to the taste
- 2 teaspoons thyme, chopped

Directions:
1. In your slow cooker, mix the celery with the stock, mustard, cream, black pepper and thyme, cover and cook on High for 3 hours.
2. Divide the celery between plates, drizzle some of the cooking juices on top and serve as a side dish.
3. Enjoy!

Nutrition Values: calories 160, fat 2, fiber 1, carbs 7, protein 4

123. Kale Side Dish

Preparation time: 10 minutes
Cooking time: 2 hours
Servings: 6
Ingredients:
- 1 pound kale, chopped
- 2 teaspoons olive oil
- 4 garlic cloves, minced
- ½ cup low-sodium veggie stock
- 1 tablespoons lemon juice
- 1 cup cherry tomatoes, halved
- Black pepper to the taste

Directions:
1. Heat up a pan with the oil over medium heat, add garlic, stir, cook for 2 minutes and transfer to your slow cooker.
2. Add kale, stock, tomatoes, black pepper and lemon juice, cover, cook on High for 2 hours.
3. Divide the whole mix between plates and serve as a side dish.
4. Enjoy!

Nutrition Values: calories 160, fat 2, fiber 3, carbs 8, protein 4

124. Spicy Eggplant

Preparation time: 10 minutes
Cooking time: 3 hours
Servings: 4
Ingredients:
- 1 eggplant, sliced
- ½ teaspoon cumin, ground
- 1 teaspoon mustard seed
- ½ teaspoon coriander, ground
- ½ teaspoon curry powder
- A pinch of nutmeg, ground
- 2 cups cherry tomatoes, halved
- ½ yellow onion, chopped
- 1 tablespoon olive oil

- 1 garlic clove, minced
- 1 teaspoon red wine vinegar
- Black pepper to the taste
- 1 tablespoon cilantro, chopped

Directions:
1. Grease the slow cooker with the oil and add eggplant slices inside.
2. Add cumin, mustard seeds, coriander, curry powder, nutmeg, tomatoes, onion, garlic, vinegar, black pepper and cilantro, cover and cook on High for 3 hours.
3. Divide between plates and serve as a side dish.
4. Enjoy!

Nutrition Values: calories 180, fat 4, fiber 5, carbs 20, protein 4

125. Corn Salad

Preparation time: 10 minutes
Cooking time: 2 hours
Servings: 6
Ingredients:
- 2 ounces prosciutto, cut into strips
- 1 teaspoon olive oil
- 2 cups corn
- ½ cup salt-free tomato sauce
- 1 teaspoon garlic, minced
- 1 green bell pepper, chopped

Directions:
1. Grease your slow cooker with the oil, add corn, prosciutto, tomato sauce, garlic and bell pepper, cover and cook on High for 2 hours.

2. Divide between plates and serve as a side dish.
3. Enjoy!

Nutrition Values: calories 109, fat 2, fiber 2, carbs 10, protein 5

126. Spiced Cabbage

Preparation time: 10 minutes
Cooking time: 4 hours
Servings: 6
Ingredients:
- 2 yellow onions, chopped
- 10 cups red cabbage, shredded
- 1 cup plums, pitted and chopped
- 1 teaspoon cinnamon powder
- 1 garlic clove, minced
- 1 teaspoon cumin seeds
- ¼ teaspoon cloves, ground
- 2 tablespoons red wine vinegar
- 1 teaspoon coriander seeds
- ½ cup water

Directions:
1. In your slow cooker, mix cabbage with onions, plums, garlic, cinnamon, cumin, cloves, vinegar, coriander and water, stir, cover and cook on Low for 4 hours.
2. Divide between plates and serve as a side dish.
3. Enjoy!

Nutrition Values: calories 197, fat 1, fiber 5, carbs 14, protein 3

SEAFOOD

127. Steamed Salmon Teriyaki

Servings: 4
Cooking time: 15 minutes
Ingredients:
- 3 green onions, minced
- 2 packet Stevia
- 1 tbsp freshly grated ginger
- 1 clove garlic, minced
- 2 tsp sesame seeds
- 1 tbsp sesame oil
- ¼ cup mirin
- 2 tbsp low sodium soy sauce
- 1/2-lb salmon filet

Directions:
1. Place a large saucepan on medium high fire. Place a trivet inside saucepan and fill pan halfway with water. Cover and bring to a boil.
2. Meanwhile in a heat-proof dish that fits inside saucepan, mix well stevia, ginger, garlic, oil, mirin, and soy sauce. Add salmon and cover well with sauce.
3. Top salmon with sesame seeds and green onions. Cover dish with foil.
4. Place on top of trivet. Cover and steam for 15 minutes.
5. Let it rest for 5 minutes in pan.
6. Serve and enjoy.

Nutrition Values:
Calories: 242.7; Carbs: 1.2g; Protein: 35.4g; Fats: 10.7g; Saturated Fat: 2.1g; Sodium: 285mg

128. Easy Steamed Alaskan Cod

Servings: 3
Cooking time: 15 minutes
Ingredients:
- 2 tbsp butter
- Pepper to taste
- 1 cup cherry tomatoes, halved
- 1 large Wild Alaskan cod filet, cut into 3 smaller pieces

Directions:
1. Place a large saucepan on medium high fire. Place a trivet inside saucepan and fill pan halfway with water. Cover and bring to a boil.
2. Meanwhile in a heat-proof dish that fits inside saucepan, add all ingredients.
3. Cover dish with a foil. Place on trivet and steam for 15 minutes.
4. Serve and enjoy.

Nutrition Values:
Calories: 132.9; Carbs: 1.9g; Protein: 12.2g; Fats: 8.5g; Saturated Fat: 4.9g; Sodium: 296mg

129. Dill and Lemon Cod Packets

Servings: 2
Cooking time: 10 minutes
Ingredients:
- 2 tsp olive oil, divided
- 4 slices lemon, divided
- 2 sprigs fresh dill, divide
- ½ tsp garlic powder, divided
- Pepper to taste
- 1/2-lb cod filets

Directions:
1. Place a large saucepan on medium high fire. Place a trivet inside saucepan and fill pan halfway with water. Cover and bring to a boil.
2. Cut two pieces of 15-inch lengths foil.
3. In one foil, place one filet in the middle. Season with pepper to taste. Sprinkle ¼ tsp garlic. Add a tsp of oil on top of filet. Top with 2 slices of lemon and a sprig of dill. Fold over the foil and seal the filet inside. Repeat process for remaining fish.
4. Place packet on trivet. Cover and steam for 10 minutes.
5. Serve and enjoy.

Nutrition Values:
Calories: 164.8; Carbs: 9.4g; Protein: 18.3g; Fats: 6g; Saturated Fat: 1g; Sodium: 347mg

130. Steamed Fish Mediterranean Style

Servings: 4
Cooking time: 15 minutes
Ingredients:
- Pepper to taste
- 1 clove garlic, smashed
- 2 tsp olive oil
- 1 bunch fresh thyme
- 2 tbsp pickled capers
- 1 cup black salt-cured olives
- 1-lb cherry tomatoes, halved
- 1 ½-lbs. cod filets

Directions:
1. Place a large saucepan on medium high fire. Place a trivet inside saucepan and fill pan halfway with water. Cover and bring to a boil.
2. Meanwhile in a heat-proof dish that fits inside saucepan, layer half of the halved cherry tomatoes. Season with pepper.
3. Add filets on top of tomatoes and season with pepper. Drizzle oil. Sprinkle 3/4s of thyme on top and the smashed garlic.
4. Cover top of fish with remaining cherry tomatoes and place dish on trivet. Cover dish with foil.
5. Cover pan and steam for 15 minutes.
6. Serve and enjoy.

Nutrition Values:
Calories: 263.2; Carbs: 21.8g; Protein: 27.8g; Fats: 7.2g; Saturated Fat: 1.1g; Sodium: 264mg

131. Steamed Veggie and Lemon Pepper Salmon

Servings: 4
Cooking time: 15 minutes

Ingredients:
- 1 carrot, peeled and julienned
- 1 red bell pepper, julienned
- 1 zucchini, julienned
- ½ lemon, sliced thinly
- 1 tsp pepper
- ½ tsp salt
- 1/2-lb salmon filet with skin on
- A dash of tarragon

Directions:
1. Place a large saucepan on medium high fire. Place a trivet inside saucepan and fill pan halfway with water. Cover and bring to a boil.
2. Meanwhile in a heat-proof dish that fits inside saucepan, add salmon with skin side down. Season with pepper. Add slices of lemon on top.
3. Place the julienned vegetables on top of salmon and season with tarragon. Cover top of fish with remaining cherry tomatoes and place dish on trivet. Cover dish with foil.
4. Cover pan and steam for 15 minutes.
5. Serve and enjoy.

Nutrition Values:
Calories: 216.2; Carbs: 4.1g; Protein: 35.1g; Fats: 6.6g; Saturated Fat: 1.5g; Sodium: 332mg

132. Steamed Fish with Scallions and Ginger

Servings: 3
Cooking time: 15 minutes
Ingredients:
- ¼ cup chopped cilantro
- ¼ cup julienned scallions
- 2 tbsp julienned ginger
- 1 tbsp peanut oil
- 1-lb Tilapia filets
- 1 tsp garlic
- 1 tsp minced ginger
- 2 tbsp rice wine
- 1 tbsp low sodium soy sauce

Directions:
1. In a heat-proof dish that fits inside saucepan, add garlic, minced ginger, rice wine, and soy sauce. Mix well. Add the Tilapia filet and marinate for half an hour, while turning over at half time.
2. Place a large saucepan on medium high fire. Place a trivet inside saucepan and fill pan halfway with water. Cover and bring to a boil.
3. Cover dish of fish with foil and place on trivet.
4. Cover pan and steam for 15 minutes.
5. Serve and enjoy.

Nutrition Values:
Calories: 219; Carbs: 4.5g; Protein: 31.8g; Fats: 8.2g; Saturated Fat: 1.9g; Sodium: 252mg

133. Steamed Tilapia with Green Chutney

Servings: 3

Cooking time: 10 minutes
Ingredients:
- 1-pound tilapia fillets, divided into 3
- ½ cup green commercial chutney

Directions:
1. Place a large saucepan on medium high fire. Place a trivet inside saucepan and fill pan halfway with water. Cover and bring to a boil.
2. Cut 3 pieces of 15-inch lengths foil.
3. In one foil, place one filet in the middle and 1/3 of chutney. Fold over the foil and seal the filet inside. Repeat process for remaining fish.
4. Place packet on trivet. Cover and steam for 10 minutes.
5. Serve and enjoy.

Nutrition Values:
Calories: 151.5; Carbs: 1.1g; Protein: 30.7g; Fats: 2.7g; Saturated Fat: .9g; Sodium: 79mg

134. Creamy Haddock with Kale

Servings: 5
Cooking time: 10 minutes
Ingredients:
- 1 tbsp olive oil
- 1 onion, chopped
- 2 cloves of garlic, minced
- 2 cups chicken broth
- 1 teaspoon crushed red pepper flakes
- 1-pound wild Haddock fillets
- ½ cup heavy cream
- 1 tablespoons basil
- 1 cup kale leaves, chopped
- Pepper to taste

Directions:
1. Place a heavy bottomed pot on medium high fire and heat pot for 3 minutes.
2. Once hot, add oil and stir around to coat pot with oil.
3. Sauté the onion and garlic for 5 minutes.
4. Add remaining ingredients, except for basil and mix well.
5. Cover, bring to a boil, lower fire to a simmer, and simmer for 5 minutes.
6. Serve and enjoy with a sprinkle of basil.

Nutrition Values:
Calories: 130.5; Carbs: 5.5g; Protein: 35.7g; Fats: 14.5g; Saturated Fat: 5.2g; Sodium: 278mg

135. Coconut Curry Sea Bass

Servings: 3
Cooking time: 15 minutes
Ingredients:
- 1 can coconut milk
- Juice of 1 lime, freshly squeezed
- 1 tablespoon red curry paste
- 1 teaspoon coconut aminos
- 1 teaspoon honey
- 2 teaspoons sriracha
- 2 cloves of garlic, minced

- 1 teaspoon ground turmeric
- 1 tablespoon curry powder
- ¼ cup fresh cilantro
- Pepper

Directions:
1. Place a heavy bottomed pot on medium high fire.
2. Mix in all ingredients.
3. Cover, bring to a boil, lower fire to a simmer, and simmer for 5 minutes.
4. Serve and enjoy.

Nutrition Values:
Calories: 241.8; Carbs: 12.8g; Protein: 3.1g; Fats: 19.8g; Saturated Fat: 17g; Sodium: 19mg

136. Stewed Cod Filet with tomatoes

Servings: 6
Cooking time: 15 minutes
Ingredients:
- 1 tbsp olive oil
- 1 onion, sliced
- 1 ½ pounds fresh cod fillets
- Pepper
- 1 lemon juice, freshly squeezed
- 1 can diced tomatoes

Directions:
1. Place a heavy bottomed pot on medium high fire and heat pot for 3 minutes.
2. Once hot, add oil and stir around to coat pot with oil.
3. Sauté the onion for 2 minutes. Stir in diced tomatoes and cook for 5 minutes.
4. Add cod filet and season with pepper.
5. Cover, bring to a boil, lower fire to a simmer, and simmer for 5 minutes.
6. Serve and enjoy with freshly squeezed lemon juice.

Nutrition Values:
Calories: 106.4; Carbs: 2.5g; Protein: 17.8g; Fats: 2.8g; Saturated Fat: .4g; Sodium: 381mg

137. Lemony Parmesan Shrimps

Servings: 4
Cooking time: 15 minutes
Ingredients:
- 1 tablespoon olive oil
- ½ cup onion, chopped
- 3 cloves of garlic, minced
- 1-pound shrimps, peeled and deveined
- ½ cup parmesan cheese, low fat
- 1 cup spinach, shredded
- ½ cup chicken broth, low sodium
- ¼ cup water
- Pepper

Directions:
1. Place a heavy bottomed pot on medium high fire and heat pot for 3 minutes.
2. Once hot, add oil and stir around to coat pot with oil.
3. Sauté the onion and garlic for 5 minutes. Stir in shrimps and cook for 2 minutes.
4. Add remaining ingredients, except for parmesan.
5. Cover, bring to a boil, lower fire to a simmer, and simmer for 5 minutes.
6. Serve and enjoy with a sprinkle of parmesan.

Nutrition Values:
Calories: 252.6; Carbs: 5.4g; Protein: 33.9g; Fats: 10.6g; Saturated Fat: 3.2g; Sodium: 344mg

138. Tuna 'n Carrots Casserole

Servings: 4
Cooking time: 12 minutes
Ingredients:
- 2 carrots, peeled and chopped
- ¼ cup diced onions
- 1 cup frozen peas
- ¾ cup milk
- 2 cans tuna in water, drained
- 1 can cream of celery soup
- 1 tbsp olive oil
- ½ cup water
- 2 eggs beaten
- Pepper

Directions:
1. Place a heavy bottomed pot on medium high fire and heat pot for 3 minutes.
2. Once hot, add oil and stir around to coat pot with oil.
3. Sauté the onion and carrots for 3 minutes.
4. Add remaining ingredients and mix well.
5. Bring to a boil while stirring constantly, cook until thickened around 5 minutes.
6. Serve and enjoy.

Nutrition Values:
Calories: 281.3; Carbs: 14.3g; Protein: 24.3g; Fats: 14.1g; Saturated Fat: 3.7g; Sodium: 275mg

139. Sweet-Ginger Scallops

Servings: 3
Cooking time: 15 minutes
Ingredients:
- 1-pound sea scallops, shells removed
- ½ cup coconut aminos
- 3 tablespoons maple syrup
- ½ teaspoon garlic powder
- ½ teaspoon ground ginger

Directions:
1. In a heat-proof dish that fits inside saucepan, add all ingredients. Mix well.
2. Place a large saucepan on medium high fire. Place a trivet inside saucepan and fill pan halfway with water. Cover and bring to a boil.
3. Cover dish of scallops with foil and place on trivet.
4. Cover pan and steam for 10 minutes. Let it rest in pan for another 5 minutes.
5. Serve and enjoy.

Nutrition Values:
Calories: 233.4; Carbs: 23.7g; Protein: 31.5g; Fats: 1.4g; Saturated Fat: .4g; Sodium: 153mg

140. Savory Lobster Roll

Servings: 6
Cooking time: 20 minutes
Ingredients:
- 1 ½ cups chicken broth, low sodium
- 2 teaspoon old bay seasoning
- 2 pounds lobster tails, raw and in the shell
- 1 lemon, halved
- 3 scallions, chopped
- 1 teaspoon celery seeds

Directions:
1. Place a heavy bottomed pot on medium high fire and add all ingredients and ½ of the lemon.
2. Cover, bring to a boil, lower fire to a simmer, and simmer for 15 minutes.
3. Let it rest for another 5 minutes.
4. Serve and enjoy with freshly squeezed lemon juice.

Nutrition Values:
Calories: 209; Carbs: 1.9g; Protein: 38.2g; Fats: 5.4g; Saturated Fat: 1.4g; Sodium: 288mg

141. Garlic 'n Tomatoes on Mussels

Servings: 6
Cooking time: 15 minutes
Ingredients:
- ¼ cup white wine
- ½ cup water
- 3 Roma tomatoes, chopped
- 2 cloves of garlic, minced
- 1 bay leaf
- 2 pounds mussels, scrubbed
- ½ cup fresh parsley, chopped
- 1 tbsp oil
- Pepper

Directions:
1. Place a heavy bottomed pot on medium high fire and heat pot for 3 minutes.
2. Once hot, add oil and stir around to coat pot with oil.
3. Sauté the garlic, bay leaf, and tomatoes for 5 minutes.
4. Add remaining ingredients, except for parsley and mussels. Mix well.
5. Add mussels.
6. Cover, bring to a boil, and boil for 5 minutes.
7. Serve and enjoy with a sprinkle of parsley and discard any unopened mussels.

Nutrition Values:
Calories: 172.8; Carbs: 10.2g; Protein: 19.5g; Fats: 6g; Saturated Fat: 1.1g; Sodium: 261mg

142. Lobster Tarragon Stew

Servings: 4
Cooking time: 30 minutes
Ingredients:

- 1 tablespoon olive oil
- 2 onions, diced
- 2 cloves of garlic, minced
- 1 carrot, chopped
- 2 lobsters, shelled
- 1-pound ripe tomatoes, chopped
- 2 tablespoon tomato paste
- 1/3 clam juice
- 1 tablespoon tarragon

Directions:
1. Place a heavy bottomed pot on medium high fire and heat pot for 3 minutes.
2. Once hot, add oil and stir around to coat pot with oil.
3. Sauté the onion, tomatoes and garlic for 10 minutes.
4. Stir in tomato paste, clam juice, and carrot. Cook for 5 minutes.
5. Add lobsters and mix well.
6. Cover and simmer for 5 minutes.
7. Serve and enjoy a sprinkle of tarragon.

Nutrition Values:
Calories: 149.9; Carbs: 13.3g; Protein: 14.5g; Fats: 4.3g; Saturated Fat: 1g; Sodium: 341mg

143. Easy Steamed Crab Legs

Servings: 4
Cooking time: 10 minutes
Ingredients:
- 2 pounds frozen crab legs
- 4 tablespoons low fat butter
- 1 tablespoon lemon juice, freshly squeezed

Directions:
1. Place a heavy bottomed pot on medium high fire, fill with 5 cups water and bring to a boil.
2. Add crab legs, cover and steam for 10 minutes. Once done, turn off fire and let it rest for 5 minutes.
3. Meanwhile, in a microwave safe bowl, melt butter. Once melted, add lemon juice and mix well.
4. Serve crab legs with lemon-butter dip on the side.

Nutrition Values:
Calories: 201.9; Carbs: 2.2g; Protein: 44g; Fats: 1.9g; Saturated Fat: .3g; Sodium: 297mg

144. Tasty Corn and Clam Stew

Servings: 4
Cooking time: 25 minutes
Ingredients:
- 1-lb clam
- 1 cup frozen corn
- ½ cup water
- 4 cloves garlic
- 1 tsp oil
- 1 tsp celery seeds
- 1 tsp Cajun seasoning

Directions:

1. Place a nonstick saucepan on medium high fire and heat pot for 3 minutes.
2. Once hot, add oil and stir around to coat pot with oil.
3. Sauté the garlic for a minute.
4. Add remaining ingredients, except for clams and mix well. Cook for 3 minutes.
5. Stir in clams.
6. Cover, bring to a boil, lower fire to a simmer, and simmer for 5 minutes.
7. Serve and enjoy. Discard any unopened clam.

Nutrition Values:
Calories: 120; Carbs: 23.2g; Protein: 2.3g; Fats: 2g; Saturated Fat: .2g; Sodium: 466mg

145. Seafood Curry Recipe from Japan

Servings: 4
Cooking time: 30 minutes
Ingredients:
- 3 onions, chopped
- 2 cloves of garlic, minced
- 1-inch ginger, grated
- 1 tsp oil
- 3 cups water
- 1 2-inch long kombu or dried kelp
- 6 shiitake mushrooms, halved
- 12 manila clams, scrubbed
- 6 ounces medium-sized shrimps, peeled and deveined
- 6 ounces bay scallops
- 1 package Japanese curry roux
- ¼ apple, sliced

Directions:
1. Place a heavy bottomed pot on medium high fire and heat pot for 3 minutes.
2. Once hot, add oil and stir around to coat pot with oil.
3. Sauté the onion, ginger and garlic for 5 minutes.
4. Add remaining ingredients and mix well.
5. Cover, bring to a boil, lower fire to a simmer, and simmer for 5 minutes. Let it rest for 5 minutes.
6. Serve and enjoy. Discard any unopened clams.

Nutrition Values:
Calories: 183.7; Carbs: 17.9g; Protein: 22.4g; Fats: 2.5g; Saturated Fat: .5g; Sodium: 294mg

146. Steamed Asparagus and Shrimps

Servings: 6
Cooking time: 25 minutes
Ingredients:
- 1-pound shrimps, peeled and deveined
- 1 bunch asparagus, trimmed
- 1 teaspoon oil
- ½ tablespoon Cajun seasoning

Directions:
1. In a heat-proof dish that fits inside saucepan, add all ingredients. Mix well.

2. Place a large saucepan on medium high fire. Place a trivet inside saucepan and fill pan halfway with water. Cover and bring to a boil.
3. Cover dish with foil and place on trivet.
4. Cover pan and steam for 10 minutes. Let it rest in pan for another 5 minutes.
5. Serve and enjoy.

Nutrition Values:
Calories: 79.8; Carbs: .4g; Protein: 15.5g; Fats: 1.8g; Saturated Fat: .3g; Sodium: 209mg

147. Coconut Milk Sauce over Crabs

Servings: 6
Cooking time: 20 minutes
Ingredients:
- 2-pounds crab quartered
- 1 can coconut milk
- 1 lemongrass stalk
- 1 thumb-size ginger, sliced
- 1 onion, chopped
- 3 cloves of garlic, minced
- Pepper

Directions:
1. Place a heavy bottomed pot on medium high fire and add all ingredients.
2. Cover, bring to a boil, lower fire to a simmer, and simmer for 10 minutes.
3. Serve and enjoy.

Nutrition Values:
Calories: 244.1; Carbs: 6.3g; Protein: 29.3g; Fats: 11.3g; Saturated Fat: 8.8g; Sodium: 356mg

148. Cajun Shrimp Boil

Servings: 4
Cooking time: 40 minutes
Ingredients:
- 2 corn on the cobs, halved
- 1/2 kielbasa sausage, sliced into 2-inch pieces
- 1 cup chicken broth, low sodium
- 1 tablespoon old bay seasoning
- 1 tsp celery seeds
- 4 garlic cloves, smashed
- 1 teaspoon crushed red peppers
- 4 small potatoes, brushed and halved
- 1 onion, chopped
- 1-pound shrimps
- 1 tbsp olive oil
- Pepper

Directions:
1. Place a heavy bottomed pot on medium high fire and heat pot for 3 minutes.
2. Once hot, add oil and stir around to coat pot with oil.
3. Sauté the garlic, onion, potatoes, and sausage for 5 minutes.
4. Stir in corn, broth, old bay, celery seeds, and red peppers. Cover and cook for 5 minutes.

5.   Stir in shrimps and cook for another 5 minutes.
6.   Serve and enjoy.
Nutrition Values:
Calories: 549.5; Carbs: 69.4g; Protein: 44.8g; Fats: 10.3g; Saturated Fat: 2.1g; Sodium: 289mg

149. Sautéed Savory Shrimps

Servings: 8
Cooking time: 15 minutes
Ingredients:
- 2 pounds shrimp, peeled and deveined
- 1 tablespoon olive oil
- 4 cloves garlic, minced
- 2 cups frozen sweet corn kernels
- ½ cup chicken stock, low sodium
- 1 tablespoon lemon juice
- Pepper
- 1 tablespoon parsley for garnish

Directions:
1.   Place a heavy bottomed pot on medium high fire and heat pot for 3 minutes.
2.   Once hot, add oil and stir around to coat pot with oil.
3.   Sauté the garlic and corn for 5 minutes.
4.   Add remaining ingredients and mix well.
5.   Cover, bring to a boil, lower fire to a simmer, and simmer for 5 minutes.
6.   Serve and enjoy.
Nutrition Values:
Calories: 180.6; Carbs: 11.4g; Protein: 25.2g; Fats: 3.8g; Saturated Fat: .6g; Sodium: 111mg

150. Sweet and Spicy Dolphinfish Filets

Servings: 2
Cooking time: 25 minutes
Ingredients:
- 2 Dolphinfish filets
- Pepper to taste
- 2 cloves of garlic, minced
- 1 thumb-size ginger, grated
- ½ lime, juiced
- 2 tablespoons honey
- 2 tablespoons sriracha
- 1 tablespoon orange juice, freshly squeezed

Directions:
1.   In a heat-proof dish that fits inside saucepan, add all ingredients. Mix well.
2.   Place a large saucepan on medium high fire. Place a trivet inside saucepan and fill pan halfway with water. Cover and bring to a boil.
3.   Cover dish with foil and place on trivet.
4.   Cover pan and steam for 10 minutes. Let it rest in pan for another 5 minutes.
5.   Serve and enjoy.
Nutrition Values:
Calories: 348.4; Carbs: 22.3g; Protein: 38.6g; Fats: 2.2g; Saturated Fat: .5g; Sodium: 183mg

151. Steamed Ginger Scallion Fish

Servings: 2
Cooking time: 30 minutes
Ingredients:
- 3 tablespoons soy sauce, low sodium
- 2 tablespoons rice wine
- 1 teaspoon minced ginger
- 1 teaspoon garlic
- 1-pound firm white fish

Directions:
1.   In a heat-proof dish that fits inside saucepan, add all ingredients. Mix well.
2.   Place a large saucepan on medium high fire. Place a trivet inside saucepan and fill pan halfway with water. Cover and bring to a boil.
3.   Cover dish with foil and place on trivet.
4.   Cover pan and steam for 10 minutes. Let it rest in pan for another 5 minutes.
5.   Serve and enjoy.
Nutrition Values:
Calories: 409.5; Carbs: 5.5g; Protein: 44.9g; Fats: 23.1g; Saturated Fat: 8.3g; Sodium: 115mg

152. Simply Steamed Alaskan Cod

Servings: 2
Cooking time: 15 minutes
Ingredients:
- 1-lb fillet wild Alaskan Cod
- 1 cup cherry tomatoes, halved
- Salt and pepper to taste
- 1 tbsp balsamic vinegar
- 1 tbsp fresh basil chopped

Directions:
1.   In a heat-proof dish that fits inside saucepan, add all ingredients except for basil. Mix well.
2.   Place a large saucepan on medium high fire. Place a trivet inside saucepan and fill pan halfway with water. Cover and bring to a boil.
3.   Cover dish with foil and place on trivet.
4.   Cover pan and steam for 10 minutes. Let it rest in pan for another 5 minutes.
5.   Serve and enjoy topped with fresh basil.
Nutrition Values:
Calories: 195.2; Carbs: 4.2g; Protein: 41g; Fats: 1.6g; Saturated Fat: .3g; Sodium: 126mg

153. Fish Jambalaya

Preparation time: 15 minutes
Servings: 2-4
Ingredients
- 1 teaspoon canola oil
- 1 jalapeno pepper, minced
- 1 small-sized leek, chopped
- 1/2 teaspoon ginger garlic paste
- 1/4 teaspoon ground cumin
- 1/4 teaspoon ground allspice
- 1/2 teaspoon oregano
- 1/4 teaspoon thyme
- 1/4 teaspoon marjoram

- 1-pound sole fish fillets, cut into bite-sized strips
- 1 large-sized ripe tomato, pureed
- 1/2 cup water
- 1/2 cup clam juice
- Kosher salt, to season
- 1 bay laurel
- 5-6 black peppercorns
- 1 cup spinach, torn into pieces

Directions

1. Heat the oil in a Dutch oven over a moderate flame.
2. Then, sauté the pepper and leek until they have softened.
3. Now, stir in the ginger-garlic paste, cumin, allspice, oregano, thyme, and marjoram; continue stirring for 30 to 40 seconds more or until aromatic.
4. Add in the fish, tomatoes, water, clam juice, salt, bay laurel, and black peppercorns.
5. Cover and decrease the temperature to medium-low. Let it simmer for 4 to 6 minutes or until the liquid has reduced slightly.
6. Stir in the spinach and let it simmer, covered, for about 2 minutes more or until it wilts. Ladle into serving bowls and serve warm.

Nutrition Values: Calories 232, Total Fat 6.7g, Carbs 3.6g, Protein 38.1g

154. Greek Sea Bass with Olive Sauce

Preparation time: 15 minutes
Servings: 2

Ingredients

- 2 sea bass fillets
- 2 tbsps. olive oil
- 1 garlic clove, minced
- A pinch of chili pepper
- 1 tbsp. green olives, pitted and sliced
- 1 lemon, juiced
- Salt to taste

Directions

1. Preheat a grill. In a small bowl mix together half of the olive oil, chili pepper, garlic, and salt and rub onto the sea bass fillets.
2. Grill the fish on both sides for 5-6 minutes until brown.
3. In a skillet over medium heat, warm the remaining olive oil and stir in the lemon juice, olives, and some salt; cook for 3-4 minutes. Plate the fillets and pour the lemon sauce over to serve.

Nutrition Values: Calories 267, Total Fat 15.6g, Carbs 1.6g, Protein 24g

155. Sardines with Green Pasta & Sun-Dried Tomatoes

Preparation time: 20 minutes
Servings: 2

Ingredients

- 2 tbsps. olive oil
- 4 cups zoodles -spiralled zucchini

- ½ pound whole fresh sardines, gutted and cleaned
- ½ cup sun-dried tomatoes, drained and chopped
- 1 tbsps. dill
- 1 garlic clove, minced

Directions

1. Preheat the oven to 350 F and line a baking sheet with parchment paper.
2. Arrange the sardines on the dish, drizzle with olive oil, sprinkle with salt and black pepper. Bake in the oven for 10 minutes until the skin is crispy.
3. Warm oil in a skillet over medium heat and stir-fry the zucchini, garlic and tomatoes for 5 minutes.
4. Adjust the seasoning.
5. Transfer the sardines to a plate and serve with the veggie pasta.

Nutrition Values: Calories 232, Total Fat 6.7g, Carbs 3.6g, Protein 38.1g

156. Saucy Cod with Mustard Greens

Preparation time: 20 minutes
Servings: 2

Ingredients

- 1 tablespoon olive oil
- 1 bell pepper, seeded and sliced
- 1 jalapeno pepper, seeded and sliced
- 2 stalks green onions, sliced
- 1 stalk green garlic, sliced
- 1/2 cup fish broth
- 2 cod fish fillets
- 1/2 teaspoon paprika
- Sea salt and ground black pepper, to season
- 1 cup mustard greens, torn into bite-sized pieces

Directions

1. Heat the olive oil in a Dutch pot over a moderate flame.
2. Now, sauté the peppers, green onions, and garlic until just tender and aromatic.
3. Add in the broth, fish fillets, paprika, salt, black pepper, and mustard greens.
4. Reduce the temperature to medium-low, cover, and let it cook for 11 to 13 minutes or until heated through.
5. Serve immediately garnished with lemon slices if desired.

Nutrition Values: Calories 171, Total Fat 7.8g, Carbs 4.8g, Protein 20.3g

157. Baked Cod with Parmesan & Almonds

Preparation time: 40 minutes
Servings: 2

Ingredients

- 2 cod fillets
- 1 cup Brussels sprouts
- 1 tbsps. butter, melted
- Salt and black pepper to taste

- 1 cup crème fraiche
- 2 tbsps. Parmesan cheese, grated
- 2 tbsps. shaved almonds

Directions
1. Toss the fish fillets and Brussels sprouts in butter and season with salt and black pepper to taste.
2. Spread in a greased baking dish.
3. Mix the crème fraiche with Parmesan cheese, pour and smear the cream on the fish.
4. Bake in the oven for 25 minutes at 400 F until golden brown on top, take the dish out, sprinkle with the almonds and bake for another 5 minutes. Best served hot.

Nutrition Values: Calories 560, Total Fat 44.7g, Carbs 5.4g, Protein 25.3g

158. Fish Tacos with Slaw, Lemon and Cilantro

Preparation time: 20 minutes
Servings: 2
Ingredients
- 1 tbsp. olive oil
- 1 tsp chili powder
- 2 halibut fillets, skinless, sliced
- 2 low carb tortillas
- Slaw
- 2 tbsps. red cabbage, shredded
- 1 tbsp. lemon juice
- Salt to taste
- ½ tbsp. extra-virgin olive oil
- ½ carrot, shredded
- 1 tbsp. cilantro, chopped

Directions
1. Combine red cabbage with salt in a bowl; massage cabbage to tenderize.
2. Add in the remaining slaw ingredient, toss to coat and set aside.
3. Rub the halibut with olive oil, chili powder and paprika.
4. Heat a grill pan over medium heat.
5. Add halibut and cook until lightly charred and cooked through, about 3 minutes per side. Divide between the tortillas.
6. Combine all slaw ingredients in a bowl. Split the slaw among the tortillas.

Nutrition Values: Calories 385, Total Fat 26g, Carbs 6.5g, Protein 23.8g

159. Fried Oysters in The Oven

Servings: 2-4
Preparation time: 20 minutes
Ingredients
- 3 tablespoons olive oil
- 1 teaspoon garlic salt
- 1 teaspoon freshly ground black pepper
- 1 teaspoon red pepper flakes
- 2 cups finely crushed pork rinds
- 24 shucked oysters

Directions

1. Preheat the oven to 400ºF.
2. In a small bowl, mix together the olive oil, garlic salt, black pepper, and red pepper flakes.
3. Put the crushed pork rinds in a separate bowl.
4. Dip each oyster first in the oil mixture to coat and then in the pork rinds, turning to coat. Arrange the coated oysters on a baking sheet in a single layer with room in between.
5. Bake in the preheated oven for 30 minutes, or until the pork rind "breading" is browned and crisp. Serve hot.

Nutrition Values: Calories: 230, Carbs: 5g, Fat: 17g, Fiber: 0g, Protein: 15g

160. Tuna with Greens and Blueberries - One Pot

Servings: 2
Preparation time: 10 minutes
Cooking time: 5 minutes
Ingredients
- ¼ cup olive
- 2 -4-ouncetuna steaks
- Salt
- Freshly ground black pepper
- Juice of 1 lemon
- 4 cups salad greens
- ¼ cup low-carb, diary-free ranch dressing - Tessemae's
- 2o blueberries

Directions
1. In a large skillet, heat the olive oil over medium-high heat.
2. Season the tuna steaks generously with salt and pepper, and add them to the skillet. Cook for 2 or 2 ½ minutes in each side to sear the outer edges.
3. Squeeze the lemon over the tuna in the pan and remove the fish
4. To serve, arrange the greens on 2 serving plates. Top each plate with one of the tuna steaks, 2 tablespoons of the ranch dressing, and 10 of the blueberries.

Nutrition Values: Calories: 549, Carbs: 7g, Fat: 41g, Fiber: 3g, Protein: 38g

161. Roasted Old Bay Prawns

Preparation time: 20 minutes
Servings: 2
Ingredients
- 3/4 pound prawns, peeled and deveined
- 1 teaspoon Old Bay seasoning mix
- 1/2 teaspoon paprika
- Coarse sea salt and ground black pepper, to taste
- 1 habanero pepper, deveined and minced
- 1 bell pepper, deveined and minced
- 1 cup pound broccoli florets
- 2 teaspoons olive oil
- 1 tablespoon fresh chives, chopped

- 2 slices lemon, for garnish
- 2 dollops of sour cream, for garnish

Directions

1. Toss the prawns with the Old Bay seasoning mix, paprika, salt, and black pepper. Arrange them on a parchment-lined roasting pan.
2. Add the bell pepper and broccoli.
3. Drizzle olive oil over everything and transfer the pan to a preheated oven.
4. Roast at 390 degrees F for 8 to 11 minutes, turning the pan halfway through the cooking time.
5. Bake until the prawns are pink and cooked through.
6. Serve with fresh chives, lemon, and sour cream.

Nutrition Values: Calories 269, Total Fat 9.6g, Carbs 7.2g, Protein 38.2g

162. Three-Minute Lobster Tail

Servings: 2
Preparation time: 5 minutes
Cooking time: 5 minutes

Ingredients

- 4 cups bone broth -or water
- 2 lobster tails

Directions

1. In a large pot, bring the broth to a boil.
2. While the broth is coming to a boil, use kitchen shears to cut the back side of the lobster shell from end to end.
3. Place the lobster in the boiling broth and bring it back to a boil. Cook the lobster for 3 minutes.
4. Drain and serve immediately.

Nutrition Values: Calories: 154, Carbs: 0g, Fat: 2g, Fiber: 0g, Protein: 32g

163. Crispy Salmon with Broccoli & Red Bell Pepper

Preparation time: 30 minutes
Servings: 2

Ingredients

- 2 salmon fillets
- Salt and black pepper to taste
- 2 tbsps. mayonnaise
- 2 tbsps. fennel seeds, crushed
- ½ head broccoli, cut in florets
- 1 red bell pepper, sliced
- 1 tbsp. olive oil
- 2 lemon wedges

Directions

1. Brush the salmon with mayonnaise and season with salt and black pepper.
2. Coat with fennel seeds, place in a lined baking dish and bake for 15 minutes at 370 F.
3. Steam the broccoli and carrot for 3-4 minutes, or until tender, in a pot over medium heat. Heat the olive oil in a saucepan and sauté the red bell pepper for 5 minutes.
4. Stir in the broccoli and turn off the heat. Let the pan sit on the warm burner for 2-3 minutes.

5. Serve with baked salmon garnished with lemon wedges.

Nutrition Values: Calories 563, Total Fat 37g, Carbs 6g, Protein 38.2g

164. Easy Baked Halibut Steaks

Preparation time: 20 minutes
Servings: 2

Ingredients

- 2 tablespoons olive oil
- 2 halibut steaks
- 1 red bell pepper, sliced
- 1 yellow onion, sliced
- 1 teaspoon garlic, smashed
- 1/2 teaspoon hot paprika
- Sea salt cracked black pepper, to your liking
- 1 dried thyme sprig, leaves crushed

Directions

1. Start by preheating your oven to 390 degrees F.
2. Then, drizzle olive oil over the halibut steaks.
3. Place the halibut in a baking dish that is previously greased with a nonstick spray.
4. Top with the bell pepper, onion, and garlic.
5. Sprinkle hot paprika, salt, black pepper, and dried thyme over everything.
6. Bake in the preheated oven for 13 to 15 minutes and serve immediately. Enjoy!

Nutrition Values: Calories 502, Total Fat 19.1g, Carbs 5.7g, Protein 72g

165. Mediterranean Tilapia Bake

Preparation time: 30 minutes
Servings: 2

Ingredients

- 2 tilapia fillets
- 2 garlic cloves, minced
- 1 tsp basil, chopped
- 1 cup canned tomatoes
- ¼ tbsp. chili powder
- 2 tbsps. white wine
- 1 tbsp. olive oil
- ½ red onion, chopped
- 2 tbsps. parsley
- 10 black olives, pitted and halved

Directions

1. Preheat oven to 350 F. Heat the olive oil in a skillet over medium heat and cook the onion and garlic for about 3 minutes.
2. Stir in tomatoes, olives, chilli powder, and white wine and bring the mixture to a boil. Reduce the heat and simmer for 5 minutes.
3. Put the tilapia in a baking dish, pour over the sauce and bake in the oven for 10-15 minutes.
4. Serve garnished with basil.

Nutrition Values: Calories 282, Total Fat 15g, Carbs 6g, Protein 23g

166. Omelet Wraps with Tuna

Preparation time: 15 minutes
Servings: 2
Ingredients
- 1 avocado, sliced
- 1 tbsp. chopped chives
- 1/3 cup canned tuna, drained
- 2 spring onions, sliced
- 4 eggs, beaten
- 4 tbsps. mascarpone cheese
- 1 tbsp. butter
- Salt and black pepper, to taste

Directions
1. In a small bowl, combine the chives and mascarpone cheese; set aside.
2. Melt the butter in a pan over medium heat.
3. Add the eggs to the pan and cook for about 3 minutes. Flip the omelet over and continue cooking for another 2 minutes until golden.
4. Season with salt and black pepper. Remove the omelet to a plate and spread the chive mixture over. Arrange the tuna, avocado, and onion slices.
5. Wrap the omelet and serve immediately.
Nutrition Values: Calories 481, Total Fat 37.9g, Carbs 6.2g, Protein 26.9g

167. Baked Trout and Asparagus Foil Packets

Preparation time: 20 minutes
Servings: 2
Ingredients
- ½ pound asparagus spears
- 1 tbsp. garlic puree
- ½ pound deboned trout, butterflied
- Salt and black pepper to taste
- 3 tbsps. olive oil
- 2 sprigs rosemary
- 2 sprigs thyme
- 2 tbsps. butter
- ½ medium red onion, sliced
- 2 lemon slices

Directions
1. Preheat the oven to 400 F. Rub the trout with garlic puree, salt and black pepper. Prepare two aluminum foil squares.
2. Place the fish on each square.
3. Divide the asparagus and onion between the squares, top with a pinch of salt and pepper, a sprig of rosemary and thyme, and 1 tbsp. of butter.
4. Also, lay the lemon slices on the fish. Wrap and close the fish packets securely, and place them on a baking sheet.
5. Bake in the oven for 15 minutes, and remove once ready.
Nutrition Values: Calories 498, Total Fat 39.3g, Carbs 4.8g, Protein 27g

168. Coconut Shrimp

Servings: 2-4
Preparation time: 20 minutes

Cooking time: 30 minutes
Ingredients
- Avocado oil spray -or other cooking oil spray
- 3 large egg whites
- 1 teaspoon cayenne
- 1 teaspoon garlic salt
- 1 teaspoon freshly ground black pepper
- ½ teaspoon Swerve granular -or another granulated alternative sweetener
- 1 cup unsweetened shredded coconut
- 24 -or soraw shrimp, peeled

Directions
1. Preheat the oven to 350ºF. Spray a large baking sheet with the avocado oil spray.
2. In a small bowl, whisk together the egg whites, cayenne, garlic salt, pepper, and sweetener.
3. Put the shredded coconut in a separate bowl.
4. One at a time, dunk the shrimp first in the egg mixture and then in the coconut, turning to coat completely.
5. Arrange the coated shrimp on the prepared baking sheet in a single layer, with room in between. Once all the shrimp have been coated, spray them lightly with avocado oil spray.
6. Bake in the preheated oven for 30 minutes, or until the coconut is golden brown.
Nutrition Values: Calories: 223, Carbs: 7g, Fat: 17g, Fiber: 4g, Protein: 13g

169. Bacon-Wrapped Scallop Cups -One Pot

Servings: 2-4
Preparation time: 10 minutes
Cooking time: 25 minutes
Ingredients
- 12 large sea scallops
- 6 strips bacon, halved to make 12 short strips
- 24 garlic cloves, peeled but left whole
- 5 tablespoons Lemon-Garlic Dressing

Directions
1. Preheat the oven to 400ºF.
2. Wrap each scallop with 1 piece of bacon. Use a toothpick to secure the bacon to the scallop. Arrange the wrapped scallops on a baking sheet.
3. Place 2 garlic cloves on top of each scallop, then top with a spoonful of the dressing. 4Bake for 25 minutes, or until the bacon is browned and crisp.
Nutrition Values: Calories: 374, Carbs: 9g, Fat: 26g, Fiber: 4g, Protein: 26g

170. Sea Bass with Vegetables and Dill Sauce

Preparation time: 25 minutes
Servings: 2
Ingredients
- 1 tablespoon olive oil

- 1 cup red onions, sliced
- 2 bell peppers, deveined and sliced
- Sea salt and cayenne pepper, to taste
- 1 teaspoon paprika
- 1-pound sea bass fillets

Dill Sauce:
- 1 tablespoon mayonnaise
- 1/4 cup Greek yogurt
- 1 tablespoon fresh dill, chopped
- 1/2 teaspoon garlic powder
- 1/2 fresh lemon, juiced

Directions
1. Toss the onions, peppers, and sea bass fillets with the olive oil, salt, cayenne pepper, and paprika. Line a baking pan with a piece of parchment paper.
2. Preheat your oven to 400 degrees F.
3. Arrange your fish and vegetables on the prepared baking pan.
4. Bake for 10 minutes; turn them over and bake for a further 10 to 12 minutes.
5. Meanwhile, make the sauce by mixing all ingredients until well combined.
6. Serve the fish and vegetables with the dill sauce on the side.

Nutrition Values: Calories 374, Total Fat 17g, Carbs 6.2g, Protein 43.2g

171. Grilled Tuna Steaks with Shirataki Pad Thai

Preparation time: 30 minutes
Servings: 2
Ingredients
- ½ pack -7-ozshirataki noodles
- 2 cups water
- 1 red bell pepper, seeded and sliced
- 2 tbsps. soy sauce, sugar-free
- 1 tbsp. ginger-garlic paste
- 1 tsp chili powder
- 1 tbsp. water
- 2 tuna steaks
- Salt and black pepper to taste
- 1 tbsp. olive oil
- 1 tbsp. parsley, chopped

Directions
1. In a colander, rinse the shirataki noodles with running cold water.
2. Bring a pot of salted water to a boil; blanch the noodles for 2 minutes.
3. Drain and set aside. Preheat a grill on medium-high.
4. Season the tuna with salt and black pepper, brush with olive oil, and grill covered.
5. Cook for 3 minutes on each side.
6. In a bowl, whisk together soy sauce, ginger-garlic paste, olive oil, chili powder, and water.
7. Add bell pepper, and dry noodles and toss to coat.

8. Assemble the noodles and tuna in serving plate and garnish with parsley.

Nutrition Values: Calories 287, Total Fat 16.2g, Carbs 6.8g, Protein 23.4g

172. Country Club Crab Cakes

Servings: 2-4
Preparation time: 30 minutes
Cooking time: 20 minutes
Ingredients
- 2 -6-ouncecans crabmeat -or 12 ounces cooked crabmeat
- 2 large eggs
- 2 tablespoons chopped fresh dill
- 1 teaspoon garlic salt
- ¼ cup olive oil

Directions
1. In a medium bowl, combine the crabmeat, eggs, dill, and garlic salt. Form the mixture into four patties.
2. In a medium skillet, heat the olive oil over medium heat. Cook the crab cakes for 3 to 4 minutes on each side, or until golden brown.

Nutrition Values: Calories: 212, Carbs: 1g, Fat: 16g, Protein: 16g

173. Coconut Fried Shrimp with Cilantro Sauce

Servings: 2
Preparation time: 15 minutes
Ingredients
- 2 tsp coconut flour
- 2 tbsps. grated Pecorino cheese
- 1 egg, beaten in a bowl
- ¼ tsp curry powder
- ½ pound shrimp, shelled
- 3 tbsps. coconut oil
- Salt to taste
- Sauce
- 2 tbsps. ghee
- 2 tbsps. cilantro leaves, chopped
- ½ onion, diced
- ½ cup coconut cream
- ½ ounce Paneer cheese, grated

Directions
1. Combine coconut flour, Pecorino cheese, curry powder, and salt in a bowl.
2. Melt the coconut oil in a skillet over medium heat.
3. Dip the shrimp in the egg first, and then coat with the dry mixture.
4. Fry until golden and crispy, about 5 minutes. In another skillet, melt the ghee.
5. Add onion and cook for 3 minutes. Add curry and cilantro and cook for 30 seconds.
6. Stir in coconut cream and Paneer cheese and cook until thickened.
7. Add the shrimp and coat well. Serve warm.

Nutrition Values: Calories: 741, Carbs: 4.3g, Fat: 64g, Protein: 34.4g

174. Shrimp Sti-fry

Servings: 2
Preparation time: 10 minutes
Cooking time: 20 minutes
Ingredients
- ¼ cup avocado oil
- ¼ cup coconut aminos
- 2 cups chopped broccoli
- 1 onion, diced
- 1 red bell pepper, chopped
- 24 cooked and peeled shrimp
- 1 -12-ouncebag riced cauliflower
- Chili sauce, for serving -Optional

Directions
1. Combine the shrimp, Cauliflower, onion, pepper, broccoli, coconut aminos, and avocado oil in a large skillet. Cook, stirring occasionally, until all the flavors are combined, about 20 minutes
2. Drizzle the chili sauce over the top and serve hot
Nutrition Values: Calories: 231, Carbs: 12g, Fat: 15g, Fiber: 5g, Protein: 12g

175. Baked Salmon with Lemon and Mush

Servings: 2
Preparation time: 10 minutes
Cooking time: 30 minutes
Ingredients
- 2 -6-ounceskin-on salmon fillets
- 1 onion, diced
- 8 ounces' mushrooms, sliced
- ¼ cup olive oil
- 1 teaspoon salt
- 1 teaspoon freshly ground black pepper
- 4 lemon slices

Directions
1. Preheat the oven to 400ºF.
2. Tear off 2 large squares of aluminum foil. Place a salmon fillet on each piece of foil and arrange the onion and mushrooms over and around the fish, dividing evenly.
3. Pour the olive oil over the fish, then season with the salt and pepper. Top each piece of fish with 2 lemon slices.
4. Wrap the foil up around the salmon and vegetables, leaving room inside the packet for heat to circulate, and bake for 30 minutes, or until the fish flakes easily with a fork. Serve hot.
Nutrition Values: Calories: 576, Carbs: 8g, Fat: 44g, Fiber: 3g, Protein: 37g

176. Pan-fried Soft Shell Crab

Servings: 2
Preparation time: 5 minutes
Cooking time: 10 minutes
Ingredients
- ½ cup olive oil
- ½ cup almond flour
- 1 teaspoon paprika
- 1 teaspoon garlic salt
- 1 teaspoon freshly ground black pepper
- 2 soft-shell crabs

Directions
1. Fill the bottom of a heavy skillet with the oil and heat over low heat.
2. While the oil is heating, in a medium bowl, mix together the almond flour, paprika, garlic salt, and pepper.
3. Dredge each crab in the flour mixture, coating both sides and shaking off any excess. Put the crabs into the hot oil in the skillet and cook for about 5 minutes per side, or until golden brown.
4. Serve hot.
Nutrition Values: Calories: 489, Carbs: 6g, Fat: 33g, Fiber: 2g, Protein: 42g

177. Chilli Cod with Chive Sauce

Servings: 2
Preparation time: 20 minutes
Ingredients
- 1 tsp chilli powder
- 2 cod fillets
- Salt and black pepper to taste
- 1 tbsp olive oil
- 1 garlic clove, minced
- 1/3 cup lemon juice
- 2 tbsps. vegetable stock
- 2 tbsps. chives, chopped

Directions
1. Preheat oven to 400 F and grease a baking dish with cooking spray.
2. Rub the cod fillets with chili powder, salt, and black pepper and lay in the baking dish.
3. Bake for 10-15 minutes until fish fillets are easily removed with a fork.
4. In a skillet over low heat, warm the olive oil and sauté the garlic for 3 minutes.
5. Add the lemon juice, vegetable stock, and chives.
6. Season with salt, black pepper, and cook for 3 minutes until the stock slightly reduces.
7. Divide fish into 2 plates, top with sauce, and serve.
Nutrition Values: Calories: 448, Carbs: 6.3g, Fat: 35.3g, Protein: 42g

178. Pan-Seared Scallops with Sausage & Mozzarella

Servings: 2-4 minutes
Preparation time: 15 minutes
Ingredients
- 2 tbsps. butter
- 12 fresh scallops, rinsed and pat dry
- 8 ounces sausage, chopped
- 1 red bell pepper, seeds removed, sliced
- 1 red onion, finely chopped

- 1 cup Grana Padano cheese, grated
- Salt and black pepper to taste

Directions

1. Melt half of the butter in a skillet over medium heat, and cook the onion and bell pepper for 5 minutes until tender.
2. Add the sausage and stir-fry for another 5 minutes.
3. Remove and set aside. Pat dry the scallops with paper towels, and season with salt and pepper.
4. Add the remaining butter to the skillet and sear the scallops for 2 minutes on each side to have a golden brown color.
5. Add the sausage mixture back, and warm through.
6. Transfer to serving platter and top with Grana Padano cheese.

Nutrition Values: Calories: 834, Carbs: 9.5g, Fat: 62g, Protein: 56g

179. Spanish Shrimp with a hint of garlic

Servings: 4
Preparation time: 5 minutes
Cooking time: 8 minutes

Ingredients:

- 1 pound large shrimp, peeled and deveined
- 2 tablespoons freshly chopped parsley
- 2 teaspoons minced garlic
- 1/4 teaspoon salt
- 1/8 teaspoon ground black pepper
- ¼teaspoon red chili flakes
- 1 teaspoon sweet Spanish paprika
- 11/2 tablespoon fresh lemon juice
- 1/3 cup olive oil
- tablespoons dry sherry

Directions:

1. Preheat a large skillet pan with oil over medium-high heat and add in garlic and red pepper flakes.
2. Cook for 2 to 3 minutes until fragrant and garlic is softened, then add shrimps and season with salt, black pepper, chili flakes and paprika.
3. Cook for additional 2 minutes or until shrimps starts turning pink.
4. Stir in wine and lemon juice and continue with additional cooking for 2 to 3 more minutes or until shrimps are cooked and cooking liquid is slightly reduced.
5. Garnish shrimps with freshly chopped parsley and remove the pan from heat.
6. Serve immediately when still warm.

180. Crusted Salmon with walnuts and rosemary

Servings: 4
Preparation time: 5 minutes
Cooking time: 12 minutes

Ingredients:

- 1 pound skinless salmon fillet
- 1/2 teaspoon minced garlic
- 1 teaspoon chopped fresh rosemary
- ½ teaspoon salt
- ¼ teaspoon crushed red pepper
- ½teaspoon honey
- ¼teaspoon lemon zest
- 1 teaspoon lemon juice
- 1 teaspoon olive oil and more as needed
- 2 teaspoons Dijon mustard
- 3 tablespoons panko breadcrumbs
- 3 tablespoons finely chopped walnuts

Directions:

1. Preheat oven to 425 degrees F.
2. Take a rimmed baking sheet, line with parchment paper and place skinless salmon fillet on it.
3. Combine together minced garlic, chopped rosemary, salt, crushed red pepper, honey, lemon zest and juice, olive oil, mustard and finely chopped walnuts.
4. Rub the mixture on fillet and then sprinkle with panko breadcrumbs.
5. Spray fish with olive oil baking spray and place the baking sheet into the oven.
6. Bake for 8 to 12 minutes or until fish is golden brown and cooked.
7. Serve immediately while still warm.

181. Mediterranean Salmon

with Fennel and Sun-Dried Tomato Couscous Salad

Servings: 4
Preparation time: 10 minutes
Cooking time: 25 minutes

Ingredients:

- 11/4pounds salmon fillets, skinned
- 1/4 teaspoon salt
- 1/4teaspoon ground black pepper
- 4 tablespoons sun-dried tomato pesto, divided
- 2 medium fennel bulbs, cut into 1/2-inch wedges
- 1 cup couscous
- 3 scallions, thinly sliced
- 1/4 cup sliced green olives
- 1 teaspoon minced garlic
- 1 tablespoons olive oil, divided
- 1 lemon
- 1 tablespoons toasted pine nuts
- ½cups chicken broth

Directions:

1. Zest lemon, set aside and then cut into 8 slices.
2. Cut salmon into four portions, season with salt and black pepper, then spread 1 ½ teaspoon pesto on each fillet.
3. Preheat a large skillet pan with oil over medium-high heat and add half of the fennel and cook for 3 minutes or until softened and nicely golden brown.

4.　　　Transfer cooked fennel to a plate, set aside and into the same pan, add remaining oil and fennel, cook for 3 minutes until nicely browned and then transfer to a plate.

5.　　　Add in couscous and thinly sliced scallion to the pan and cook for 2 minutes or until lightly browned.

6.　　　Add in olives, garlic, nuts, lemon zest, remaining pesto, chicken broth and stir until well combined.

7.　　　Add fennel and salmon, top with lemon wedges and then reduce the heat to medium-low, covering the pan, cook for additional 10 to 15 minutes or until cooked completely.

8.　　　Serve while still warm.

182. Cod with Roasted Tomatoes – Mediterranean style

Servings: 4
Preparation time: 10 minutes
Cooking time: 12 minutes

Ingredients:

- 4 skinless cod fillets, about 4-ounce
- 3 cups cherry tomatoes
- 2 tablespoons sliced pitted olives
- 2 teaspoons capers
- 2 cloves of garlic, peeled and sliced thinly
- 1/4 teaspoon garlic powder
- ½ teaspoon salt
- 1/4teaspoon ground black pepper
- 1/4 teaspoon paprika
- 2 teaspoons fresh oregano
- 1 teaspoon fresh thyme
- 1 tablespoon olive oil and more as needed

Fresh oregano leaves

Directions:

1.　　　Preheat oven to 450 degrees F.

2.　　　In a bowl mix together garlic powder, salt, black pepper, paprika, oregano, and thyme and rub half of this mixture over both sides of cod fillets.

3.　　　Take a 15x10x1 inch baking pan, line with aluminum foil, grease well with olive oil and place seasoned cod fillets on it.

4.　　　Assemble tomatoes and garlic on the other side of the pan.

5.　　　Add oil into remaining oregano mixture, drizzle over tomatoes and mix until well coated.

6.　　　Place the baking pan into the oven and bake for 8 to 12 minutes or until fish is cooked, stirring tomatoes halfway through the cooking process.

7.　　　When baked, remove baking pan from the oven, stir in olives and capers into cooked tomatoes and garlic.

8.　　　Garnish with oregano leaves and serve while still warm.

183. Shrimp Piccata with Zucchini Noodles

Servings: 4
Preparation time: 40 minutes
Cooking time: 10 minutes

Ingredients:

- 1 pound shrimp, peeled and deveined
- 2 ½ pounds zucchini, trimmed
- 2 tablespoons chopped fresh parsley
- 2 tablespoons capers, rinsed
- 1 tablespoon cornstarch
- 1 teaspoon minced garlic
- 1/2teaspoon salt
- 2 tablespoons unsalted butter
- 1/4 cup lemon juice
- 1/3 cup white wine
- 2 tablespoons olive oil, divided
- 1 cup chicken broth

Directions:

1.　　　Using a vegetable peeler cut zucchini into thin strips and place in a colander, season with salt, toss until well coated and let rest for 15 to 30 minutes to realize all juices.

2.　　　Meanwhile, preheat a large skillet pan with oil and butter and add in garlic.

3.　　　Cook for 30 seconds or until fragrant and slightly softened and then add in shrimps and cook for 1 more minute.

4.　　　Combine together cornstarch and chicken broth in a small bowl or glass and add in to shrimps alongside with capers, lemon juice, and wine.

5.　　　Mix well and simmer for additional 5 more minutes or until shrimps are cooked and set aside

6.　　　Drain zucchini noodles from their water and gently squeeze to remove any excess liquid.

7.　　　Preheat large skillet pan with oil over medium-high heat and add in zucchini noodles and toss until well coated and slightly golden brown.

8.　　　Cook for about 3 minutes and garnish with parsley.

9.　　　Serve zucchini with shrimps in a serving platter.

184. Mediterranean Fish Soup

Servings: 6
Preparation time: 5 minutes
Cooking time: 4 hours and 30 minutes

Ingredients:

- 1 pound cod fillets, cubed
- 1 pound medium shrimp, peeled and deveined
- 1 medium white onion, peeled and roughly chopped
- ½of medium green bell pepper, chopped
- 2 ½ounces mushrooms
- 14.5 ounce diced tomatoes, drained
- ¼cup sliced black olives
- 1 teaspoon minced garlic
- 1/8 teaspoon ground black pepper
- teaspoon dried basil
- bay leaves
- 1/4 teaspoon fennel seed, crushed
- 1/2 cup orange juice
- 1/2 cup dry white wine

- 8-ounce tomato sauce
- 28-ounce chicken broth

Directions:

1. Turn on your 6-quart slow cooker on low heat setting and place in chopped onion, green bell pepper, mushrooms, olives, garlic, black pepper, basil, bay leaves, crushed fennel seeds, orange juice, white wine, tomato sauce and chicken broth. Stir well until mixed and combined.
2. Shut slow cooker with its lid, plug in and cook for 4 to 4 hours and 30 minutes or until vegetables are tender-crisp.
3. Then add shrimps and cod to vegetables and cook for additional 20 to 30 minutes or until shrimps are pink and cooked,.

185. Rich Mediterranean Avocado and Tuna Tapas

Servings: 4
Preparation time: 10 minutes
Cooking time: 0 minutes
Ingredients:

- 12 ounce cooked tuna
- 2 medium avocados
- 3 green onions, thinly sliced and more for garnishing
- 1/2 of medium red bell pepper, chopped
- 1/8 teaspoon garlic salt
- 1/8 teaspoon ground black pepper
- 1 tablespoon mayonnaise
- 1/8 teaspoon apple cider vinegar

Directions:

1. In a bowl place in cooked tuna, green onions, red bell pepper, garlic salt, ground black pepper, mayonnaise and apple cider vinegar and stir well until well combined.
2. Cut avocados into half each, remove its stone and stuff with prepared tuna salad.
3. Garnish with green onions and serve immediately.
4. Per Serving: Calories: 294; Total Fat: 18.2g; Protein: 23.9g; Carbs: llg; Fiber: 7.4g; Sugar: 2g

186. Mediterranean Spanish Cod

Servings: 6
Preparation time: 5 minutes
Cooking time: 13 minutes
Ingredients:

- 6 cod fillets, each about 4-ounce
- 1/4 cup marinated Italian vegetable salad
- 15 cherry tomatoes, halved
- 1/2 cup chopped green olives
- 1/4 cup finely chopped white onion
- 2 tablespoons chopped garlic
- 1/8 teaspoon ground black pepper
- 1/8 teaspoon paprika
- 1/8 teaspoon cayenne pepper
- 1 tablespoon olive oil
- 1 tablespoon unsalted butter

- 1 cup tomato sauce

Directions:

1. Preheat a large skillet pan with butter and oil over medium heat and add in onion and garlic.
2. Cook for 3 to 5 minutes or until onions are softened and slightly browned
3. Then add in tomatoes and tomato sauce, stir until well combined and bring the whole mixture to simmer.
4. Meanwhile, drain the salad and chop it on a cutting board.
5. In the simmering skillet pan add in the salad, olives, season with black pepper, cayenne pepper and paprika, toss slightly and add cod fillets.
6. Cook for 5 to 8 minutes or until cod is completely cooked .
7. Serve immediately in a serving plate.

187. Lemon Garlic Salmon with Asparagus

Preparation Time: 15 minutes
Servings: 3
Ingredients:

- Trimmed asparagus - 1 bunch
- Olive oil - 1 tbsp
- Minced garlic - 2 cloves
- Salmon - 1 pound
- Salted butter - 1 tbsp
- Salt and pepper -optional
- Juice and zest of lemon - 1 small

Directions:

1. Cut the salmon into 3 equal sized fillets
2. Heat a pan and melt the butter and olive oil
3. Place the 3 fillets on the pan.
4. Slowly add the asparagus
5. Cook for 4 minutes on each side then sprinkle salt and pepper
6. Add the lemon zest and garlic in the pan then cook till the garlic is brown.
7. Remove from heat and pour the lemon juice into the meal.
8. Best served hot.

188. Easy Zucchini and Tuna Super Bowl

Preparation Time: 5 minutes
Servings: 1
Ingredients:

- Lime juice - 1 small sized
- Thai peanut dressing
- Red onion diced - 2 tbsp
- Red cabbage chopped - ¼ cup
- Thinly cut carrot - 1
- Chickpeas roasted -¼ cup
- Quinoa cooked - ½ cup -cold/room temp
- Spiralized zucchini - ½ cup
- Tuna - 1 can 5.05 oz
- Cilantro -optional

Directions:

1. Take a medium sized bowl and place the cooked quinoa.

2. Pour in the chickpeas, carrot, zucchini, red onion, red cabbage, and Tuna into the bowl
3. Garnish with cilantro then add the lime juice in
4. Add Thai dressing in and enjoy.

189. Shrimp and Spinach Tortellini

Preparation Time: 20 minutes
Servings: 5
Ingredients:
- Olive oil - 4 tbsp
- Chopped spinach - 6 cups
- Shrimps - 1 pound
- Three cheese tortellini - 1 pack 20 oz
- Pesto with basil - 1 tub 7 oz
- Pine nuts - ⅓ cup -optional
- Parmesan cheese - shredded -optional

Directions:
1. Carefully follow the pasta cooking Directions: on the package and start preparing the pasta
2. Prepare the shrimps by removing the tails.
3. Place a large skillet on medium heat then add 2 tbsp of olive oil in
4. Pour the pine nuts in and roast for 3 minutes until brown
5. Add 2 tbsp of olive oil in the skillet then slowly pour in the spinach then cook for 4 minutes
6. Pour the shrimps in and cook for 4 minutes till pink
7. Drain the pasta but save ¼ of the water
8. In a large pot pour the pasta water then add the pesto and basil.
9. Stir for a minute till smooth then pour in the pasta and shrimp with spinach dish into the pot
10. Sprinkle with parmesan cheese and serve while hot.

190. Oven-baked Garlic Salmon in foil

Preparation Time: 40 minutes
Servings: 4
Ingredients:
- Crushed garlic - 15 cloves
- Squash - 2
- Sliced green onions - 2 large
- Thyme springs - 4
- Sweet paprika - 1 tsp
- Salt and pepper -optional
- Chopped parsley - ½ cup
- Lemon juice - 1 lemon
- Lemon slices - 1 medium-sized
- Butter - 2 tbsp
- Extra virgin oil
- Salmon - 4 fillets 5 oz each
- Tomato - 1 large

Directions:
1. Cut the squash and tomato into small bite-sized cubes
2. Preheat the oven to 400 degrees

3. Spread oil on the fillets on all sides then gently place them on four separate foils- 12" by 17"
4. Take ½ of the crushed garlic and rub it evenly all over the fillets.
5. Add salt and thyme
6. Melt the butter then in a separate bowl, add the butter, remaining garlic, ⅓ cup olive oil, lemon juice, paprika, salt and pepper
7. Take the tomato, squash, and onion and mix then pour the sauce in
8. Divide and place on to the salmon fillets then wrap the foil til sealed
9. Bake in 400 degrees for 20-25 minutes
10. Remove from the oven and serve with the lemon wedges

191. Mouth-Watering Oysters Rockefeller

Preparation Time: 45 minutes
Servings: 3-5
Ingredients:
- Heavy cream - 1 cup
- Minced garlic - 3 cloves
- Pernod - 3 tbsp
- Chopped spinach - 4 cups
- Shucked oysters - 12
- Grated Pecorino Romano cheese - ¾ cup
- Salted butter - 2 tbsp
- Minced shallot - 1 small
- Salt and pepper -optional

Directions:
1. Heat butter on a medium pan then slowly add shallot and garlic and cook for 2 minutes.
2. Remove the pan from heat, gently add Pernod. Return on medium heat, simmer till the alcohol has evaporated.
3. Pour the heavy cream in and simmer till it is thickened and reduced.
4. Pour the spinach in and cook then add ⅓ of the cheese in.
5. Place the oysters on a baking tray.
6. Put a teaspoon of the dish into the oysters and top off with the rest of the cheese.
7. Place them on low heat in a broiler and let it stay till the cheese turns brown and the oysters are cooked to perfection.

192. Healthy crab and coconut soup

Preparation Time: 35 minutes
Servings: 5
Ingredients:
- Spinach - 5 cups
- Peeled and cubed potato - 1 medium
- Chopped bacon - 4 slices
- Diced yellow onion - 1 medium
- Crushed garlic - 2 cloves
- Chopped tomatoes- 2 cups
- Minced thyme leaves - 1 Tsp
- Crabmeat - 8 oz
- Chicken stock - 4 cups

- Coconut milk - 1 can
- Salt and pepper-optional

Directions:
1. On a pot or in an oven, brown the bacon.
2. In a large pot, add onions and cook for 4 minutes then add the crushed garlic and leave it for a minute.
3. Gently add the potatoes, thyme, salt, and pepper into the pot.
4. Pour the chicken stock and begin to stir then add the tomatoes and leave it to boil for 10 minutes until the potatoes are soft.
5. Pour the coconut milk in, followed by the spinach and cook till wilted then remove from heat.
6. Add the crabmeat in and gently stir to avoid breaking it apart.
7. Best served hot with scallions and lime.

193. Creamy Salmon Mac N Cheese

Preparation Time: 45 minutes
Servings: 2-3
Ingredients:
- Spinach - 2 ½ cups
- Salmon - 5 oz
- Macaroni shells - 8 oz
- Goat cheese - 1 tbsp
- Heavy cream - 2 cups
- Shredded mozzarella - 1 cup
- Crushed potato chips - 1 ½ cup
- Salt and pepper-optional

Directions:
1. Start cooking the macaroni shells according to the Directions: on the package.
2. Turn on the oven and preheat at 375 degrees
3. In a large pan, boil the heavy cream on low heat.
4. Slowly pour in the mozzarella and whisk away while adding the goat cheese and some salt and pepper.
5. Once the pasta is ready, drain it and add the heavy cream and cheese mixture on top.
6. Add the spinach and packaged salmon in and cook on low heat until the spinach is wilted.
7. Remove from heat, place in a baking dish then sprinkle the crushed potato chips on top and bake for 25 minutes until the top is browned.
8. Remove from the oven and serve hot.

194. Easy Spinach and Salmon wraps

Preparation Time: 10 minutes
Servings: 1
Ingredients:
- Smoked salmon - 1 oz.
- Ground pepper-optional
- Egg whites - 4
- Green onions - 3 -green part chopped
- Baby spinach - 1 handful
- Mustard - 1 tbsp

Directions:

1. In a bowl mix green onion, mustard, pepper and egg whites
2. Heat a nonstick pan on medium heat
3. Slowly pour the mixture on the pan and spread into a circle.
4. Let it cook for 4 minutes to remain intact before turning it.
5. Remove from the pan and place on a flat plate then place the spinach and salmon then wrap.
6. You can add other fillings of your choice to the wrap.

195. Shrimp and Spinach dip

Preparation Time: 35 minutes
Servings: 16
Ingredients:
- Cooked shrimp - 1 lb. -roughly chopped and tails removed
- Artichoke hearts - 1 cup -marinated, chopped and drained
- Baby spinach - 4 cups -chopped
- Salted butter -¼ cup
- Mayonnaise - ½ cup
- Cream cheese - 12 oz
- Thinly cut onion - ½ large
- Parmesan cheese - 1 ¼ cup -grated
- Greek yogurt - ½ cup
- Bread or crackers
- Salt and pepper-optional

Directions:
1. On medium heat, melt the butter on a large skillet and add the onion then cook for 5 minutes
2. Preheat the oven to 425 degrees
3. Pour the spinach into the skillet and cook for a minute
4. Remove and place the onions and spinach in a separate bowl then add heavy cream onto the large skillet and cook for 2 minutes.
5. Gently add the onions and spinach and stir.
6. Add the 1 cup Parmesan, yogurt, mayonnaise, shrimp, artichoke hearts, salt, and pepper and mix properly.
7. Sprinkle the remaining cheese on top then bake for 20 minutes then remove from heat and serve with the bread or crackers

DeliciousTuna Lemon Noodle Salad

Preparation Time: 10 minutes
Servings: 1
Ingredients:
- Cooked elbow noodles - ½ cup
- Tuna - 1 can
- Spinach - 1 cup
- lemon pepper salt
- lemon juice - ½ small lemon

Directions:
1. On medium heat, cook the spinach for two minutes until wilted
2. In a medium bowl add tuna, spinach and noodles then mix

3.   Pour the lemon juice and salt to your desired taste

Tuna and spinach power bowl

Preparation Time: 20 minutes
Servings: 6
Ingredients:
- Beans, great northern or cannellini -15oz - rinsed and drained
- Chopped spinach - 12 cups
- Tuna in olive oil,-6 oz -undrained
- Olive oil - 3 tbsp
- Onion - 1 cup -chopped
- Capers - ¼ cup
- Olives - 1/2 cup-sliced and drained
- Red pepper crushed - ¼ Tsp
- 3 garlic cloves, minced - 1 ½ Tsp
- Sugar - 2 Tsp
- Black pepper - ¼ Tsp
- Salt - ¼ Tsp

Directions:
1.   In a pot boil, the spinach for 2 minutes to soften it then drain.
2.   Heat olive oil in a medium-sized pot and pour the onions in then cook for 5 minutes.
3.   Add the garlic and cook for a minute.
4.   Take the olives, red pepper and capers and add into the pot for a minute
5.   Pour the sugar and spinach into the pot, stir, cover the lip of the pot and cook for 8 minutes.

6.   Remove from heat, place in a bowl and mix with beans and tuna.
7.   Season as desired and enjoy

198. Sunflower Kale salad with Baked Honey Salmon

Preparation Time: 25 minutes
Servings: 6
Ingredients:
- Salmon - 32 oz
- Smart vegetable Salad Kits -Sunflower Kale- 1-2 Eat
- 4 cloves minced garlic - 4 cloves
- Melted butter - 3 tbsp
- Lemon juice - 1 small
- Honey - 3 tbsp
- salt and pepper -optional

Directions:
1.   Cover a baking tray with aluminum foil and place the salmon-skin side up
2.   Turn the oven to 375 degrees to preheat
3.   Mix the butter, lemon juice, honey, and garlic in a bowl then pour on top of the salmon.
4.   Lift the sides of the foil to avoid spilling.
5.   Sprinkle pepper and salt to desired taste on the salmon
6.   Bake for 18 minutes till the salmon easily flakes then broil for 5 minutes while closely observing to avoid overcooking
7.   Read the Directions: on the Smart sunflower kale salad and prepare
8.   Serve the salmon on top of the salad

POULTRY

199. Easy Chicken Skillet

Preparation time: 10 minutes
Cooking time: 20 minutes
Servings: 4
Ingredients:
- 2 tablespoons olive oil
- 4 chicken breasts, skinless and boneless
- A pinch of black pepper
- 2 tablespoons low-fat butter
- ½ teaspoon oregano, dried
- 3 garlic cloves, minced
- 2 cups baby spinach
- 14 ounces canned artichokes, no-salt-added, chopped
- ½ cup roasted red peppers, chopped
- 1 cup coconut cream
- ¾ cup low-fat mozzarella, shredded
- ¼ cup low-fat parmesan, grated

Directions:
1.   Heat up a pan with the oil over medium-high heat, add chicken, season with black pepper and oregano, cook for 6 minutes on each side and transfer to a bowl.
2.   Heat up the same pan with the butter over medium-high heat, add garlic, spinach, artichokes and red peppers, stir and cook for 3 minutes more.
3.   Return chicken breasts, also add mozzarella, parmesan and coconut cream, toss, bring to a simmer, cook for 5 minutes more, divide into bowls and serve.
4.   Enjoy!
Nutrition Values: calories 211, fat 4, fiber 5, carbs 14, protein 11

200. Chicken And Onion Mix

Preparation time: 10 minutes
Cooking time: 45 minutes
Servings: 4
Ingredients:
- 3 tablespoons olive oil
- 1 yellow onion, roughly chopped
- 2 teaspoons thyme, chopped
- 2 garlic cloves, minced
- A pinch of black pepper
- 4 chicken breasts, skinless, boneless and cubed
- ½ teaspoon oregano, dried
- 1 and ½ cup low-sodium beef stock
- 1 tablespoon parsley, chopped

Directions:
1.   Heat up a pan with 2 tablespoons olive oil over medium-low heat, add the onion, black pepper and thyme, toss and cook for 24 minutes.
2.   Add garlic, cook for 1 more minute and transfer to a bowl.
3.   Clean the pan, heat it up with the rest of the oil over medium-high heat, add chicken, black pepper, and oregano, stir and cook for 8 minutes more.
4.   Add beef, add the onion mix and the parsley, toss, cook for 10 minutes, divide into bowls and serve.
5.   Enjoy!
Nutrition Values: calories 231, fat 4, fiber 7, carbs 14, protein 15

201. Balsamic Chicken Mix

Preparation time: 10 minutes
Cooking time: 35 minutes
Servings: 4
Ingredients:
- 1 tablespoon olive oil
- 1 pound chicken thighs, bone-in, skin-on
- ½ cup cranberries
- 2 garlic cloves, minced
- 1/3 cup balsamic vinegar
- 2 teaspoons thyme, chopped
- 1 teaspoon rosemary, chopped
- Zest of 1 orange, grated

Directions:
1.   Heat up a pan with the oil over medium-high heat, add chicken thighs skin side down, cook for 5 minutes and transfer to a plate.
2.   Heat up the same pan over medium heat, add cranberries, garlic, vinegar, thyme, rosemary and orange zest, toss and bring to a simmer.
3.   Return chicken to the pan as well, cook everything for 10 minutes, introduce the pan in the oven and bake at 325 degrees F for 25 minutes.
4.   Divide between plates and serve.
5.   Enjoy!
Nutrition Values: calories 235, fat 5, fiber 6, carbs 14, protein 15

202. Asian Glazed Chicken

Preparation time: 10 minutes
Cooking time: 30 minutes
Servings: 4
Ingredients:
- 8 chicken thighs, boneless and skinless
- 1/3 cup coconut aminos
- ½ cup balsamic vinegar
- 3 tablespoon garlic, minced
- ¼ cup olive oil
- A pinch of black pepper
- 1 tablespoon green onion, chopped
- 3 tablespoons garlic chili sauce

Directions:
1.   Put the oil in a baking dish, add chicken, aminos, vinegar, garlic, black pepper, onion and chili sauce, toss well, introduce in the oven and bake at 425 degrees F for 30 minutes.
2.   Divide the chicken and the sauce between plates and serve.
3.   Enjoy!
Nutrition Values: calories 254, fat 12, fiber 6, carbs 15, protein 20

203. Easy Greek Chicken

Preparation time: 10 minutes
Cooking time: 15 minutes
Servings: 4
Ingredients:
• 1 pound chicken breasts, skinless and boneless
• A pinch of black pepper
• 1 tablespoon olive oil
• 2 garlic cloves, minced
• 1 teaspoon oregano, dried
• 1 cup coconut milk
• 1 tablespoon lemon juice
• 1 teaspoon lemon zest, grated
• 1 and ½ cups cherry tomatoes, halved
• ½ cup kalamata olives, pitted and sliced
• ¼ cup dill, chopped
• 1 cucumber, sliced
Directions:
1. Heat up a pan with the oil over medium-high heat, add chicken and cook for 4 minutes on each side.
2. Add black pepper, garlic, oregano, milk, lemon juice, lemon zest, tomatoes, olives, dill and cucumber, toss, cook for 10 minutes more, divide between plates and serve.
3. Enjoy!
Nutrition Values: calories 241, fat 4, fiber 8, carbs 15, protein 16

204. Summer Chicken Mix

Preparation time: 10 minutes
Cooking time: 27 minutes
Servings: 4
Ingredients:
• 1 tablespoon olive oil
• 4 chicken breasts, skinless and boneless
• A pinch of black pepper
• 1 shallot, chopped
• 2 garlic cloves, minced
• 4 peaches, sliced
• ¼ cup balsamic vinegar
• ¼ cup basil, chopped
Directions:
1. Heat up a pan with the oil over medium-high heat, add chicken, season with black pepper, cook for 8 minutes on each side and transfer to a plate.
2. Heat up the same pan over medium-high heat, add shallot and garlic, stir and cook for 2 minutes.
3. Add peaches, stir and cook for 5 minutes more.
4. Add the vinegar, return the chicken, also add the basil, toss, cook for 3-4 minutes more, divide everything between plates and serve.
5. Enjoy!
Nutrition Values: calories 241, fat 4, fiber 7, carbs 15, protein 15

205. Cajun Chicken

Preparation time: 10 minutes
Cooking time: 20 minutes
Servings: 4
Ingredients:
• 1 tablespoon olive oil
• 1 pound chicken breast, skinless and boneless
• ½ teaspoon oregano, dried
• A pinch of black pepper
• ¼ cup low-sodium veggie stock
• 2 cups cherry tomatoes, halved
• 4 green onions, chopped
• 1 tablespoon Cajun seasoning
• 3 garlic cloves, minced
• ½ teaspoon sweet paprika
• 2/3 cup coconut cream
• 2 tablespoons lemon juice
Directions:
1. Heat up a pan with the oil over medium-high heat, add chicken and a pinch of black pepper and cook for 5 minutes on each side.
2. Add oregano, stock, green onions, Cajun seasoning, garlic, paprika, cream and lemon juice, toss, cook for 10 minutes, divide into bowls and serve.
3. Enjoy!
Nutrition Values: calories 233, fat 4, fiber 6, carbs 15, protein 20

206. Chicken And Veggies

Preparation time: 10 minutes
Cooking time: 25 minutes
Servings: 4
Ingredients:
1. 4 chicken breasts, skinless, boneless and cubed
2. 2 tablespoons olive oil
3. ½ teaspoon Italian seasoning
4. A pinch of black pepper
5. ½ cup yellow onion, chopped
6. 14 ounces canned tomatoes, no-salt-added, drained and chopped
7. 16 ounces cauliflower florets
Directions:
1. Heat up a pan with the oil over medium-high heat, add chicken, black pepper, onion and Italian seasoning, toss and cook for 5 minutes.
2. Add tomatoes and cauliflower, toss, cover the pan and cook over medium heat for 20 minutes.
3. Toss again, divide everything between plates and serve.
4. Enjoy!
Nutrition Values: calories 310, fat 6, fiber 4, carbs 14, protein 20

207. Chicken And Broccoli

Preparation time: 10 minutes
Cooking time: 25 minutes

Servings: 4

Ingredients:
- 1 tablespoon olive oil
- 4 chicken breasts, skinless and boneless
- 1 cup red onions, chopped
- 2 garlic cloves, minced
- 2 cups broccoli florets
- ½ cup coconut cream

Directions:
1.   Heat up a pan with the oil over medium-high heat, add chicken breasts and cook for 5 minutes on each side.
2.   Add onions and garlic, stir and cook for 5 minutes more.
3.   Add oregano, broccoli and cream, toss everything, cook for 10 minutes more, divide between plates and serve.
4.   Enjoy!

Nutrition Values: calories 287, fat 10, fiber 2, carbs 14, protein 19

208. Artichoke And Spinach Chicken

Preparation time: 10 minutes
Cooking time: 20 minutes
Servings: 4

Ingredients:
- 2 tablespoons olive oil
- 10 ounces baby spinach
- 14 ounces artichoke hearts, chopped
- 4 chicken breasts, boneless and skinless
- 28 ounces tomato sauce, no-salt-added
- ½ teaspoon red pepper flakes, crushed

Directions:
1.   Heat up a pan with the oil over medium-high heat, add chicken and red pepper flakes and cook for 5 minutes on each side.
2.   Add spinach, artichokes and tomato sauce, toss, cook for 10 minutes more, divide between plates and serve.
3.   Enjoy!

Nutrition Values: calories 212, fat 3, fiber 7, carbs 16, protein 20

209. Pumpkin And Black Beans Chicken

Preparation time: 10 minutes
Cooking time: 25 minutes
Servings: 4

Ingredients:
- 1 pound chicken breasts, skinless and boneless
- 2 cups water
- 1 tablespoon olive oil
- 1 cup coconut milk
- ½ cup pumpkin flesh
- 15 ounces canned black beans, no-salt-added, drained and rinsed
- 1 tablespoon cilantro, chopped

Directions:

1.   Heat up a pan with the oil over medium-high heat, add the chicken and cook for 5 minutes.
2.   Add the water, milk, pumpkin and black beans, toss, cover the pan, reduce heat to medium and cook for 20 minutes.
3.   Add cilantro, toss, divide between plates and serve.
4.   Enjoy!

Nutrition Values: calories 254, fat 6, fiber 4, carbs 16, protein 22

210. Chutney Chicken Mix

Preparation time: 10 minutes
Cooking time: 10 minutes
Servings: 4

Ingredients:
- 4 chicken breast halves, skinless and boneless
- 2 tablespoons lime juice
- 2 tablespoons olive oil
- 4 tablespoons mango chutney
- ½ teaspoon ginger, grated
- 1 avocado, peeled, pitted and chopped
- 8 cups micro greens
- A pinch of black pepper

Directions:
1.   In a bowl, mix chicken breasts with oil with chutney, lime juice and ginger and toss to coat.
2.   Heat up your kitchen grill over medium-high heat, add chicken, cook for 5 minutes on each side, cut into thin strips and put in a salad bowl.
3.   Add avocado, black pepper and greens, drizzle the chutney dressing, toss to coat and serve.
4.   Enjoy!

Nutrition Values: calories 210, fat 3, fiber 4, carbs 12, protein 9

211. Chicken And Sweet Potato Soup

Preparation time: 10 minutes
Cooking time: 20 minutes
Servings: 6

Ingredients:
- 2 chicken breasts, skinless, boneless and cubed
- 1 yellow onion, chopped
- 2 tablespoons olive oil
- 1 garlic clove, minced
- 4 sweet potatoes, cubed
- 2 carrots, chopped
- ½ teaspoon ginger, grated
- ½ teaspoon cumin, ground
- A pinch of black pepper
- 20 ounces low-sodium veggie stock

Directions:
1.   Heat up a pot with the oil over medium-high heat, add onion and garlic, stir and cook for 5 minutes.
2.   Add carrots and potatoes, stir and cook for 5 minutes.

3.   Add ginger, cumin, stock, pepper and chicken, stir, bring to a boil, reduce heat to medium, simmer for 10 minutes, ladle into soup bowls and serve.
4.   Enjoy!
Nutrition Values: calories 209, fat 5, fiber 5, carbs 13, protein 9

212. Chicken And Dill Soup

Preparation time: 10 minutes
Cooking time:: 1 hour and 20 minutes
Servings: 6
Ingredients:
- 1 whole chicken
- 1 pound carrots, sliced
- 6 cups low-sodium veggie stock
- 1 cup yellow onion, chopped
- A pinch of salt and black pepper
- 2 teaspoons dill, chopped
- ½ cup red onion, chopped

Directions:
1.   Put chicken in a pot, add water to cover, bring to a boil over medium heat, cook for 1 hour, transfer to a cutting board, discard bones, shred the meat, strain the soup, return it to the pot, heat it up over medium heat and add the chicken.
2.   Also add the carrots, yellow onion, red onion, a pinch of salt, black pepper and the dill, cook for 15 minutes, ladle into bowls and serve.
3.   Enjoy!
Nutrition Values: calories 202, fat 6, fiber 4, carbs 8, protein 12

213. Cilantro Serrano Chicken Soup

Preparation time: 10 minutes
Cooking time: 1 hour
Servings: 4
Ingredients:
- 4 chicken thighs, skin and bone in
- 1 cup cilantro, chopped
- 2 small Serrano peppers, chopped
- 4 and ¼ cups low-sodium veggie stock
- 2 whole garlic cloves+ 2 garlic cloves, minced
- 2 tablespoons olive oil
- ½ red bell pepper chopped
- ½ yellow onion, chopped
- A pinch of salt and black pepper

Directions:
1.   Put cilantro in your food processor, add Serrano peppers, 2 whole garlic cloves and ¼ cup stock, blend very well and transfer to a bowl.
2.   Heat up a pot with the olive oil over medium-high heat, add chicken thighs, cook for 5 minutes on each side and transfer to a bowl.
3.   Return pot to medium heat, add onion, stir and cook for 5 minutes.
4.   Add bell pepper, salt, pepper, minced garlic, cilantro paste, chicken and the rest of the stock, toss,

bring to a simmer over medium heat, cook for 40 minutes, ladle into bowls and serve
5.   Enjoy!
Nutrition Values: calories 291, fat 5, fiber 8, carbs 10, protein 12

214. Leek And Chicken Soup

Preparation time: 15 minutes
Cooking time:: 1 hour and 20 minutes
Yield: 4
Ingredients:
- 1 whole chicken, cut into medium pieces
- A pinch of salt and black pepper
- 12 cups low-sodium veggie stock
- 3 leek, roughly chopped
- 3 tablespoons olive oil
- 2 cups yellow onion, chopped
- ½ cup lemon juice

Directions:
1.   Put chicken in a pot, add the stock, a pinch of salt and black pepper, stir, bring to a boil over medium heat and skim foam.
2.   Add leeks, toss and simmer for 1 hour.
3.   Heat up a pan with the oil over medium heat, add onion, stir and cook for 5 minutes.
4.   Add this to the pot, also add the lemon juice, toss, cook for 20 minutes more, ladle into bowls and serve.
5.   Enjoy!
Nutrition Values: calories 199, fat 3, fiber 5, carbs 6, protein 11

215. Collard Greens And Chicken Soup

Preparation time: 10 minutes
Cooking time: 30 minutes
Servings: 4
Ingredients:
- 4 cups low-sodium chicken stock
- 1 garlic clove, minced
- 1 yellow onion, chopped
- 8 ounces chicken breast skinless, boneless and chopped
- 2 cups collard greens, chopped
- A pinch of salt and black pepper
- 2 tablespoons ginger, grated

Directions:
1.   Put the stock in a pot, add garlic, chicken and onion, stir, bring to a boil over medium heat and simmer for 20 minutes.
2.   Add collard greens, salt, pepper and ginger, stir and cook for 10 more minutes, ladle into bowls and serve.
3.   Enjoy!
Nutrition Values: calories 199, fat 5, fiber 5, carbs 8, protein 12

216. Chicken, Scallions And Avocado Soup

Preparation time: 10 minutes
Cooking time: 25 minutes
Servings: 4

Ingredients:
- 2 cups chicken breast, skinless, boneless, cooked and shredded
- 2 avocados, peeled, pitted and chopped
- 5 cups low-sodium veggie stock
- 1 and ½ cups scallions, chopped
- 2 garlic cloves, minced
- ½ cup cilantro, chopped
- A pinch of salt and black pepper
- 2 teaspoons olive oil

Directions:
1. Heat up a pot with the oil over medium heat, add 1 cup scallions and garlic, stir and cook for 5 minutes.
2. Add stock, salt and pepper, bring to a boil, reduce heat to low, cover and simmer for 20 minutes.
3. Divide chicken, the rest of the scallions and avocado in bowls, add soup, top with chopped cilantro and serve.
4. Enjoy!

Nutrition Values: calories 205, fat 5, fiber 6, carbs 14, protein 8

217. Coconut Chicken And Mushrooms

Preparation time: 10 minutes
Cooking time: 52 minutes
Servings: 8
Ingredients:
- 3 tablespoons olive oil
- 8 chicken thighs
- A pinch of salt and black pepper
- 3 garlic cloves, minced
- 8 ounces mushrooms, halved
- 1 cup coconut cream
- ½ teaspoon basil, dried
- ½ teaspoon oregano, dried
- 1 tablespoon mustard

Directions:
1. Heat up a pot with 2 tablespoons oil over medium-high heat, add chicken, salt and pepper, brown for 3 minutes on each side and transfer to a plate.
2. Heat up the same pot with the rest of the oil over medium heat, add mushroom and garlic, stir and cook for 6 minutes.
3. Add salt, pepper, oregano, basil and chicken, stir and bake in the oven at 400 degrees F for 30 minutes.
4. Add cream and mustard, stir, simmer for 10 minutes more, divide everything between plates and serve.
5. Enjoy!

Nutrition Values: calories 269, fat 5, fiber 6, carbs 13, protein 12

218. Chicken Chili

Preparation time: 10 minutes
Cooking time: 1 hour and 10 minutes
Servings: 6
Ingredients:
- 1 cup coconut flour
- 8 lemon tea bags
- A pinch of salt and black pepper
- 4 pounds chicken breast, skinless, boneless and cubed
- 4 ounces olive oil
- 4 ounces celery, chopped
- 3 garlic cloves, minced
- 2 yellow onion, chopped
- 2 red bell pepper, chopped
- 7 ounces poblano pepper, chopped
- 1-quart low-sodium stock veggie stock
- 1 teaspoon chili powder
- ¼ cup cilantro, chopped

Directions:
1. Dredge the chicken pieces in coconut flour.
2. Heat up a pot with the oil over medium-high heat, add chicken, cook for 5 minutes on each side and transfer to a bowl.
3. Heat up the pot again over medium-high heat, add onion, celery, garlic, bell pepper and poblano pepper, stir and cook for 2 minutes.
4. Add stock, chili powder, salt, pepper, chicken and tea bags, stir, bring to a simmer, reduce heat to medium-low, cover and cook for 1 hour.
5. Discard tea bags, add cilantro, stir, ladle into bowls and serve.
6. Enjoy!

Nutrition Values: calories 205, fat 8, fiber 3, carbs 12, protein 6

219. Chicken, Spinach And Asparagus Soup

Preparation time: 10 minutes
Cooking time: 30 minutes
Servings: 6
Ingredients:
- 2 chicken breasts, cooked, skinless, boneless and shredded
- 1 tablespoon olive oil
- A pinch of salt and black pepper
- 1 yellow onion, finely chopped
- 2 carrots, chopped
- 3 garlic cloves, minced
- 4 cups spinach
- 12 asparagus spears, chopped
- 6 cups low-sodium veggie stock
- Zest of ½ lime, grated
- 1 handful cilantro, chopped

Directions:
1. Heat up a pot with the oil over medium heat, add onions, stir and cook for 5 minutes.
2. Add carrots, garlic and asparagus, stir and cook for 5 minutes.
3. Add spinach, salt, pepper, stock and chicken, stir and cook for 20 minutes.
4. Add lime zest and cilantro, stir soup again, ladle into bowls and serve..
5. Enjoy!

Nutrition Values: calories 245, fat 2, fiber 3, carbs 5, protein 6

220. Chicken And Broccoli Salad

Preparation time: 10 minutes
Cooking time: 10 minutes
Servings: 4
Ingredients:
- 3 medium chicken breasts, skinless, boneless and cut into thin strips
- 12 ounces broccoli florets, roughly chopped
- 5 tablespoon olive oil
- A pinch of salt and black pepper
- 2 tablespoon vinegar
- 1 and ½ cups peaches, pitted and sliced
- 1 tablespoon chives, chopped
- 2 bacon slices, cooked and crumbled

Directions:
1. In a salad bowl, mix 4 tablespoon oil with vinegar, salt, pepper, broccoli and peaches and toss.
2. Heat up a pan with the rest of the oil over medium-high heat, add chicken, season with salt and pepper, cook for 5 minutes on each side, transfer to the salad bowl, add bacon and chives, toss and serve.
3. Enjoy!
Nutrition Values: calories 210, fat 12, fiber 3, carbs 10, protein 23

221. Garlicky Zucchini-Turkey Casserole

Servings: 4
Cooking time: 40 minutes
Ingredients:
- 1 tablespoon oil
- 1 white onion, chopped
- 2 cloves of garlic, minced
- 1-pound cooked turkey meat, shredded
- A dash of rosemary
- 1 zucchini, chopped
- 1 carrot, peeled and chopped
- ½ cup water
- Pepper to taste

Directions:
1. Preheat oven to 400oF.
2. Grease an oven safe casserole dish with oil.
3. Mix onion, garlic, turkey, pepper, salt, and rosemary in a bowl.
4. Pour into prepared casserole dish.
5. Sprinkle carrot on top, followed by zucchini, and then pour water over mixture.
6. Cover dish with a foil and bake for 25 minutes or until bubbly hot.
7. Remove foil and return to oven and broil top for 2 minutes on high.
8. Let it rest for 10 minutes.
9. Serve and enjoy.
Nutrition Values:
Calories: 250; Carbs: 5.7g; Protein: 32.9g; Fats: 10.0g; Saturated Fat: 2.8g; Sodium: 88 mg

222. Casserole a La Chicken Enchilada

Servings: 10
Cooking time: 6 hours
Ingredients:
- 5 pitted dates
- 3 tablespoons olive oil
- ¼ cup chili powder
- 1 cup water
- 1 cup tomato paste
- 1 teaspoon ground cumin
- 1 teaspoon dried oregano
- Salt and pepper to taste
- 2 pounds chicken breasts, cut into strips
- 1 sweet potato, scrubbed and chopped

Directions:
1. In a blender or food processor, place the dates, olive oil, chili powder, water, tomato paste, cumin, and oregano. Season with salt and pepper to taste. Pulse until smooth. This will be the enchilada sauce.
2. On the Crock-Pot, place the chicken breasts and sweet potatoes on bottom of pot.
3. Pour over chicken the enchilada sauce.
4. Close the lid and press the low settings and adjust the cooking time to 6 hours.
5. Serve and enjoy.
Nutrition Values:
Calories: 240; Carbs: 12.2g; Protein: 30.2g; Fats: 8.0g; Saturated Fat: 2.7g; Sodium: 204mg

223. Cilantro-Coconut Chicken Stew

Servings: 8
Cooking time: 30 minutes
Ingredients:
- 1 whole chicken, around 2-lbs
- 1 can light coconut milk
- 1 cup water
- ½ fresh cilantro, chopped
- 1 tablespoon ginger
- 1 teaspoon cumin
- 1 teaspoon coriander
- ½ teaspoon salt
- ½ teaspoon curry
- 1 lemon, juice extracted

Directions:
1. Place a heavy bottomed pot on medium high fire.
2. Add all ingredients except for coconut milk. Mix well.
3. Bring to a boil. Once boiling, lower fire to a simmer and cook for 20 minutes.
4. Stir in coconut milk. Continue simmering for another 10 minutes.
5. Serve and enjoy.
Nutrition Values:
Calories: 194; Carbs: 2.3g; Protein: 23.8g; Fats: 9.9g; Saturated Fat: 6.7g; Sodium: 236mg

224. Turkey Legs in Thai Sauce

Servings: 6

Cooking time: 30 minutes
Ingredients:
- 1 ½ pounds large turkey legs
- 1 can light coconut milk
- 1 cup water
- 1 ½ teaspoon lemon juice
- ¼ cup cilantro, chopped
- Pepper to taste

Directions:
1. Place a heavy bottomed pot on medium high fire.
2. Add all ingredients except for coconut milk. Mix well.
3. Bring to a boil. Once boiling, lower fire to a simmer and cook for 20 minutes.
4. Stir in coconut milk. Continue simmering for another 10 minutes.
5. Serve and enjoy.

Nutrition Values:
Calories: 236; Carbs: 2.5g; Protein: 23.0g; Fats: 14.8g; Saturated Fat: 3.8g; Sodium: 90mg

225. Filling Turkey Chili Recipe

Servings: 6
Cooking time: 25 minutes
Ingredients:
- 1 tablespoon olive oil
- 1-pound ground turkey
- 1 onion, chopped
- 1 green bell pepper, seeded and chopped
- 3 carrots, peeled and chopped
- 2 stalks of celery, sliced thinly
- 1 cup chopped tomatoes
- 3 poblano chilies, chopped
- ½ cup water
- 3 tablespoons chili powder
- 1 ½ teaspoons ground cumin
- Pepper to taste

Directions:
1. Place a heavy bottomed pot on medium high fire and heat for 3 minutes.
2. Add oil, swirl to coat bottom and sides of pot, and heat for a minute.
3. Stir in turkey. Brown and crumble for 8 minutes. Season generously with pepper. Discard excess fat.
4. Add all ingredients. Mix well.
5. Bring to a boil. Once boiling, lower fire to a simmer and cook for 10 minutes.
6. Serve and enjoy.

Nutrition Values:
Calories: 175; Carbs: 8.7g; Protein: 16.4g; Fats: 9.1g; Saturated Fat: 2.0g; Sodium: 188mg

226. Chicken Meatloaf with a Tropical Twist

Servings: 4
Cooking time: 45 minutes
Ingredients:

- 1/8 teaspoon salt
- 1/8 teaspoon pepper
- 2 eggs
- ¼ cup parsley, chopped
- ¼ cup coconut flakes
- ½ tablespoons jalapeno, seeded and diced
- ½ cups diced mango
- 1 cup yellow bell pepper, diced
- 1-pound ground chicken
- 1 tablespoon oil

Directions:
- Preheat oven to 400oF and lightly grease a loaf pan with oil.
- In a large bowl, mix remaining ingredients.
- Evenly spread in prepared pan and cover pan with foil.
- Pop in the oven and bake for 30 minutes.
- Remove foil and broil top for 3 minutes.
- Let it sit for 10 minutes.
- Serve and enjoy.

Nutrition Values:
Calories: 301; Carbs: 8.0g; Protein: 25.0g; Fats: 19.0g; Saturated Fat: 4.6g; Sodium: 215mg

227. Chicken-Mushroom Casserole

Servings: 3
Cooking time: 35 minutes
Ingredients:
- 2 tbsp chopped fresh parsley
- 4 slices Muenster cheese
- 1 garlic clove, minced
- 1-lb sliced fresh mushrooms
- 1 cup water
- 1 18-oz can creamy mushroom soup, low sodium
- 1 chicken breast, sliced thinly
- ¼ tsp pepper
- 2 tbsp all-purpose flour

Directions:
1. Place a nonstick saucepan on medium high fire and heat for 3 minutes.
2. Add oil and swirl pan to coat sides and bottom with oil Heat for a minute.
3. Add chicken and sauté until no longer pink, around 5 minutes. Season with pepper and transfer to a plate.
4. In same pan, add flour and sauté for 3 minutes. Add garlic and sauté for a minute more.
5. Stir in mushrooms and cook for 5 minutes until water comes out of it.
6. Add remaining ingredients, except for cheese and parsley. Mix well. Return chicken to pan.
7. Bring to a simmer, cover and cook for 10 minutes while mixing frequently.
8. Place cheese on top and let it rest while covered for 5 minutes.
9. Serve and enjoy with a sprinkle of parsley.

Nutrition Values:

Calories: 346; Carbs: 14.7g; Protein: 36.4g; Fats: 16.3g; Saturated Fat: 6.8g; Sodium: 109mg

228. Pineapple Chicken Hawaiian Style

Servings: 6
Cooking time: 40 minutes
Ingredients:
- 2 tbsp cornstarch
- 1 small yellow bell pepper, cut into 1-inch pieces
- 1 small red bell pepper, cut into 1-inch pieces
- 1 20-oz can pineapple chunks, drained and ¼ cup liquid reserved
- 1 cup honey BBQ sauce
- 2 cloves garlic, chopped finely
- 1.5-lbs boneless, skinless chicken thighs
- 1 tsp oil

Directions:
1. Place a heavy bottomed pot on medium high fire and heat pot for 3 minutes.
2. Once hot, add oil and stir around to coat pot with oil.
3. Add chicken and cook for 4 minutes per side.
4. Meanwhile, in a bowl mix cornstarch with ¼ cup water and set aside
5. Add pineapple chunks to pot and sauté for 2 minutes.
6. Stir in reserved liquid form pineapple, BBQ sauce, and garlic. Mix well and bring to a boil.
7. Cover, lower fire to a simmer and simmer for 8 minutes.
8. Stir in bell peppers and cornstarch slurry. Continue mixing and cooking until sauce has thickened, around 5 minutes.
9. Serve and enjoy.

Nutrition Values:
Calories: 402; Carbs: 45.9g; Protein: 28.7g; Fats: 11.6g; Saturated Fat: 3.0g; Sodium: 285mg

229. Honey Sesame Chicken

Servings: 4
Cooking time: 20 minutes
Ingredients:
- 1 tbsp toasted sesame seeds
- 2 green onions, chopped
- 3 tbsp water
- 2 tbsp cornstarch
- ¼ tsp red pepper flakes
- ½ cup honey
- 2 tsp sesame oil
- ¼ ketchup
- 2 tbsp soy sauce
- 2 garlic cloves, minced
- ½ cup onion, diced
- 1 tsp olive oil
- Pepper to taste

- 2 medium boneless, skinless chicken breasts, chopped into 1-inch cubes

Directions:
1. Place a heavy bottomed pot on medium high fire and heat pot for 3 minutes.
2. Meanwhile season chicken generously with pepper.
3. Once hot, add oil and stir around to coat pot with oil.
4. Stir in garlic and onion. Cook for 3 minutes.
5. Add chicken and cook for 5 minutes.
6. Stir in red pepper flakes, ketchup, and soy sauce. Mix well.
7. Cover, bring to a boil, lower fire to a simmer, and simmer for 5 minutes.
8. Meanwhile, in a bowl mix cornstarch with water and set aside
9. Stir in honey and sesame oil. Pour the cornstarch slurry and continue mixing while cooking until sauce has thickened, around 5 minutes.
10. Serve and enjoy with a sprinkle of green onions.

Nutrition Values:
Calories: 228; Carbs: 44.7g; Protein: 3.9g; Fats: 5.4g; Saturated Fat: 0.8g; Sodium: 304mg

230. Chicken Cooked the Italian Way

Servings: 6
Cooking time: 25 minutes
Ingredients:
- ¼ cup loosely packed fresh Italian parsley, chopped coarsely
- ½ cup loosely packed fresh basil leaves, sliced thinly
- ¼ tsp black pepper
- ½ cup pitted green olives
- 2 cups cherry tomatoes
- 1 tbsp tomato paste
- 3 garlic cloves, smashed and peeled
- ½-lb cremini mushroom, quartered
- 2 medium carrot, chopped coarsely
- 1 small onion, chopped coarsely
- 1 tsp olive oil
- 6 boneless, skinless chicken thighs

Directions:
1. Place a heavy bottomed pot on medium high fire and heat pot for 3 minutes.
2. Meanwhile season chicken generously with pepper.
3. Once hot, add oil and stir around to coat pot with oil.
4. Pan fry chicken for 4 minutes per side and transfer to a plate.
5. Add mushrooms, carrots, and onions to pot. Season with pepper. Sauté for 5 minutes.
6. Add tomato paste and garlic. Sauté for 2 minutes.
7. Add olives, cherry tomatoes, and return chicken. Mix well.

8. Cover, bring to a boil, lower fire to a simmer, and simmer for 10 minutes.
9. Stir in the fresh herbs.
10. Serve and enjoy.
Nutrition Values:
Calories: 241; Carbs: 7.7g; Protein: 21.5g; Fats: 13.9g; Saturated Fat: 3.7g; Sodium: 403mg

231. Italian Chicken Cacciatore

Servings: 6
Cooking time: 30-40minutes
Ingredients:
*   ¼ cup balsamic vinegar
*   1 tsp fresh thyme
*   2 tbsp parsley
*   1 14.5-oz can low sodium diced tomatoes, pulsed in a blender
*   1 14.5-oz can low sodium diced tomatoes in juice
*   1 cup chicken broth
*   1 bay leaf
*   2 tbsp fresh basil, chopped
*   ¼ tsp red pepper flakes
*   1 tsp dried oregano
*   2 large garlic cloves, minced
*   ½-lb mushrooms, sliced
*   1 red bell pepper, diced
*   3 carrots, peeled and diced
*   1 medium onion, sliced thinly
*   1 tbsp extra virgin olive oil
*   2 tsp ground pepper
*   6 chicken thighs, pat dry with paper towels
Directions:
1. Place a heavy bottomed pot on medium high fire and heat pot for 3 minutes.
2. Meanwhile season chicken generously with pepper.
3. Once hot, add oil and stir around to coat pot with oil.
4. Brown chicken for 5 minutes per side. If needed cook in batches and place on a plate.
5. Add mushroom and onion. Sauté for 5 minutes.
6. Stir in pepper flakes, oregano, and garlic. Cook for a minute.
7. Stir in thyme and bay leaf. Cook for another minute.
8. Pour in tomatoes, chicken broth, bell pepper, carrots, and the chicken. Mix well.
9. Cover, bring to a boil, lower fire to a simmer, and simmer for 10 minutes.
10. Serve and enjoy with a sprinkle of parsley.
Nutrition Values:
Calories: 412; Carbs: 43.0g; Protein: 37.0g; Fats: 13.0g; Saturated Fat: 3.6g; Sodium: 364mg

232. Oregano-Basil Chicken Breast

Servings: 4
Cooking time: 25 minutes
Ingredients:

*   1/2 cup water
*   1/8 tsp dried basil
*   1/8 tsp dried oregano
*   2 tbsp balsamic vinegar
*   Black pepper to taste
*   2 boneless, skinless chicken breasts
*   1 tbsp oil
Directions:
1. Place a heavy bottomed pot on medium high fire and heat pot for 3 minutes.
2. Meanwhile season chicken generously with pepper.
3. Once hot, add oil and stir around to coat pot with oil.
4. Add chicken breasts to hot pot and cook for 5 minutes per side.
5. Add remaining ingredients to pot.
6. Cover, bring to a boil, lower fire to a simmer, and simmer for 10 minutes.
7. Serve and enjoy.
Nutrition Values:
Calories: 142; Carbs: 2.5g; Protein: 19.1g; Fats: 5.8g; Saturated Fat: 1.0g; Sodium: 305mg

233. Filipino Style Chicken Adobo

Servings: 8
Cooking time: 35 minutes
Ingredients:
*   4 dried bay leaves
*   1 tsp ground black peppercorn
*   1 large sweet onion, chopped
*   10 cloves garlic, smashed
*   ¼ cup vinegar
*   2 tbsp coconut aminos
*   1.5-lbs chicken breast, boneless and skinless, cut into 2-inch cubes
Directions:
1. Place a heavy bottomed pot on medium high fire and heat pot for 3 minutes.
2. Once hot, add oil and stir around to coat pot with oil.
3. Add garlic and sauté for 2 minutes or until lightly browned.
4. Add half of onions and sauté until soft, around 4 minutes.
5. Stir in chicken and cook for 10 minutes.
6. Add remaining ingredients, except for onions.
7. Cover, bring to a boil, lower fire to a simmer, and simmer for 15 minutes.
8. Stir in remaining onions.
9. Serve and enjoy.
Nutrition Values:
Calories: 169; Carbs: 3.1g; Protein: 23.5g; Fats: 6.3g; Saturated Fat: 1.8g; Sodium: 328mg

234. Stewed Chicken & Dried Cherries

Servings: 6
Cooking time: 25 minutes
Ingredients:

- 1 tablespoon olive oil
- 1 cup shredded chicken meat
- 1 onion, chopped
- 2 teaspoons chili powder
- 1 teaspoon sambal oelek
- 1 tablespoon coconut aminos
- 2 cans cannellini beans, drained and rinsed
- ½ cup dried cherries
- 2 cups chicken broth, low sodium
- Pepper to taste
- 2 tablespoons chopped parsley

Directions:
1. Place a heavy bottomed pot on medium high fire and heat pot for 3 minutes.
2. Once hot, add oil and stir around to coat pot with oil. sauté the chicken meat, onions, chili powder, and sambal oelek for 5 minutes. Season with coconut aminos.
3. Stir in the cannellini beans and cherries.
4. Add the broth and season with pepper.
5. Cover, bring to a boil, lower fire to a simmer, and simmer for 15 minutes.
6. Serve and enjoy with a sprinkle of parsley.

Nutrition Values:
Calories: 278; Carbs: 33.1g; Protein: 16.8g; Fats: 9.0g; Saturated Fat: 1.6g; Sodium: 264mg

235. Chicken 'n Ginger Congee

Servings: 8
Cooking time: 45 minutes
Ingredients:
- 8 cups water
- 3 boneless chicken thighs, sliced thinly
- 1 cup rice, uncooked
- 4 thick slices of ginger, smashed
- ½ teaspoon salt
- 4 cloves garlic, peeled and minced
- ½ cup scallions, chopped
- 3 tablespoons ginger, minced
- ½ cup cilantro leaves
- 1 tsp olive oil
- Pepper to taste

Directions:
1. Place a heavy bottomed pot on medium high fire and heat pot for 3 minutes.
2. Meanwhile season chicken generously with pepper.
3. Once hot, add oil and stir around to coat pot with oil.
4. Sauté garlic and ginger for 3 minutes. Add chicken and sauté for 3 minutes.
5. Add 4 cups water and remaining ingredients except for cilantro and scallions. Mix well.
6. Cover, bring to a boil and boil for 5 minutes.
7. Stir in remaining water and bring to a simmer and simmer for 25 minutes. Continue cooking until rice is soft and tender.
8. Stir in cilantro.

9. Serve and enjoy with a sprinkle of pepper and scallions.
Nutrition Values:
Calories: 152; Carbs: 19.7g; Protein: 9.1g; Fats: 3.9g; Saturated Fat: 0.9g; Sodium: 280mg

236. Broccoli-Chicken Rice

Servings: 5
Cooking time: 35 minutes
Ingredients:
- 1 tsp olive oil
- 1-pound boneless chicken breasts, sliced thinly
- 2 cloves of garlic, minced
- 1 onion, chopped
- Pepper to taste
- 1 1/3 cups long grain rice
- 1 1/3 cups chicken broth, low sodium
- ½ cup skim milk
- 1 cup broccoli florets
- ½ cup low fat cheddar cheese, grated

Directions:
1. Place a heavy bottomed pot on medium high fire and heat pot for 3 minutes.
2. Meanwhile season chicken generously with pepper.
3. Once hot, add oil and stir around to coat pot with oil.
4. Sauté garlic and onion for 3 minutes. Add chicken and cook for another 3 minutes.
5. Add rice and stir fry for 3 minutes.
6. Stir in chicken broth and season with pepper. Cover and simmer for 10 minutes or until water is fully absorbed.
7. Add broccoli florets and skim milk. Cover and simmer for another 5 minutes.
8. Sprinkle cheese on top, cover and let it sit for 5 minutes.
9. Serve and enjoy.

Nutrition Values:
Calories: 462; Carbs: 43.3g; Protein: 43.0g; Fats: 12.0g; Saturated Fat: 3.8g; Sodium: 413mg

237. Cajun Chicken and Rice

Servings: 5
Cooking time: 35 minutes
Ingredients:
- 1 tablespoon oil
- 1 onion, diced
- 3 cloves of garlic, minced
- 1-pound chicken breasts, sliced
- 1 tablespoon Cajun seasoning
- 1 tablespoon tomato paste
- 2 cups chicken broth, low sodium
- 1 ½ cups white rice, rinsed
- 1 bell pepper, chopped

Directions:
1. Place a heavy bottomed pot on medium high fire and heat pot for 3 minutes.

2. Once hot, add oil and stir around to coat pot with oil.
3. Sauté the onion and garlic until fragrant, around 3 minutes.
4. Stir in the chicken breasts and tomato paste. Season with Cajun seasoning. Sauté for 5 minutes.
5. Add broth and deglaze pot. Stir in rice.
6. Cover, bring to a boil, lower fire to a simmer, and simmer for 5 minutes.
7. Stir in bell pepper. Continue simmering for another 10 minutes or until rice is absorbed.
8. Turn off fire and let rice sit for 5 minutes.
9. Serve and enjoy.

Nutrition Values:
Calories: 389; Carbs: 50.4g; Protein: 30.8g; Fats: 5.8g; Saturated Fat: 3.2g; Sodium: 189mg

238. Chicken-Rice Pilaf

Servings: 6
Cooking time: 30 minutes
Ingredients:
- 2 cups uncooked rice, rinsed
- 2 ½ cups, chicken stock low sodium
- 1 tablespoon rice wine
- 1 teaspoon olive oil
- 1 cup leftover chicken meat
- 2 small potatoes, peeled and quartered
- 2 carrots, chopped
- 1-pound white mushrooms, halved
- 1-pound green beans, chopped
- 3 cups kale, chopped
- 2 tablespoons soy sauce
- 1 tablespoon oyster sauce

Directions:
1. Place a heavy bottomed pot on medium high fire and heat pot for 3 minutes.
2. Once hot, add oil and stir around to coat pot with oil.
3. Sauté the rice wine, chicken meat, potatoes, carrots, mushrooms, green beans, soy sauce, and oyster sauce. Mix well and cook for 5 minutes.
4. Add rice and chicken stock.
5. Cover, bring to a boil, lower fire to a simmer, and simmer for 15 minutes or until water is absorbed.
6. Stir in kale and fluff rice. Let it rest for 5 minutes.
7. Serve and enjoy.

Nutrition Values:
Calories: 396; Carbs: 73.6g; Protein: 16.3g; Fats: 4.3g; Saturated Fat: 0.9g; Sodium: 204mg

239. Chicken and Jasmine Rice

Servings: 6
Cooking time: 30 minutes
Ingredients:
- 1 tablespoon olive oil
- 3 small shallots, diced
- 2 cloves of garlic, minced
- 1-pound boneless, skinless chicken thighs, sliced thinly
- Pepper to taste
- 3 carrots, diced
- 1 ½ cups white jasmine rice, rinsed and drained
- 2 cups low sodium chicken stock
- 2 tablespoons thyme leaves

Directions:
1. Place a heavy bottomed pot on medium high fire and heat pot for 3 minutes.
2. Once hot, add oil and stir around to coat pot with oil.
3. Sauté the shallots and garlic until fragrant, around 3 minutes.
4. Stir in the chicken breasts and thyme leaves. Season with pepper. Sauté for 5 minutes.
5. Add broth and deglaze pot. Stir in rice and carrots.
6. Cover, bring to a boil, lower fire to a simmer, and simmer for 12 minutes.
7. Turn off fire and let rice sit for 5 minutes.
8. Fluff rice, serve and enjoy.

Nutrition Values:
Calories: 213; Carbs: 27.1g; Protein: 10.1g; Fats: 7.9g; Saturated Fat: 1.8g; Sodium: 324mg

240. Stewed Chicken Enchiladas

Servings: 6
Cooking time: 20 minutes
Ingredients:
- 1 tablespoon coconut oil
- 1 onion, chopped
- 3 cloves of garlic, minced
- 1.5-pounds chicken breasts
- 1 green bell pepper, chopped
- 1 can jalapenos, chopped
- 1 can green chilies, chopped
- 1 can diced tomatoes, no salt added
- 1 can tomato sauce, no salt added
- 1 tablespoon cumin
- 1 tablespoon chili powder
- 2 teaspoons dried oregano
- Pepper to taste

Directions:
- Place a heavy bottomed pot on medium high fire and heat pot for 3 minutes.
- Once hot, add oil and stir around to coat pot with oil.
- Sauté the onion and garlic until fragrant, around 3 minutes.
- Stir in the chicken. Season with pepper. Sauté for 5 minutes.
- Add remaining ingredients and deglaze pot.
- Cover, bring to a boil, lower fire to a simmer, and simmer for 12 minutes.
- Serve and enjoy.

Nutrition Values:

Calories: 265; Carbs: 10.3g; Protein: 25.8g; Fats: 13.8g; Saturated Fat: 5.1g; Sodium: 159mg

241. Creamy Thai Coconut Chicken Soup

Servings: 4
Cooking time: 35 minutes
Ingredients:
- 2 tablespoons oil
- 1 onion, quartered
- 1-pound chicken breasts, skin and bones removed
- 2 tablespoons Thai red curry paste
- 1 red bell pepper, cut into strips
- 6 slices ginger
- 6 kaffir lime leaves
- 3 cups chicken broth
- 1 tablespoon coconut aminos
- 1 tablespoon sugar
- ¾ cup coconut milk
- 2 ½ tablespoons lime juice
- Cilantro leaves for serving

Directions:
1. Place a heavy bottomed pot on medium high fire and heat pot for 3 minutes.
2. Once hot, add oil and stir around to coat pot with oil.
3. Brown chicken for 5 minutes per side. Transfer to a chopping board and cut into 1-inch cubes.
4. Sauté the onion, garlic and chicken for 5 minutes.
5. Add the red curry paste, bell pepper, galangal, and kaffir limes.
6. After 30 seconds, add the chicken broth, fish sauce, and sugar.
7. Cover, bring to a boil, lower fire to a simmer, and simmer for 10 minutes.
8. Stir in lime juice and coconut milk. Cook for 5 minutes.
9. Serve and enjoy.

Nutrition Values:
Calories: 380; Carbs: 16.1g; Protein: 25.7g; Fats: 25.0g; Saturated Fat: 10.5g; Sodium: 85mg

242. Chicken Tortilla Soup

Servings: 4
Cooking time: 20 minutes
Ingredients:
1 tablespoon olive oil
- 1 onion, chopped
- 2 cloves of garlic, minced
- 2 tablespoons fresh cilantro, chopped
- 1 large ripe tomato, chopped
- 1 can black beans, drained and rinsed
- 1 cup frozen corn
- 4 cups chicken broth, low sodium
- 2 teaspoons chili powder
- 1 teaspoon cumin powder
- 1 bay leaf

- Pepper to taste
- 3 cooked chicken breasts, shredded
- 2 cooked corn tortillas, crumbled

Directions:
1. Place a heavy bottomed pot on medium high fire and heat pot for 3 minutes.
2. Once hot, add oil and stir around to coat pot with oil.
3. Sauté the onion, tomato and garlic for 5 minutes.
4. Stir in remaining ingredients except for tortillas.
5. Cover, bring to a boil, lower fire to a simmer, and simmer for 10 minutes.
6. Serve and enjoy with a sprinkle of crumbled tortillas.

Nutrition Values:
Calories: 453; Carbs: 40.1; Protein: 50.1g; Fats: 10.0g; Saturated Fat: 2.1g; Sodium: 303mg

243. Chipotle Beans 'n Chicken Soup

Servings: 8
Cooking time: 20 minutes
Ingredients:
- 1 tablespoon coconut oil
- 1 onion, chopped
- 3 cloves of garlic, minced
- 1 teaspoon chipotle seasoning
- ½ taco seasoning
- 6 cups sweet potatoes, peeled and chopped
- 6 cups chicken soup
- 3 cans cannellini beans, drained and rinsed well
- 4 cups cooked chicken, shredded
- Pepper

Directions:
1. Place a heavy bottomed pot on medium high fire and heat pot for 3 minutes.
2. Once hot, add oil and stir around to coat pot with oil.
3. Sauté the onion and garlic for 5 minutes.
4. Add remaining ingredients and mix well.
5. Cover, bring to a boil, lower fire to a simmer, and simmer for 10 minutes.
6. Serve and enjoy.

Nutrition Values:
Calories: 277; Carbs: 26.8g; Protein: 26.7g; Fats: 7.1g; Saturated Fat: 2.5g; Sodium: 305mg

244. Chicken 'n Potatoes the French Way

Servings: 8
Cooking time: 25 minutes
Ingredients:
- 1 tablespoon olive oil
- 4 chicken thighs, skinless and boneless
- 2 cloves of garlic, minced
- 1 onion, chopped
- 1 teaspoon onion powder
- 1 teaspoon garlic powder

- 2 teaspoons white sugar
- ¼ cup Dijon mustard
- 1 teaspoon rosemary
- 1 teaspoon thyme
- ½ pound baby potatoes, scrubbed and halved
- Pepper to taste
- 1 cup chicken stock, low sodium
- 2 tablespoons flour + 2 tablespoons skim milk

Directions:

1. Place a heavy bottomed pot on medium high fire and heat pot for 3 minutes.
2. Once hot, add oil and stir around to coat pot with oil.
3. Brown chicken for 5 minutes per side. Transfer to a chopping board and cut into 1-inch cubes.
4. Sauté the onion and garlic for 3 minutes.
5. Add onion powder, chicken, garlic powder, white sugar, rosemary, thyme, and pepper.
6. After 30 seconds, add the chicken broth and Dijon mustard.
7. Cover, bring to a boil, lower fire to a simmer, and simmer for 5 minutes.
8. Stir in the milk mixture and continue stirring until thickened, around 5 minutes.
9. Serve and enjoy.

Nutrition Values:

Calories: 285; Carbs: 9.6g; Protein: 18.4g; Fats: 19.0g; Saturated Fat: 5.0g; Sodium: 214mg

MEAT

245. Grilled Flank Steak with Lime Vinaigrette

Servings: 6
Cooking Time: 10 minutes
Ingredients:
- 2 tablespoons lime juice, freshly squeezed
- 2 tablespoons extra virgin olive oil
- ½ teaspoon ground black pepper
- ¼ cup chopped fresh cilantro
- 1 tablespoon ground cumin
- ¼ teaspoon red pepper flakes
- ¾ pound flank steak

Directions:
1. Heat the grill to low medium heat.
2. In a food processor, place all ingredients except for the cumin, red pepper flakes, andflank steak. Pulse until smooth. This will be the vinaigrette sauce. Set aside.
3. Season the flank steak with ground cumin and red pepper flakes and allow to marinate for at least 10 minutes.
4. Place the steak on the grill rack and cook for 5 minutes on each side. Cut into the center to check the doneness of the meat. You can also insert a meat thermometer to check the internal temperature.
5. Remove from the grill and allow to stand for 5 minutes.
6. Slice the steak to 2 inches long and toss the vinaigrette to flavor the meat.
7. Serve with salad if desired.
Nutrition Values:
Calories per Serving:103 ; Protein: 13g; Carbs: 1g; Fat: 5g; Saturated Fat: 1g; Sodium: 73mg

246. Asian Pork Tenderloin

Servings: 4
Cooking Time: 15 minutes
Ingredients:
- 2 tablespoons sesame seeds
- 1 teaspoon ground coriander
- 1/8 teaspoon cayenne pepper
- 1/8 teaspoon celery seed
- ½ teaspoon minced onion
- ¼ teaspoon ground cumin
- 1/8 teaspoon ground cinnamon
- 1 tablespoon sesame oil
- 1-pound pork tenderloin sliced into 4 equal portions

Directions:
1. Preheat the oven to 4000F.
2. In a skillet, toast the sesame seeds over low heat and set aside. Allow the sesame seeds to cool.
3. In a bowl, combine the rest of the ingredients expect for the pork tenderloin. Stir in the toasted sesame seeds.
4. Place the pork tenderloin in a baking dish and rub the spices on both sides.

5. Place the baking dish with the pork in the oven and bake for 15 minutes or until the internal temperature of the meat reaches to 1700F.
6. Serve warm.
Nutrition Values:
Calories: 248; Protein: 26g; Carbs: 0g; Fat: 16g; Saturated Fat: 5g; Sodium: 57mg

247. Simple Beef Brisket and Tomato Soup

Servings: 8
Cooking Time: 3 hours
Ingredients:
- 1 tablespoon olive oil
- 2 ½ pounds beef brisket, trimmed of fat and cut into 8 equal parts
- A dash of ground black pepper
- 1 ½ cups chopped onions
- 4 clovs of garlic, smashed
- 1 teaspoon dried thyme
- 1 cup ripe roma tomatoes, chopped
- ¼ cup red wine vinegar
- 1 cup beef stock, low sodium or home made

Directions:
1. In a heavy pot, heat the oil over medium-high heat.
2. Season the brisket with ground black pepper and place in the pot.
3. Cook while stirring constantly until the beef turns brown on all sides.
4. Stir in the onions and cook until fragrant. Add in the garlic and thyme and cook for another minute until fragrant.
5. Pour in the rest of the ingredients and bring to a boil.
6. Cook until the beef is tender. This may take about 3 hours or more.
Nutrition Values:
Calories: 229; Protein: 31g; Carbs: 6g; Fat: 9g; Saturated Fat: 3g; Sodium: 184mg

248. Beef Stew with Fennel And Shallots

Servings: 6
Cooking Time: 40 minutes
Ingredients:
- 1 tablespoon olive oil
- 1-pound boneless lean beef stew meat, trimmed from fat and cut into cubes
- ½ fennel bulb, trimmed and sliced thinly
- 3 large shallots, chopped
- ¾ teaspoons ground black pepper
- 2 fresh thyme sprigs
- 1 bay leaf
- 3 cups low sodium beef broth
- ½ cup red wine
- 4 large carrots, peeled and cut into chunks
- 4 large white potatoes, peeled and cut into chunks

- 3 portobello mushrooms, cleaned and cut into chunks
- 1/3 cup Italian parsley, chopped

Directions:
1. Heat oil in a pot over medium heat and stir in the beef cubes for 5 minutes or until all sides turn brown.
2. Stir in the fennel, shallots, black pepper, and thyme for one minute or until the ingredients become fragrant.
3. Stir in the bay leaf, broth, red wine, carrots, white potatoes and mushrooms.
4. Bring to a boil and cook for 30 minutes or until everything is tender.
5. Stir in the parsley last.

Nutrition Values:
Calories: 244; Protein: 21g; Carbs: 22g; Fat: 8g; Saturated Fat: 2g; Sodium: 184mg

249. Rustic Beef and Barley Soup

Servings: 6
Cooking Time: 40 minutes
Ingredients:
- 1 teaspoon olive oil
- 1-pound beef round steak, sliced into strips
- 2 cups yellow onion, chopped
- 1 cup diced celery
- 4 cloves of garlic, chopped
- 1 cup diced roma tomatoes
- ½ cup diced sweet potato
- ½ cup diced mushrooms
- 1 cup diced carrots
- ¼ cup uncooked barley
- 3 cups low sodium vegetable stock
- 1 teaspoon dried sage
- 1 tpaprika
- A dash of black pepper to taste
- 1 cup chopped kale

Directions:
1. In a large pot, heat the oil over medium flame and stir in the beef. Cook for 5 minutes while stirring constantly until all sides turn brown.
2. Stir in the onion, celery, and garlic until fragrant.
3. Add in the rest of the ingredients except for the kale.
4. Bring to a boil and cook for 30 minutes until everything is tender.
5. Stir in the kale last and cook for another 5 minutes.

Nutrition Values:
Calories per Serving:246 ; Protein: 21g; Carbs: 24g; Fat: 4g; Saturated Fat: 1g; Sodium: 13mg

250. Beef Stroganoff

Servings: 4
Cooking Time: 25 minutes
Ingredients:
- ½ cup chopped onion

- ½ pound boneless beef round steak, cut into ¾ inch thick
- 4 cups pasta noodles
- ½ cup fat-free cream of mushroom soup
- ½ cup water
- ½ teaspoon paprika
- ½ cup fat-free sour cream

Directions:
1. In a non-stick frying pan, saute the onions over low to medium heat without oil while stirring constantly for about 5 minutes.
2. Stir in the beef and cook for another 5 minutes until the beef is tender and turn brown on all sides. Set aside.
3. In a large pot, fill it with water until ¾ full and bring to a boil. Cook the noodles until done accoring to package instructions. Drain the noodles and set aside.
4. In a saucepan, whisk the mushroom soup and water. Bring to a boil over medium heat and stir constantly until the sauce has reduced. Add in paprika and sour cream.
5. Assemble the stroganoff by placing the pasta in a bowl and pouring over the sauce. Top with the meat.
6. Serve warm.

Nutrition Values:
Calories: 273; Protein: 20g; Carbs: 37g; Fat: 5g; Saturated Fat: 2g; Sodium: 193mg

251. Curried Pork Tenderloin in Apple Cider

Servings: 6
Cooking Time: 26 minutes
Ingredients:
- 16 ounces pork tenderloin, cut into 6 pieces
- 1 ½ tablespoons curry powder
- 1 tablespoon extra virgin olive oil
- 2 medium onions, chopped
- 2 cups apple cider, organic and unsweetened
- 1 tart apple, peeled and chopped into chunks

Directions:
1. In a bowl, season the pork with the curry powder and set aside.
2. Heat oil in a pot over medium flame.
3. Saute the onions for one minute until fragrant.
4. Stir in the seasoned pork tenderloin and cook for 5 minutes or until lightly golden.
5. Add in the apple cider and apple chunks.
6. Close the lid and bring to a boil.
7. Allow to simmer for 20 minutes.

Nutrition Values:
Calories: 244; Protein: 24g; Carbs: 18g; Fat: 8g; Saturated Fat: 2g; Sodium: 70mg

252. Pork Medallions with Five Spice Powder

Servings: 4
Cooking Time: 25 minutes
Ingredients:
- 1 tablespoon olive oil
- 3 cloves of garlic, minded
- 1-pound pork tenderloin, fat trimmed
- 2 tablespoon low-sodium soy sauce
- 1 tablespoon green onion, minced
- ¾ teaspoon five spice powder
- ½ cup water
- ¼ cup dry white wine
- 1/3 cup chopped onion
- ½ head green cabbage, thinly sliced and wilted
- 1 tablespoon chopped fresh parsley

Directions:
1. In a bowl, combine the olive oil, garlic, pork tenderloin, soy sauce, green onion, and five spice powder. Mix until well combined and allow to marinate in the fridge for at least two hours.
2. Heat the oven to 4000F.
3. Remove the pork from the marinade and pat dry.
4. On a skillet, sear the meat on all sides until slightly brown before transferring into a heat-proof baking dish.
5. Place inside the oven and roast the pork for 20 minutes.
6. Meanwhile, pour the water, dry white wine, and onions in the skillet where you seared the pork and deglaze. Allow to simmer until the sauce has reduced.
7. Serve the pork medallions with wilted cabbages and drizzle the sauce on top.

Nutrition Values:
Calories: 219; Protein: 25g; Carbs: 5g; Fat: 11g; Saturated Fat: 2g; Sodium: 296mg

253. Grilled Pork Fajitas

Servings: 8
Cooking Time: 15 minutes
Ingredients:
- ½ teaspoon paprika
- ½ teaspoon oregano
- ¼ teaspoon ground coriander
- ¼ teaspoon garlic powder
- 1 tablespoon chili powder
- 1-pound pork tenderloin, fat trimmed and cut into large strips
- 1 onion, sliced
- 8 whole wheat flour tortillas, warmed
- 4 medium tomatoes, chopped
- 4 cups shredded lettuce

Directions:
1. In a bowl, mix the paprika, oregano, coriander, garlic powder, and chili powder.
2. Sprinkle the spice mixture on the pork tenderloin strips and toss to coat the meat with the spices.
3. Prepare the grill and heat to 4000F.
4. Place the meat and onion in a grill basket and broil for 20 minutes or until all sides have browned.
5. Assemble the fajitas by placing in the center of the tortillas the grilled pork and onions. Add in the tomatoes and lettuce before rolling the fajitas.

Nutrition Values:
Calories: 250; Protein: 20g; Carbs: 29g; Fat: 6g; Saturated Fat: 2g; Sodium: 234mg

254. New York Strip Steak with Mushroom Sauce

Servings: 2
Cooking Time: 20 minutes
Ingredients:
- 2 New York Strip steaks -4 ounces each, trimmed from fat
- 3 cloves of garlic, minced
- 2 ounces shiitake mushrooms, sliced
- 2 ounces button mushrooms, sliced
- ¼ teaspoon thyme
- ¼ teaspoon rosemary
- ¼ cup low sodium beef broth

Directions:
1. Heat the grill to 3500F.
2. Position the grill rack 6 inches from the heat source.
3. Grill the steaks for 10 minutes on each side or until slightly pink on the inside.
4. Meanwhile, prepare the sauce. In a small nonstick pan, water saute the garlic, mushrooms, thyme and rosemary for a minute. Pour in the broth and bring to a boil. Allow the sauce to simmer until the liquid is reduced.
5. Top the steaks with the mushroom sauce.
6. Serve warm.

Nutrition Values:
Calories: 270; Protein: 23g; Carbs: 4g; Fat: 6g; Saturated Fat: 2g; Sodium: 96 mg

255. Pork Chops with Black Currant Jam

Servings: 6
Cooking Time: 20 minutes
Ingredients:
- ¼ cup black currant jam
- 2 tablespoons Dijon mustard
- 1 teaspoon olive oil
- 6 center cut pork loin chops, trimmed from fat
- 1/3 cup wine vinegar
- 1/8 teaspoon ground black pepper
- 6 orange slices

Directions:
1. In a small bowl, mix together the jam and mustard. Set aside.

2. In a nonstick pan, heat the oil over medium flames and sear the pork chops for 5 minutes on each side or until all sides turn brown.

3. Brush the pork chops with the mustard mixture and turn the flame to low. Cook for two more minutes on each side. Set aside.

4. Using the same frying pan, pour in the wine vinegar to deglaze the pan. Season with ground black pepper and allow to simmer for at least 5 minutes or until the vinegar has reduced.

5. Pour over the pork chops and garnish with orange slices on top.

Nutrition Values:
Calories: 198; Protein: 25g; Carbs: 11g; Fat: 6g; Saturated Fat: 2g; Sodium: 188mg

256. Pork Medallion with Herbes de Provence

Servings: 2
Cooking Time: 15 minutes
Ingredients:
- 8 ounces of pork medallion, trimmed from fat
- Freshly ground black pepper to taste
- ½ teaspoon Herbes de Provence
- ¼ cup dry white wine

Directions:
1. Season the meat with black pepper.

2. Place the meat in between sheets of wax paper and pound on a mallet until about ¼ inch thick.

3. In a nonstick skillet, sear the pork over medium heat for 5 minutes on each side or until the meat is slightly brown.

4. Remove meat from the skillet and sprinkle with herbes de Provence.

5. Using the same skillet, pour the wine and scrape the sides to deglaze. Allow to simmer until the wine is reduced.

6. Pour the wine sauce over the pork.

7. Serve immediately.

Nutrition Values:
Calories: 120; Protein: 24g; Carbs: 1g; Fat: 2g; Saturated Fat: 0.5g; Sodium: 62mg

257. Pork Tenderloin with Apples And Balsamic Vinegar

Servings: 4
Cooking Time: 25 minutes
Ingredients:
- 1 tablespoon olive oil
- 1-pound pork tenderloin, trimmed from fat
- Freshly ground black pepper
- 2 cups chopped onion
- 2 cups chopped apple
- 1 ½ tablespoons fresh rosemary, chopped
- 1 cup low sodium chicken broth
- 1 ½ tablespoons balsamic vinegar

Directions:
1. Heat the oven to 4500F.

2. Heat the oil in a large skillet over medium flame.

3. Sear the pork and season with black pepper. Cook the pork for 3 minutes until all sides turn light brown. Remove from the heat and place in a baking pan.

4. Roast the pork for 15 minutes.

5. Meanwhile, place the onion, apples, and rosemary on the skillet where the pork is seared.Continue stirring for 5 minutes. Pour in broth and balsamic vinegar and allow to simmer until the sauce thickens.

6. Serve the roasted pork with the onion and apple sauce.

Nutrition Values:
Calories: 240; Protein: 26g; Carbs: 17g; Fat: 6g; Saturated Fat: 1g; Sodium: 83mg

258. Pork Tenderloin with Apples And Blue Cheese

Servings: 4
Cooking Time: 25 minutes
Ingredients:
- 1-pound pork tenderloin, trimmed from fat
- ½ teaspoon white pepper
- 2 teaspoons black pepper
- ¼ teaspoon cayenne pepper
- 1 teaspoon paprika
- 2 apples, sliced
- ½ cup unsweetened apple juice
- ¼ cup crumbled blue cheese

Directions:
1. Heat the oven to 3500F.

2. Season the tenderloin with white pepper, black pepper, cayenne pepper, and paprika.

3. Heat a non-stick pan over medium flame and sear the meat for 3 minutes on each side. Transfer to a bakind dish and roast in the oven for 20 minutes or until the internal temperature is at 1550F. Remove from the oven to cool.

4. While the pork is roasting, prepare the sauce. Using the same skillet used to sear the meat, saute the apples for 3 minutes. Add the apple juice and allow the sauce to thicken for at least 10 minutes.

5. Serve the pork with the apple sauce and sprinkle with blue cheese on top.

Nutrition Values:
Calories: 235; Protein: 26g; Carbs: 17; Fat: 3g; Saturated Fat: 1g; Sodium: 145mg

259. Pork Tenderloin with Fennel Sauce

Servings: 4
Cooking Time: 30 minutes
Ingredients:
- 4 pork tenderloin fillets, trimmed from fat and cut into 4 portions
- 1 tablespoon olive oil
- 1 teapsoon fennel seeds
- 1 fennel bulb, cored and sliced thinly
- 1 sweet onion, sliced thinly

- ½ cup dry white wine
- 12 ounces low sodium chicken broth
- 1 orange, sliced for ganish

Directions:
1. Place the pork slices in between wax paper and pound with a mallet to about ¼-inch thick.
2. Heat oil in a skillet and fry the fennel seeds for 3 minutes or until fragrant.
3. Stir in the pork and cook on all sides for 3 minutes or until golden brown. Remove the pork from the skillet and set aside.
4. Using the same skillet, add the fennel bulb slices and onion.Saute for 5 minutes then set aside.
5. Add the wine and chicken broth in the skillet and bring to a boil until the sauce reduces in half.
6. Return the pork to the skillet and cook for another 5 minutes.
7. Serve the pork with sauce and vegetables.

Nutrition Values:
Calories: 276; Protein: 29g; Carbs: 13g; Fat: 12g; Saturated Fat:3 g; Sodium: 122mg

260. Spicy Beef Kebabs

Servings: 8
Cooking Time: 10 minutes
Ingredients:
- 2 yellow onions, minced
- 2 tablespoons fresh lemon juice
- 1 ½ pounds lean ground beef, minced
- ¼ cup bulgur, soaked in water for 30 minutes then rinsed
- ¼ cup chopped pine nuts
- 2 cloves of garlic, minced
- 1 teaspoon ground cumin
- ½ teaspoon ground cinnamon
- ½ teaspoon ground cardamom
- ½ teaspoon freshly ground black pepper
- 16 wooden skewers, soaked in water for 30 minutes

Directions:
1. In a mixing bowl, combine all ingredients except for the skewers. Mix well unt
2. Form a sausage from the meat mixture and thread it into the skewers. If the sausage is crumbly, add a tablespoon of water at a time until it holds well together. Refrigerate the skewered meat sausages until ready to cook.
3. Heat the grill to 3500F and place the grill rack 6 inches from the heat source.
4. Place the skewerd kebabs on the grill and broil for 5 minutes on each side.
5. Serve with yogurt if desired.

Nutrition Values:
Calories: 219; Protein: 23g; Carbs: 3g; Fat: 12g; Saturated Fat: 3g; Sodium: 53mg

261. Spicy Beef Curry

Servings: 6
Cooking Time: 40 minutes

Ingredients:
- 1 medium serrano pepper, cut into thirds
- 4 cloves of garlic, minced
- 1 2-inch piece ginger, peeled and chopped
- 1 yellow onion, chopped
- 2 tablespoons ground coriander
- 2 teaspoons ground cumin
- ½ teaspoon ground turmeric
- 2 teaspoons garam masala
- 1 tablespoon olive oil
- pounds beef, cut into chunks
- 1 cup ripe tomatoes, diced
- 2 cups water
- 1 cup fresh cilantro for garnish

Directions:
1. In a food processor, pulse the serrano peppers, garlic, ginger, onion, coriander, cumin, turmeric, and garam masala until well-combined.
2. Heat oil over medium heat in a skillet and saute the spice mixture for 2 minutes or until fragrant.
3. Stir in the beef and allow to cook while stirring constantly for three minutes or until the beef turns brown.
4. Stir in the tomatoes and saute for another three minutes.
5. Add in the water and bring to a boil.
6. Once boiling, turn the heat to low and allow to simmer for thirty minutes or until the meat is tender.
7. Add cilantro last before serving.

Nutrition Values:
Calories: 181; Protein: 16g; Carbs: 5g; Fat: 8g; Saturated Fat: 2g; Sodium: 74mg

262. Pork Tenderloin with Apples And Sweet Potatoes

Servings: 4
Cooking Time: 30 minutes
Ingredients:
- ¾ cup apple cider
- ¼ cup apple cider vinegar
- 2 tablespoons maple syrup
- ¼ teaspoon smoked paprika powder
- 1 teaspoon grated ginger
- ¼ teaspoon groun black pepper
- 2 teaspoons olive oil
- 1 12-ounce pork tenderloin
- 1 large sweet potato, cut into cubes
- 1 large apple, cored and into cubes

Directions:
1. Preheat the oven to 3750F.
2. In a bowl, combine the apple cider, apple cider vinegar, maple syrup, smoked paprika, ginger, and black pepper. Set aside.
3. Heat the oil in a large skillet and sear the meat for 3 minutes on both sides.

4. Transfer the pork in a baking dish and place the sweet potatoes and apples around the pork. Pour in the apple cider sauce.
5. Place inside the oven and cook for 20 minutes.
Nutrition Values:
Calories: 267; Protein: 23.5g; Carbs:31 g; Fat: 5g; Saturated Fat: 0.5g; Sodium: 69mg

263. Mexican Beef and Veggie Skillet

Servings: 4
Cook Time:15 minutes
Ingredients:
- ½ pound lean ground beef
- ¾ cup chopped onion
- ½ cup bell pepper -any color, seeded and chopped
- ½ tablespoon chili powder
- 1 tablespoon oregano
- 1 cup tomatoes, chopped
- 1 cup frozen vegetable mix, chopped
- 2 cups water
- 1/2 cup shredded Mexican cheese blend

Directions:
1. Place the beef in a large skillet and add onions. Sauté for 3 minutes or until the beef has slightly rendered its fat.
2. Stir in the bell pepper, chili powder, and oregano and cook for another minute.
3. Add in the tomatoes, vegetable mix and water.
4. Close the lid and bring to a simmer for 10 minutes.
5. Before serving, stir in cheese last.
Nutrition Values:
Calories: 222; Protein: 20g; Carbs11 g; Fat: 10g; Saturated Fat: 5g; Sodium: 132mg

264. Garlic Lime Marinated Pork Chops

Servings: 4
Cooking Time: 10 minutes
Ingredients:
- 4 6-ounce lean boneless pork chops, trimmed from fat
- 4 cloves of garlic, crushed
- 1 teaspoon cumin
- 1 teaspoon chili powder
- 1 teaspoon paprika
- A dash of black pepper to taste
- Juice from ½ lime
- Zest from ½ lime

Directions:
1. In a bowl, season the pork with the rest of the ingredients.
2. Allow to marinate inside the fridge for at least 2 hours.
3. Place the pork chops in a baking dish or broiler pan and grill for 5 minutes on each side until golden brown.
4. Serve with salad if desired.

Nutrition Values:
Calories: 233; Protein: 38.5g; Carbs: 4g; Fat: 6g; Saturated Fat: 1g; Sodium: 105mg

265. Oriental Stir Fry

Servings: 4
Cooking Time: 20 minutes
Ingredients:
- 4 ounces pork loin, cut into thin strips
- 1 tablespoon ginger, minced
- 1 clove of garlic, chopped
- 1 ½ cups sliced onions
- 1 medium carrot, sliced thinly
- 2 medium green bell peppers, seeded and cut into thick strips
- 1 cup sliced celery
- 1 cup dried plums, pitted and halved
- 2 tablespoons low sodium soy sauce
- ¼ cup cold water + 2 tablespoons cornstarch

Directions:
1. In a skillet, sauté the pork on medium heat until it has slightly rendered fat.
2. Stir in the ginger, garlic, and onions until fragrant.
3. Stir in the carrots, green bell peppers, celery, and plums.
4. Season with soy sauce.
5. Close the lid and adjust the flame to low. Cook for 10 minutes while stirring every 3 minutes.
6. Open the lid and adjust the flame to medium. Stir in the cornstarch slurry and cook for another 5 minutes until the sauce thickens.
Nutrition Values:
Calories: 145; Protein: 9g; Carbs: 21g; Fat: 3g; Saturated Fat: 0.4g; Sodium: 106mg

266. Cocoa-Crusted Pork Tenderloin

Servings: 2
Cooking Time: 25 minutes
Ingredients:
- 1-pound pork tenderloin, trimmed from fat
- 1 tablespoon cocoa powder
- 1 teaspoon instant coffee powder
- ½ teaspoon ground cinnamon
- ½ teaspoon chili powder
- 1 tablespoon olive oil

Directions:
1. In a bowl, dust the pork tenderloin with cocoa powder, coffee, cinnamon, and chili powder.
2. In a skillet, heat the oil and sear the meat for 5 minutes on both sides over low to medium flame.
3. Transfer the pork in a bakind dish and cook in the oven for 15 minutes in a 3500F-preheated oven.
Nutrition Values:
Calories: 395; Protein: 60g; Carbs: 2g; Fat: 15g; Saturated Fat: 4g; Sodium: 150mg

267. Beef Kabobs with Pineapples

Servings: 6
Cooking Time: 10 minutes
Ingredients:
- 1 ½ pounds beef shoulder steaks, cut into thick chunks
- A dash of ground black pepper
- 2 tablespoons olive oil
- 2 tablespoons lime juice
- 2 cloves of garlic, minced
- ½ teaspoon ground cumin
- 1 cup pineapple chunks
- 12 wooden skewers, soaked in water for 30 minutes

Directions:
1. In a bowl, combine the beef, black pepper, olive oil, lime juice, garlic, and cumin until well-incorporated.
2. Place inside the fridge and allow to marinate for at least 3 hours.
3. Thread one chunk of beef and a chunk of pineapple alternately through the wooden skewer. Do two or three alternating layers.
4. Heat the grill to 3500F and place the grill rack 6 inches away from the charcoal.
5. Grill the kabobs for 5 minutes on each side.

Nutrition Values:
Calories: 243; Protein: 24g; Carbs:11 g; Fat: 11g; Saturated Fat: 1g; Sodium: 71mg

268. Asian Beef and Zucchini Noodles

Servings: 4
Cooking Time: 15 minutes
Ingredients:
- ½ pound lean ground beef
- 1 tablespoon minced ginger
- 2 cloves of garlic, minced
- 16 ounces Asian-style vegetable package, frozen
- 2 cups low sodium beef broth
- 1 large zucchini, spiralized or thinly sliced
- 2 green onions, sliced thinly

Directions:
1. In a large skillet, saute the beef with minced ginger and garlic for three minutes while constantly stirring.
2. Stir in the vegetable package and the beef broth.
3. Bring to a boil for 10 minutes.
4. Assemble the dish by putting the zucchini in a bowl.
5. Pour in the soup and garnish with green onions.

Nutrition Values:
Calories: 271; Protein: 23g; Carbs:21 g; Fat: 5g; Saturated Fat: 3g; Sodium: 138mg

269. Exotic Thai Steak

Servings: 4

Cooking Time: 20 minutes
Ingredients:
- 1-pound London broil, trimmed from fat
- 2 tablespoons light fish sauce
- 1 tablespoon olive oil
- 2 cloves of garlic, minced
- ½ teaspoon grated ginger
- ½ cup chopped coriander
- ¼ cup white vinegar
- 2 tablespoons honey

Directions:
1. Place in a Ziploc bag all ingredients and allow to marinate in the fridge for at least 3 hours.
2. Heat the grill to low heat.
3. Place the meat on the grill rack and allow to cook for 10 minutes on each side or until the internal temperature reaches 1750F.
4. Slice the London broil and serve with vegetables.

Nutrition Values:
Calories: 219; Protein: 23g; Carbs: 9g; Fat: 5g; Saturated Fat: 1g; Sodium: 100mg

270. Sweet and Spicy Edamame Beef Stew

Servings: 6
Cooking Time: 20 minutes
Ingredients:
- 1 tablespoon olive oil
- 8 ounces sirloin steak, trimmed from fat
- 2 teaspoon ginger, finely chopped
- 3 cloves of garlic, minced
- 3 cups packaged vegetable of your choice
- 1 cup shelled sweet soybeans or edamame
- 3 tablespoons hoisin sauce
- 2 tablespoons rice vinegar
- 1 teaspoon red chili paste

Directions:
1. In a non-stick pan, heat the oil over medium flame.
2. Saute the sirloin steak for 3 minutes while stirring constantly.
3. Stir in the ginger and garlic and saute for 1 minute.
4. Add in the rest of the ingredients.
5. Close the lid and allow to simmer for 10 minutes until the vegetables are cooked.

Nutrition Values:
Calories: 205; Protein: 14g; Carbs: 17g; Fat: 4g; Saturated Fat: 1g; Sodium: 146mg

271. Filling Sirloin Soup

Servings: 4
Cooking Time: 15 minutes
Ingredients:
- 1 tablespoon oil
- 1 small onion, diced
- 3 cloves of garlic, minced
- 1-pound lean ground sirloin
- 3 cups low sodium beef broth

- 1 bag frozen vegetables of your choce
- Black pepper to taste

Directions:
1. In a large saucepan, heat the oil over medium heat and saute the onion and garlic until fragrant.
2. Stir in the lean ground sirloin and cook for 3 minutes until lightly golden.
3. Add in the rest of the ingredients and bring the broth to a boil for 10 minutes.
4. Serve warm.

Nutrition Values:
Calories: 245; Protein: 29g; Carbs: 22g; Fat: 4g; Saturated Fat: 1g; Sodium: 152mg

272. Roast Rack of Lamb

Servings: 8
Cooking Time: 30 minutes
Ingredients:
- 2 1-poundFrench-style lamb rib roast, trimmed from fat
- 1 cup dry red wine
- 2 cloves of garlic, minced
- 1 teaspoon freshly grated nutmeg
- 1 tablespoon olive oil
- 1 tablespoon chopped rosemary
- 3 tablespoons dried cranberries, chopped

Directions:
1. In a reseable plastic, place the lamb and add in red wine, garlic, nutmeg, olive oil, and rosemary. Seal the bag and turn it to coat the lamb with the spices. Marinate inside the fridge for at least 4 hours while turning the bag occasionally.
2. Preheat the oven to 4500F and remove the lamb from the marinade. Reserve the juices.
3. Place the lamb bone side down on a roasting pan lined with foil.
4. Pour the reserved marinade over the roasting pan.
5. Roast for 30 minutes until the lamb turns slightly golden. Turn the lamb every 10 minutes and baste with the sauce.
6. Once cooked, take out the lamb from the oven and slice.
7. Serve with chopped cranberries on top.

Nutrition Values:
Calories: 241; Protein: 25; Carbs: 1g; Fat: 12g; Saturated Fat: 3g; Sodium: 46mg

273. Garlic Pork Mix

Preparation time: 10 minutes
Cooking time: 45 minutes
Servings: 8
Ingredients:
- 2 pounds pork meat, boneless and cubed
- 1 red onion, chopped
- 1 tablespoon olive oil
- 3 garlic cloves, minced
- 1 cup low-sodium beef stock
- 2 tablespoons sweet paprika

- Black pepper to the taste
- 1 tablespoon chives, chopped

Directions:
1. Heat up a pan with the oil over medium heat, add the onion and the meat, toss and brown for 5 minutes.
2. Add the rest of the ingredients, toss, reduce heat to medium, cover and cook for 40 minutes.
3. Divide the mix between plates and serve.

Nutrition Values: calories 407, fat 35.4, fiber 1, carbs 5, protein 14.9

274. Paprika Pork with Carrots

Preparation time: 10 minutes
Cooking time: 30 minutes
Servings: 4
Ingredients:
- 1 pound pork stew meat, cubed
- ¼ cup low-sodium veggie stock
- 2 carrots, peeled and sliced
- 2 tablespoons olive oil
- 1 red onion, sliced
- 2 teaspoons sweet paprika
- Black pepper to the taste

Directions:
1. Heat up a pan with the oil over medium heat, add the onion, stir and sauté for 5 minutes.
2. Add the meat, toss and brown for 5 minutes more.
3. Add the rest of the ingredients, bring to a simmer and cook over medium heat for 20 minutes.
4. Divide the mix between plates and serve.

Nutrition Values: calories 328, fat 18.1, fiber 1.8, carbs 6.4, protein 34

275. Ginger Pork and Onions

Preparation time: 10 minutes
Cooking time: 35 minutes
Servings: 4
Ingredients:
- 2 red onions, sliced
- 2 green onions, chopped
- 1 tablespoon olive oil
- 2 teaspoons ginger, grated
- 4 pork chops
- 3 garlic cloves, chopped
- Black pepper to the taste
- 1 carrot, chopped
- 1 cup low sodium beef stock
- 2 tablespoons tomato paste
- 1 tablespoon cilantro, chopped

Directions:
1. Heat up a pan with the oil over medium heat, add the green and red onions, toss and sauté them for 3 minutes.
2. Add the garlic and the ginger, toss and cook for 2 minutes more.
3. Add the pork chops and cook them for 2 minutes on each side.

4.	Add the rest of the ingredients, bring to a simmer and cook over medium heat for 25 minutes more.
5.	Divide the mix between plates and serve.
Nutrition Values: calories 332, fat 23.6, fiber 2.3, carbs 10.1, protein 19.9

276. Cumin Pork

Preparation time: 10 minutes
Cooking time: 45 minutes
Servings: 4
Ingredients:
- ½ cup low-sodium beef stock
- 2 tablespoons olive oil
- 2 pounds pork stew meat, cubed
- 1 teaspoon coriander, ground
- 2 teaspoons cumin, ground
- Black pepper to the taste
- 1 cup cherry tomatoes, halved
- 4 garlic cloves, minced
- 1 tablespoon cilantro, chopped

Directions:
1.	Heat up a pan with the oil over medium heat, add the garlic and the meat, toss and brown for 5 minutes.
2.	Add the stock and the other ingredients, bring to a simmer and cook over medium heat for 40 minutes.
3.	Divide everything between plates and serve.
Nutrition Values: calories 559, fat 29.3, fiber 0.7, carbs 3.2, protein 67.4

277. Pork and Greens Mix

Preparation time: 10 minutes
Cooking time: 20 minutes
Servings: 4
Ingredients:
- 2 tablespoons balsamic vinegar
- 1/3 cup coconut aminos
- 1 tablespoon olive oil
- 4 ounces mixed salad greens
- 1 cup cherry tomatoes, halved
- 4 ounces pork stew meat, cut into strips
- 1 tablespoon chives, chopped

Directions:
1.	Heat up a pan with the oil over medium heat, add the pork, aminos and the vinegar, toss and cook for 15 minutes.
2.	Add the salad greens and the other ingredients, toss, cook for 5 minutes more, divide between plates and serve.
Nutrition Values: calories 125, fat 6.4, fiber 0.6, carbs 6.8, protein 9.1

278. Thyme Pork Pan

Preparation time: 10 minutes
Cooking time: 25 minutes
Servings: 4
Ingredients:
- 1 pound pork butt, trimmed and cubed

- 1 tablespoon olive oil
- 1 yellow onion, chopped
- 3 garlic cloves, minced
- 1 tablespoon thyme, dried
- 1 cup low-sodium chicken stock
- 2 tablespoons low-sodium tomato paste
- 1 tablespoon cilantro, chopped

Directions:
1.	Heat up a pan with the oil over medium-high heat, add the onion and the garlic, toss and cook for 5 minutes.
2.	Add the meat, toss and cook for 5 more minutes.
3.	Add the rest of the ingredients, toss, bring to a simmer, reduce heat to medium and cook the mix for 15 minutes more.
4.	Divide the mix between plates and serve right away.
Nutrition Values: calories 281, fat 11.2, fiber 1.4, carbs 6.8, protein 37.1

279. Marjoram Pork and Zucchinis

Preparation time: 10 minutes
Cooking time: 30 minutes
Servings: 4
Ingredients:
- 2 pounds pork loin boneless, trimmed and cubed
- 2 tablespoons avocado oil
- ¾ cup low-sodium veggie stock
- ½ tablespoon garlic powder
- 1 tablespoon marjoram, chopped
- 2 zucchinis, roughly cubed
- 1 teaspoon sweet paprika
- Black pepper to the taste

Directions:
1.	Heat up a pan with the oil over medium-high heat, add the meat, garlic powder and the marjoram, toss and cook for 10 minutes.
2.	Add the zucchinis and the other ingredients, toss, bring to a simmer, reduce heat to medium and cook the mix for 20 minutes more.
3.	Divide everything between plates and serve.
Nutrition Values: calories 359, fat 9.1, fiber 2.1, carbs 5.7, protein 61.4

280. Spiced Pork

Preparation time: 10 minutes
Cooking time: 8 hours
Servings: 4
Ingredients:
- 3 tablespoons olive oil
- 2 pounds pork shoulder roast
- 2 teaspoons sweet paprika
- 1 teaspoon garlic powder
- 1 teaspoon onion powder
- 1 teaspoon nutmeg, ground
- 1 teaspoon allspice, ground
- Black pepper to the taste

- 1 cup low-sodium veggie stock

Directions:

1. In your slow cooker, combine the roast with the oil and the other ingredients, toss, put the lid on and cook on Low for 8 hours.
2. Slice the roast, divide it between plates and serve with the cooking juices drizzled on top.

Nutrition Values: calories 689, fat 57.1, fiber 1, carbs 3.2, protein 38.8

281. Coconut Pork and Celery

Preparation time: 10 minutes
Cooking time: 35 minutes
Servings: 4

Ingredients:

- 2 pounds pork stew meat, cubed
- 2 tablespoons olive oil
- 1 cup low-sodium veggie stock
- 1 celery stalk, chopped
- 1 teaspoon black peppercorns
- 2 shallots, chopped
- 1 tablespoon chives, chopped
- 1 cup coconut cream
- Black pepper to the taste

Directions:

1. Heat up a pan with the oil over medium heat, add the shallots and the meat, toss and brown for 5 minutes.
2. Add the celery and the other ingredients, toss, bring to a simmer and cook over medium heat for 30 minutes more.
3. Divide everything between plates and serve right away.

Nutrition Values: calories 690, fat 43.3, fiber 1.8, carbs 5.7, protein 6.2

282. Pork and Tomatoes Mix

Preparation time: 10 minutes
Cooking time: 30 minutes
Servings: 4

Ingredients:

- 2 garlic cloves, minced
- 2 pounds pork stew meat, ground
- 2 cups cherry tomatoes, halved
- 1 tablespoon olive oil
- Black pepper to the taste
- 1 red onion, chopped
- ½ cup low-sodium veggie stock
- 2 tablespoons low-sodium tomato paste
- 1 tablespoon parsley, chopped

Directions:

1. Heat up a pan with the oil over medium heat, add the onion and the garlic, toss and sauté for 5 minutes.
2. Add the meat and brown it for 5 minutes more.
3. Add the rest of the ingredients, toss, bring to a simmer, cook over medium heat for 20 minutes more, divide into bowls and serve.

Nutrition Values: calories 558, fat 25.6, fiber 2.4, carbs 10.1, protein 68.7

283. Sage Pork Chops

Preparation time: 10 minutes
Cooking time: 35 minutes
Servings: 4

Ingredients:

- 4 pork chops
- 2 tablespoons olive oil
- 1 teaspoon smoked paprika
- 1 tablespoon sage, chopped
- 2 garlic cloves, minced
- 1 tablespoon lemon juice
- Black pepper to the taste

Directions:

1. In a baking dish, combine the pork chops with the oil and the other ingredients, toss, introduce in the oven and bake at 400 degrees F for 35 minutes.
2. Divide the pork chops between plates and serve with a side salad.

Nutrition Values: calories 263, fat 12.4, fiber 6, carbs 22.2, protein 16

284. Thai Pork and Eggplant

Preparation time: 10 minutes
Cooking time: 30 minutes
Servings: 4

Ingredients:

- 1 pound pork stew meat, cubed
- 1 eggplant, cubed
- 1 tablespoon coconut aminos
- 1 teaspoon five spice
- 2 garlic cloves, minced
- 2 Thai chilies, chopped
- 2 tablespoons olive oil
- 2 tablespoons low-sodium tomato paste
- 1 tablespoon cilantro, chopped
- ½ cup low-sodium veggie stock

Directions:

1. Heat up a pan with the oil over medium-high heat, add the garlic, chilies and the meat and brown for 6 minutes.
2. Add the eggplant and the other ingredients, bring to a simmer and cook over medium heat for 24 minutes.
3. Divide the mix between plates and serve.

Nutrition Values: calories 320, fat 13.4, fiber 5.2, carbs 22.8, protein 14

285. Pork and Lime Scallions

Preparation time: 10 minutes
Cooking time: 30 minutes
Servings: 4

Ingredients:

- 2 tablespoons lime juice
- 4 scallions, chopped
- 1 pound pork stew meat, cubed
- 2 garlic cloves, minced

- 2 tablespoons olive oil
- Black pepper to the taste
- ½ cup low-sodium veggie stock
- 1 tablespoon cilantro, chopped

Directions:
1. Heat up a pan with the oil over medium heat, add the scallions and the garlic, toss and cook for 5 minutes.
2. Add the meat, toss and cook for 5 minutes more.
3. Add the rest of the ingredients, bring to a simmer and cook over medium heat for 20 minutes.
4. Divide the mix between plates and serve.

Nutrition Values: calories 273, fat 22.4, fiber 5, carbs 12.5, protein 18

286. Balsamic Pork

Preparation time: 10 minutes
Cooking time: 30 minutes
Servings: 4
Ingredients:
- 1 red onion, sliced
- 1 pound pork stew meat, cubed
- 2 red chilies, chopped
- 2 tablespoons balsamic vinegar
- ½ cup coriander leaves, chopped
- Black pepper to the taste
- 2 tablespoons olive oil
- 1 tablespoon low-sodium tomato sauce

Directions:
1. Heat up a pan with the oil over medium heat, add the onion and the chilies, toss and cook for 5 minutes.
2. Add the meat, toss and cook for 5 minutes more.
3. Add the rest of the ingredients, toss, bring to a simmer and cook over medium heat for 20 minutes more.
4. Divide everything between plates and serve right away.

Nutrition Values: calories 331, fat 13.3, fiber 5, carbs 22.7, protein 17

287. Pesto Pork

Preparation time: 10 minutes
Cooking time: 36 minutes
Servings: 4
Ingredients:
- 2 tablespoons olive oil
- 2 spring onions, chopped
- 1 pound pork chops
- 2 tablespoons basil pesto
- 1 cup cherry tomatoes, cubed
- 2 tablespoons low-sodium tomato paste
- ½ cup parsley, chopped
- ½ cup low-sodium veggie stock
- Black pepper to the taste

Directions:

1. Heat up a pan with the olive oil over medium-high heat, add the spring onions and the pork chops, and brown for 3 minutes on each side.
2. Add the pesto and the other ingredients, toss gently, bring to a simmer and cook over medium heat for 30 minutes more.
3. Divide everything between plates and serve.

Nutrition Values: calories 293, fat 11.3, fiber 4.2, carbs 22.2, protein 14

288. Pork and Parsley Peppers

Preparation time: 10 minutes
Cooking time: 1 hour
Servings: 4
Ingredients:
- 1 green bell pepper, chopped
- 1 red bell pepper, chopped
- 1 yellow bell pepper, chopped
- 1 red onion, chopped
- 1 pound pork chops
- 1 tablespoon olive oil
- Black pepper to the taste
- 26 ounces canned tomatoes, no-salt-added and chopped
- 2 tablespoons parsley, chopped

Directions:
1. Grease a roasting pan with the oil, arrange the pork chops inside and add the other ingredients on top.
2. Bake at 390 degrees F for 1 hour, divide everything between plates and serve.

Nutrition Values: calories 284, fat 11.6, fiber 2.6, carbs 22.2, protein 14

289. Cumin Lamb Mix

Preparation time: 10 minutes
Cooking time: 25 minutes
Servings: 4
Ingredients:
- 1 tablespoon olive oil
- 1 red onion, chopped
- 1 cup cherry tomatoes, halved
- 1 pound lamb stew meat, ground
- 1 tablespoon chili powder
- Black pepper to the taste
- 2 teaspoons cumin, ground
- 1 cup low-sodium veggie stock
- 2 tablespoons cilantro, chopped

Directions:
1. Heat up the a pan with the oil over medium-high heat, add the onion, lamb and chili powder, toss and cook for 10 minutes.
2. Add the rest of the ingredients, toss, cook over medium heat for 15 minutes more.
3. Divide into bowls and serve.

Nutrition Values: calories 320, fat 12,7, fiber 6, carbs 14.3, protein 22

290. Pork with Radishes and Green Beans

Preparation time: 10 minutes

Cooking time: 35 minutes
Servings: 4
Ingredients:
- 1 pound pork stew meat, cubed
- 1 cup radishes, cubed
- ½ pound green beans, trimmed and halved
- 1 yellow onion, chopped
- 1 tablespoon olive oil
- 2 garlic cloves, minced
- 1 cup canned tomatoes, no-salt-added and chopped
- 2 teaspoons oregano, dried
- Black pepper to the taste

Directions:
1. Heat up a pan with the oil over medium-high heat, add the onion and the garlic, toss and cook for 5 minutes.
2. Add the meat, toss and cook for 5 minutes more.
3. Add the rest of the ingredients, bring to a simmer and cook over medium heat for 25 minutes.
4. Divide everything into bowls and serve.

Nutrition Values: calories 289, fat 12, fiber 8, carbs 13.2, protein 20

291. Fennel Lamb and Mushrooms

Preparation time: 10 minutes
Cooking time: 40 minutes
Servings: 4
Ingredients:
- 1 pound lamb shoulder, boneless and cubed
- 8 white mushrooms, halved
- 2 tablespoons olive oil
- 1 yellow onion, chopped
- 2 garlic cloves, minced
- 1 an ½ tablespoons fennel powder
- Black pepper to the taste
- A bunch of scallions, chopped
- 1 cup low-sodium veggie stock

Directions:
1. Heat up a pan with the oil over medium heat, add the onion and the garlic, toss and cook for 5 minutes.
2. Add the meat and the mushrooms, toss and cook for 5 minutes more.
3. Add the other ingredients, toss, bring to a simmer and cook over medium heat for 30 minutes.
4. Divide the mix into bowls and serve.

Nutrition Values: calories 290, fat 15.3, fiber 7, carbs 14.9, protein 14

292. Pork and Spinach Pan

Preparation time: 10 minutes
Cooking time: 30 minutes
Servings: 4
Ingredients:
- 1 pound pork, ground
- 2 tablespoons olive oil
- 1 red onion, chopped

- ½ pound baby spinach
- 4 garlic cloves, minced
- ½ cup low-sodium veggie stock
- ½ cup canned tomatoes, no-salt-added, chopped
- Black pepper to the taste
- 1 tablespoon chives, chopped

Directions:
1. Heat up a pan with the oil over medium-high heat, add the onion and the garlic, toss and cook for 5 minutes.
2. Add the meat, toss and brown for 5 minutes more.
3. Add the rest of the ingredients except the spinach, toss, bring to a simmer, reduce heat to medium and cook for 15 minutes.
4. Add the spinach, toss, cook the mix for another 5 minutes, divide everything into bowls and serve.

Nutrition Values: calories 270, fat 12, fiber 6, carbs 22.2, protein 23

293. Pork with Avocados

Preparation time: 10 minutes
Cooking time: 15 minutes
Servings: 4
Ingredients:
- 2 cups baby spinach
- 1 pound pork steak, cut into strips
- 1 tablespoon olive oil
- 1 cup cherry tomatoes, halved
- 2 avocados, peeled, pitted and cut into wedges
- 1 tablespoon balsamic vinegar
- ½ cup low-sodium veggie stock

Directions:
1. Heat up a pan with the oil over medium-high heat, add the meat, toss and cook for 10 minutes.
2. Add the spinach and the other ingredients, toss, cook for 5 minutes more, divide into bowls and serve.

Nutrition Values: calories 390, fat 12.5, fiber 4, carbs 16.8, protein 13.5

294. Pork and Apples Mix

Preparation time: 10 minutes
Cooking time: 40 minutes
Servings: 4
Ingredients:
- 2 pounds pork stew meat, cut into strips
- 2 green apples, cored and cut into wedges
- 2 garlic cloves, minced
- 2 shallots, chopped
- 1 tablespoon sweet paprika
- ½ teaspoon chili powder
- 2 tablespoons avocado oil
- 1 cup low-sodium chicken stock
- Black pepper to the taste
- A pinch of red chili pepper flakes

Directions:
1. Heat up a pan with the oil over medium heat, add the shallots and the garlic, toss and sauté for 5 minutes.
2. Add the meat and brown for another 5 minutes.
3. Add the apples and the other ingredients, toss, bring to a simmer and cook over medium heat for 30 minutes more.
4. Divide everything between plates and serve.
Nutrition Values: calories 365, fat 7, fiber 6, carbs 15.6, protein 32.4

295. Cinnamon Pork Chops

Preparation time: 10 minutes
Cooking time: 1 hour and 10 minutes
Servings: 4
Ingredients:
- 4 pork chops
- 2 tablespoons olive oil
- 2 garlic cloves, minced
- ¼ cup low-sodium veggie stock
- 1 tablespoon cinnamon powder
- Black pepper to the taste
- 1 teaspoon chili powder
- ½ teaspoon onion powder

Directions:
1. In a roasting pan, combine the pork chops with the oil and the other ingredients, toss, introduce in the oven and bake at 390 degrees F for 1 hour and 10 minutes.
2. Divide the pork chops between plates and serve with a side salad.
Nutrition Values: calories 288, fat 5.5, fiber 6, carbs 12.7, protein 23

296. Coconut Pork Chops

Preparation time: 10 minutes
Cooking time: 20 minutes
Servings: 4
Ingredients:
- 2 tablespoons olive oil
- 4 pork chops
- 1 yellow onion, chopped
- 1 tablespoon chili powder
- 1 cup coconut milk
- ¼ cup cilantro, chopped

Directions:
1. Heat up a pan with the oil over medium-high heat, add the onion and the chili powder, toss and sauté for 5 minutes.
2. Add the pork chops and brown them for 2 minutes on each side.
3. Add the coconut milk, toss, bring to a simmer and cook over medium heat for 11 minutes more.
4. Add the cilantro, toss, divide everything into bowls and serve.
Nutrition Values: calories 310, fat 8, fiber 6, carbs 16.7, protein 22.1

297. Pork with Peaches Mix

Preparation time: 10 minutes
Cooking time: 25 minutes
Servings: 4
Ingredients:
- 2 pounds pork tenderloin, roughly cubed
- 2 peaches, stones removed and cut into quarters
- ¼ teaspoon onion powder
- 2 tablespoons olive oil
- ¼ teaspoon smoked paprika
- ¼ cup low-sodium veggie stock
- Black pepper to the taste

Directions:
1. Heat up a pan with the oil over medium heat, add the meat, toss and cook for 10 minutes.
2. Add the peaches and the other ingredients, toss, bring to a simmer and cook over medium heat for 15 minutes more.
3. Divide the whole mix between plates and serve.
Nutrition Values: calories 290, fat 11.8, fiber 5.4, carbs 13.7, protein 24

298. Cocoa Lamb and Radishes

Preparation time: 10 minutes
Cooking time: 35 minutes
Servings: 4
Ingredients:
- ½ cup low-sodium veggie stock
- 1 pound lamb stew meat, cubed
- 1 cup radishes, cubed
- 1 tablespoon cocoa powder
- Black pepper to the taste
- 1 yellow onion, chopped
- 1 tablespoon olive oil
- 2 garlic cloves, minced
- 1 tablespoon parsley, chopped

Directions:
1. Heat up a pan with the oil over medium-high heat, add the onion and the garlic, toss and sauté for 5 minutes.
2. Add the meat, toss and brown for 2 minutes on each side.
3. Add the stock and the other ingredients, toss, bring to a simmer and cook over medium heat for 25 minutes more.
4. Divide everything between plates and serve.
Nutrition Values: calories 340, fat 12.4, fiber 9.3, carbs 33.14, protein 20

299. Beef And Sauerkraut Soup Recipe

Preparation Time: 1hour 30 minutes
Servings: 8
Ingredients:
- 1 pound beef; ground
- 14 ounces beef stock
- 2 cups chicken stock
- 3 teaspoons olive oil

- 2 cups water
- 1 tablespoon gluten free Worcestershire sauce
- 4 bay leaves
- 1 onion; chopped.
- 1 tablespoon stevia
- 1 teaspoon sage; dried
- 1 tablespoon garlic; minced
- 14 ounces canned tomatoes and juice
- 14 ounces sauerkraut; chopped.
- 3 tablespoons parsley; chopped.
- Salt and black pepper to the taste.

Directions:

1. Heat up a pan with 1 teaspoon oil over medium heat; add beef; stir and brown for 10 minutes
2. Meanwhile; in a pot, mix chicken and beef stock with sauerkraut, stevia, canned tomatoes, Worcestershire sauce, parsley, sage and bay leaves; stir and bring to a simmer over medium heat.
3. Add beef to soup; stir and continue simmering.
4. Heat up the same pan with the rest of the oil over medium heat; add onions; stir and cook for 2 minutes.
5. Add garlic; stir, cook for 1 minute more and add this to the soup.
6. Reduce heat to soup and simmer it for 1 hour.
7. Add salt, pepper and water; stir and cook for 15 minutes more
8. Divide into bowls and serve

Nutrition Values: Calories: 250; Fat : 5; Fiber : 1; Carbs : 3; Protein : 12

300. Meatballs And Mushroom Sauce

Preparation Time: 35 minutes
Servings: 6
Ingredients:

- 2 pounds beef; ground
- 1 tablespoon coconut aminos
- 1/2 teaspoon garlic powder
- 1 tablespoon parsley; chopped.
- 1 tablespoon onion flakes
- 1/4 cup beef stock
- ¾ cup almond flour
- Salt and black pepper to the taste.
- For the sauce:
- 1 cup yellow onion; chopped.
- 2 cups mushrooms; sliced
- 1/2 teaspoon coconut aminos
- 1/4 cup sour cream
- 1/2 cup beef stock
- 2 tablespoons bacon fat
- 2 tablespoons ghee
- Salt and black pepper to the taste.

Directions:

1. In a bowl, mix beef with salt, pepper, garlic powder, 1 tablespoons coconut aminos, 1/4 cup beef stock, almond flour, parsley and onion flakes; stir well, shape 6 patties, place them on a baking sheet, introduce in the oven at 375 degrees F and bake for 18 minutes
2. Meanwhile; heat up a pan with the ghee and the bacon fat over medium heat; add mushrooms; stir and cook for 4 minutes
3. Add onions; stir and cook for 4 minutes more
4. Add 1/2 teaspoon coconut aminos, sour cream and 1/2 cup beef stock; stir well and bring to a simmer.
5. Take off heat; add salt and pepper and stir well.
6. Divide beef patties between plates and serve with mushroom sauce on top.

Nutrition Values: Calories: 435; Fat : 23; Fiber : 4; Carbs : 6; Protein : 32

301. Lamb Casserole

Preparation Time: 1 hour 50 minutes
Servings: 2
Ingredients:

- 2 carrots; chopped.
- 1/2 tablespoon rosemary; chopped.
- 1/2 cauliflower; florets separated
- 1/2 celeriac; chopped.
- 2 garlic cloves; minced
- 1¼ cups lamb stock
- 1 red onion; chopped.
- 1 leek; chopped.
- 1 tablespoon olive oil
- 1 celery stick; chopped.
- 1 tablespoon mint sauce
- 1 teaspoon stevia
- 1 tablespoon tomato puree
- 2 tablespoons ghee
- 10 ounces lamb fillet; cut into medium pieces
- Salt and black pepper to the taste.

Directions:

1. Heat up a pot with the oil over medium heat; add garlic, onion and celery; stir and cook for 5 minutes
2. Add lamb pieces; stir and cook for 3 minutes
3. Add carrot, leek, rosemary, stock, tomato puree, mint sauce and stevia; stir, bring to a boil, cover and cook for 1 hour and 30 minutes
4. Heat up a pot with water over medium heat; add celeriac, cover and simmer for 10 minutes
5. Add cauliflower florets, cook for 15 minutes, drain everything and mix with salt, pepper and ghee
6. Mash using a potato masher and divide mash between plates
7. Add lamb and veggies mix on top and serve

Nutrition Values: Calories: 324; Fat : 4; Fiber : 5; Carbs : 8; Protein : 20

302. Thai Beef Recipe

Preparation Time: 20 minutes
Servings: 6
Ingredients:
- 1 pound beef steak; cut into strips
- 1 cup beef stock
- 1½ teaspoons lemon pepper
- 4 tablespoons peanut butter
- 1/4 teaspoon garlic powder
- 1/4 teaspoon onion powder
- 1 tablespoon coconut aminos
- 1 green bell pepper; chopped.
- 3 green onions; chopped.
- Salt and black pepper to the taste.

Directions:
1. In a bowl, mix peanut butter with stock, aminos and lemon pepper; stir well and leave aside
2. Heat up a pan over medium high heat; add beef, season with salt, pepper, onion and garlic powder and cook for 7 minutes
3. Add green pepper; stir and cook for 3 minutes more
4. Add peanut sauce you've made at the beginning and green onions; stir, cook for 1 minute more, divide between plates and serve

Nutrition Values: Calories: 224; Fat : 15; Fiber : 1; Carbs : 3; Protein : 19

303. Goulash

Preparation Time: 30 minutes
Servings: 5
Ingredients:
- 2 ounces bell pepper; chopped.
- 2 cups cauliflower florets
- 1/4 teaspoon garlic powder
- 1½ pounds beef; ground
- 14 ounces canned tomatoes and their juice
- 1 tablespoon tomato paste
- 14 ounces water
- 1/4 cup onion; chopped.
- Salt and black pepper to the taste.

Directions:
1. Heat up a pan over medium heat; add beef; stir and brown for 5 minutes
2. Add onion and bell pepper; stir and cook for 4 minutes more
3. Add cauliflower, tomatoes and their juice and water; stir, bring to a simmer, cover pan and cook for 5 minutes
4. Add tomato paste, garlic powder, salt and pepper; stir, take off heat; divide into bowls and serve

Nutrition Values: Calories: 275; Fat : 7; Fiber : 2; Carbs : 4; Protein : 10

304. Lamb And Mustard Sauce

Preparation Time: 30 minutes
Servings: 4
Ingredients:
- 2/3 cup heavy cream
- 1/2 cup beef stock
- 1 tablespoon mustard
- 2 teaspoons gluten free Worcestershire sauce
- 1½ pounds lamb chops
- 2 tablespoons olive oil
- 1 tablespoon fresh rosemary; chopped.
- 2 garlic cloves; minced
- 1 teaspoon erythritol
- 2 tablespoons ghee
- A spring of rosemary
- A spring of thyme
- 1 tablespoon shallot; chopped.
- 2 teaspoons lemon juice
- Salt and black pepper to the taste.

Directions:
1. In a bowl, mix 1 tablespoon oil with garlic, salt, pepper and rosemary and whisk well.
2. Add lamb chops, toss to coat and leave aside for a few minutes
3. Heat up a pan with the rest of the oil over medium high heat; add lamb chops, reduce heat to medium, cook them for 7 minutes, flip, cook them for 7 minutes more, transfer to a plate and keep them warm.
4. Return pan to medium heat; add shallots; stir and cook for 3 minutes
5. Add stock; stir and cook for 1 minute
6. Add Worcestershire sauce, mustard, erythritol, cream, rosemary and thyme spring; stir and cook for 8 minutes
7. Add lemon juice, salt, pepper and the ghee, discard rosemary and thyme; stir well and take off heat.
8. Divide lamb chops on plates, drizzle the sauce over them and serve

Nutrition Values: Calories: 435; Fat : 30; Fiber : 4; Carbs : 5; Protein : 32

305. Beef Zucchini Cups

Preparation Time: 45 minutes
Servings: 4
Ingredients:
- 1 pound beef; ground
- 2 garlic cloves; minced
- 1 teaspoon cumin; ground
- 1 tablespoon coconut oil
- 1/2 cup red onion; chopped.
- 1/2 cup cheddar cheese; shredded
- 1½ cupsenchilada sauce
- 1 teaspoon smoked paprika
- 3 zucchinis; sliced in halves lengthwise and insides scooped out
- 1/4 cup cilantro; chopped.
- Some chopped avocado for serving
- Some green onions; chopped for serving
- Some tomatoes; chopped for serving
- Salt and black pepper to the taste.

Directions:

1. Heat up a pan with the oil over medium high heat; add red onions; stir and cook for 2 minutes
2. Add beef; stir and brown for a couple of minutes
3. Add paprika, salt, pepper, cumin and garlic; stir and cook for 2 minutes
4. Place zucchini halves in a baking pan, stuff each with beef, pour enchilada sauce on top and sprinkle cheddar cheese
5. Bake covered in the oven at 350 degrees F for 20 minutes
6. Uncover the pan, sprinkle cilantro and bake for 5 minutes more
7. Sprinkle avocado, green onions and tomatoes on top, divide between plates and serve
Nutrition Values: Calories: 222; Fat : 10; Fiber : 2; Carbs : 8; Protein : 21

306. Beef And Tzatziki

Preparation Time: 25 minutes
Servings: 6
Ingredients:
- 17 ounces beef; ground
- 7 ounces cherry tomatoes; cut in halves
- 1/4 cup almond milk
- 1 yellow onion; grated
- 5 bread slices; torn
- 1 egg; whisked
- 1/4 cup olive oil
- 1 cucumber; thinly sliced
- 1 cup baby spinach
- 1½ tablespoons lemon juice
- 1/4 cup parsley; chopped.
- 2 garlic cloves; minced
- 1/4 cup mint; chopped.
- 2½ teaspoons oregano; dried
- 7 ounces jarred tzatziki
- Salt and black pepper to the taste.

Directions:
1. Put torn bread in a bowl, add milk and leave aside for 3 minutes
2. Squeeze bread, chop and put into a bowl.
3. Add beef, egg, salt, pepper, oregano, mint, parsley, garlic and onion and stir well.
4. Shape balls from this mix and place on a working surface
5. Heat up a pan with half of the oil over medium high heat; add meatballs, cook them for 8 minutes flipping them from time to time and transfer them all to a tray.
6. In a salad bowl, mix spinach with cucumber and tomato.
7. Add meatballs, the rest of the oil, some salt, pepper and lemon juice
8. Also add tzatziki, toss to coat and serve
Nutrition Values: Calories: 200; Fat : 4; Fiber : 1; Carbs : 3; Protein : 7

307. Beef And Tomato Stuffed Squash

Preparation Time: 1 hour 10 minutes
Servings: 2
Ingredients:
- 28 ounces canned tomatoes; chopped.
- 2 pounds spaghetti squash; pricked with a fork
- 1/2 teaspoon thyme; dried
- 1 pound beef; ground
- 1 green bell pepper; chopped.
- 3 garlic cloves; minced
- 1 yellow onion; chopped.
- 1 Portobello mushroom; sliced
- 1 teaspoon oregano; dried
- 1/4 teaspoon cayenne pepper
- Salt and black pepper to the taste.

Directions:
1. Place spaghetti squash on a lined baking sheet, introduce in the oven at 400 degrees F and bake for 40 minutes
2. Cut in half, leave aside to cool down, remove seeds and leave aside
3. Heat up a pan over medium high heat; add meat, garlic, onion and mushroom; stir and cook until meat browns
4. Add salt, pepper, thyme, oregano, cayenne, tomatoes and green pepper; stir and cook for 10 minutes
5. Stuff squash halves with this beef mix, introduce in the oven at 400 degrees F and bake for 10 minutes
6. Divide between 2 plates and serve
Nutrition Values: Calories: 260; Fat : 7; Fiber : 2; Carbs : 4; Protein : 10

308. Braised Lamb Chops

Preparation Time: 2 hours 30 minutes
Servings: 4
Ingredients:
- 1 teaspoon garlic powder
- 1 shallot; chopped.
- 1 cup white wine
- 1 bay leaf
- 2 cups beef stock
- 8 lamb chops
- Some chopped parsley for serving
- 2 teaspoons mint; crushed.
- A drizzle of olive oil
- Juice of 1/2 lemon
- Salt and black pepper to the taste.

For the sauce:
- 2 cups cranberries
- 1/2 teaspoon rosemary; chopped.
- 1 teaspoon ginger; grated
- 1 cup water
- 1/2 cup swerve
- 1 teaspoon mint; dried
- Juice of 1/2 lemon
- 1 teaspoon harissa paste

Directions:

1.   In a bowl, mix lamb chops with salt, pepper, 1 teaspoon garlic powder and 2 teaspoons mint and rub well.
2.   Heat up a pan with a drizzle of oil over medium high heat; add lamb chops, brown them on all sides and transfer to a plate
3.   Heat up the same pan again over medium high heat; add shallots; stir and cook for 1 minute
4.   Add wine and bay leaf; stir and cook for 4 minutes
5.   Add 2 cups beef stock, parsley and juice from 1/2 lemon; stir and simmer for 5 minutes
6.   Return lamb; stir and cook for 10 minutes
7.   Cover pan and introduce it in the oven at 350 degrees F for 2 hours
8.   Meanwhile; heat up a pan over medium high heat; add cranberries, swerve, rosemary, 1 teaspoon mint, juice from 1/2 lemon, ginger, water and harissa paste; stir, bring to a simmer for 15 minutes
9.   Take lamb chops out of the oven, divide them between plates, drizzle the cranberry sauce over them and serve
Nutrition Values: Calories: 450; Fat : 34; Fiber : 2; Carbs : 6; Protein : 26

309. Lamb With Fennel

Preparation Time: 50 minutes
Servings: 4
Ingredients:
*   12 ounces lamb racks
*   1 tablespoon swerve
*   4 figs; cut in halves
*   2 fennel bulbs; sliced
*   2 tablespoons olive oil
*   1/8 cup apple cider vinegar
*   Salt and black pepper to the taste.
Directions:
1.   In a bowl, mix fennel with figs, vinegar, swerve and oil, toss to coat well and transfer to a baking dish.
2.   Season with salt and pepper, introduce in the oven at 400 degrees F and bake for 15 minutes
3.   Season lamb with salt and pepper, place into a heated pan over medium high heat and cook for a couple of minutes
4.   Add lamb to the baking dish with the fennel and figs, introduce in the oven and bake for 20 minutes more
5.   Divide everything between plates and serve
Nutrition Values: Calories: 230; Fat : 3; Fiber : 3; Carbs : 5; Protein : 10

310. Beef And Eggplant Casserole

Preparation Time: 4 hours 30 minutes
Servings: 12
Ingredients:
*   2 pounds beef; ground
*   2 cups mozzarella; grated
*   1 tablespoon olive oil
*   2 cups eggplant; chopped.
*   16 ounces tomato sauce
*   1 teaspoon oregano; dried
*   2 teaspoons mustard
*   2 tablespoons parsley; chopped.
*   2 teaspoons gluten free Worcestershire sauce
*   28 ounces canned tomatoes; chopped.
*   Salt and black pepper to the taste.
Directions:
1.   Season eggplant pieces with salt and pepper, leave them aside for 30 minutes, squeeze water a bit, put them into a bowl, add the olive oil and toss them to coat.
2.   In another bowl, mix beef with salt, pepper, mustard and Worcestershire sauce and stir well.
3.   Press them on the bottom of a crock pot.
4.   Add eggplant and spread.
5.   Also add tomatoes, tomato sauce, parsley, oregano and mozzarella.
6.   Cover Crockpot and cook on Low for 4 hours
7.   Divide casserole between plates and serve hot.
Nutrition Values: Calories: 200; Fat : 12; Fiber : 2; Carbs : 6; Protein : 15

311. Burgundy Beef Stew Recipe

Preparation Time: 3 hours 10 minutes
Servings: 7
Ingredients:
*   2 pounds beef chuck roast; cubed
*   15 ounces canned tomatoes; chopped.
*   2 yellow onions; chopped.
*   3 tablespoons almond flour
*   1 cup water
*   4 carrots; chopped.
*   1 cup beef stock
*   1 tablespoon thyme; chopped.
*   1/2 teaspoon mustard powder
*   1/2 pounds mushrooms; sliced
*   2 celery ribs; chopped.
*   Salt and black pepper to the taste.
Directions:
1.   Heat up an oven proof pot over medium high heat; add beef cubes; stir and brown them for a couple of minutes on each side
2.   Add tomatoes, mushrooms, onions, carrots, celery, salt, pepper mustard, stock and thyme and stir.
3.   In a bowl mix water with flour and stir well.
4.   Add this to the pot; stir well, introduce in the oven and bake at 325 degrees F for 3 hours
5.   Stir every half an hour. Divide into bowls and serve
Nutrition Values: Calories: 275; Fat : 13; Fiber : 4; Carbs : 7; Protein : 28

312. Beef Roast

Preparation Time: 1 hour 25 minutes

Servings: 4

Ingredients:
- 3½ pounds beef roast
- 1 ounce onion soup mix
- 1/2 cup Italian dressing
- 12 ounces beef stock
- 4 ounces mushrooms; sliced

Directions:
1. In a bowl, mix stock with onion soup mix and Italian dressing and stir.
2. Put beef roast in a pan, add mushrooms, stock mix, cover with tin foil, introduce in the oven at 300 degrees F and bake for 1 hour and 15 minutes
3. Leave roast to cool down a bit, slice and serve with the gravy on top.

Nutrition Values: Calories: 700; Fat : 56; Fiber : 2; Carbs : 10; Protein : 70

313. Lamb

Preparation Time: 8 hours 10 minutes
Servings: 6

Ingredients:
- 2 pounds lamb leg
- 6 mint leaves
- 1 tablespoon maple extract
- 2 tablespoons mustard
- 1/4 cup olive oil
- 1 teaspoon garlic; minced
- A pinch of rosemary; dried
- 4 thyme spring
- Salt and black pepper to the taste.

Directions:
1. Put the oil in your slow cooker.
2. Add lamb, salt, pepper, maple extract, mustard, rosemary and garlic, rub well, cover and cook on Low for 7 hours
3. Add mint and thyme and cook for 1 more hour.
4. Leave lamb to cool down a bit before slicing and serving with pan juices on top.

Nutrition Values: Calories: 400; Fat : 34; Fiber : 1; Carbs : 3; Protein : 26

VEGETABLES

314. Cauliflower Pizza Crust

Preparation time: 15 minutes
Cooking time: 20 minutes
Servings:6
Ingredients:
- 2 cups cauliflower, chopped
- 1 egg, whisked
- 1 teaspoon butter
- 1 teaspoon dried basil
- 1 teaspoon salt
- 6 oz Cheddar cheese, shredded
- 1 tablespoon heavy cream

Directions:
1. Place the cauliflower in the food processor and blend until you get cauliflower rice.
2. Then squeeze the juice from the cauliflower rice.
3. Line the baking tray with the parchment and then spread parchment with the butter.
4. Place the cauliflower rice in the tray in the shape of the pizza crust.
5. Bake the cauliflower pizza crust for 10 minutes at 365F.
6. Meanwhile, mix up together salt, shredded Cheddar cheese, heavy cream, and egg.
7. When the cauliflower crust is cooked, spread it with cheese mixture and flatten gently it.
8. Bake the meal for 10 minutes more at 375F.
9. When the pizza crust is cooked, cut it into 6 servings.
Nutrition Values: calories 147, fat 11.7, fiber 0.8, carbs 2.3, protein 8.7

315. Zucchini Ravioli

Preparation time: 20 minutes
Cooking time: 15 minutes
Servings:4
Ingredients:
- 1 zucchini, trimmed
- 2 tablespoons ricotta cheese
- ½ cup spinach, chopped
- 1 teaspoon olive oil
- ½ teaspoon salt
- 1/3 cup marinara sauce
- 4 oz Parmesan, grated

Directions:
1. Slice the zucchini with the help of the peeler to get long slices.
2. Then take 4 zucchini slices and make the cross from them.
3. Repeat the same steps with all remaining zucchini slices.
4. After this, place chopped spinach in the skillet.
5. Add salt and olive oil. Mix up spinach and cook it for 5 minutes. Stir it from time to time.
6. After this, mix up spinach with ricotta and stir well.
7. Pour marinara sauce in the casserole dish.
8. Place the ricotta mixture in the center of every zucchini cross and fold up them.
9. Transfer zucchini balls -ravioliin the casserole to dish on the marinara sauce.
10. Sprinkle the zucchini ravioli over with grated Parmesan and transfer the casserole dish in the preheated to the 395F oven. Cook the meal for 15 minutes.
Nutrition Values: calories 141, fat 8.9, fiber 1.2, carbs 5.9, protein 11.1

316. Vegetable Crackers

Preparation time: 20 minutes
Cooking time: 20 minutes
Servings:4
Ingredients:
- 1 cup cauliflower
- 1 tablespoon flax meal
- 1 teaspoon chia seeds
- 1 teaspoon ground cumin
- 1 teaspoon salt
- ½ teaspoon ground paprika
- 1 tablespoon rice flour
- 1 teaspoon nutritional yeast
- 1 cup water, for the steamer

Directions:
1. Chop the cauliflower roughly.
2. Pour water in the steamer and insert steamer rack. Place the cauliflower in the rack and close the lid.
3. Preheat the steamer and steam cauliflower for 5 minutes.
4. After this, place the vegetables in the food processor and blend well.
5. Transfer the blended cauliflower in the cheesecloth and squeeze the liquid from it.
6. Then transfer the cauliflower in the bowl.
7. Add all ingredients from the list above and mix up well.
8. Line the baking tray with the parchment and place cauliflower mixture over it.
9. Cover it with the second parchment sheet.
10. Roll up the cauliflower mixture into the rectangular.
11. Remove the upper parchment sheet and cut the cauliflower mixture into the crackers.
12. Transfer the tray in the preheated to the 365F oven.
13. Cook crackers for 15 minutes.
14. Chill the crackers well remove from the baking tray.
Nutrition Values: calories 35, fat 1.3, fiber 2.1, carbs 5.2, protein 1.8

317. Crunchy Okra Bites

Preparation time: 10 minutes
Cooking time: 12 minutes
Servings:2
Ingredients:
- 1 cup okra, roughly sliced
- ¼ cup almond flour
- 1 tablespoon coconut flakes
- 1 teaspoon chili powder
- ½ teaspoon salt
- 3 eggs, whisked

Directions:
1. In the mixing bowl,mix up together almond flour, coconut flakes, chili powder, and salt.
2. Place the sliced okra into the whisked egg and mix up well.
3. Then coat every okra bite into the almond flour mixture.
4. Line the tray with the parchment.
5. Place the okra bites into the tray to make the okra layer.
6. Preheat the oven to 375F.
7. Place the tray with okra bites in the oven and cook for 12 minutes.
8. Chill the hot okra bites little before serving.

Nutrition Values: calories 147, fat 9.5, fiber 2.7, carbs 6.1, protein 10.3

318. Arugula-Tomato Salad

Preparation time: 15 minutes
Servings:6
Ingredients:
- 2 cups arugula, chopped
- 1 cup lettuce, chopped
- ½ cup cherry tomatoes
- ¼ cup fresh basil
- 1 tablespoon olive oil
- ½ teaspoon chili flakes
- 5 oz Mozzarella cheese balls, cherry size

Directions:
1. Make the salad dressing: blend the fresh basil until smooth and add olive oil and chili flakes. Pulse the mixture for 5 seconds.
2. After this, place arugula and lettuce into the salad bowl.
3. Cut the cherry tomatoes into the halves and add in the salad bowl.
4. Then add Mozzarella cheese balls and shake the salad well.
5. Pour the salad dressing over the salad.

Nutrition Values: calories 93, fat 8.3, fiber 0.4, carbs 1.1, protein 4.5

319. Basil Bake

Preparation time: 15 minutes
Cooking time: 25 minutes
Servings:4
Ingredients:
- ½ cup fresh basil
- 4 tablespoons coconut oil
- 1 zucchini, sliced

- 2 oz Parmesan, grated
- 1 tablespoon walnuts, chopped
- ½ teaspoon salt
- 2 tomatoes, sliced

Directions:
1. Melt coconut oil and transfer it in the blender.
2. Add fresh basil, walnuts, and salt. Blend the mixture until smooth. Add grated Parmesan and stir it. The pesto sauce is cooked.
3. Place the sliced zucchini and tomatoes into the casserole dish one-by-one.
4. Then top it with pesto sauce.
5. Cover the casserole dish with the foil and transfer in the oven.
6. Bake the meal for 25 minutes at 375F.
7. Then discard the foil and remove the basil bake from the oven.

Nutrition Values: calories 194, fat 18, fiber 1.5, carbs 4.8, protein 6.2

320. Roasted Bok Choy with Chili Sauce

Preparation time: 10 minutes
Cooking time: 10 minutes
Servings:2
Ingredients:
- 8 oz bok choy
- 4 tablespoons chili sauce
- 2 tablespoons almond butter
- 1 teaspoon dried dill

Directions:
1. Slice bok choy into halves and place in the big bowl.
2. Add chili sauce and dried dill and mix up well.
3. Place the almond butter in the skillet and melt it.
4. Add the chili bok choy and roast it for 5 minutes from each side over the medium-low heat.
5. Gently transfer the cooked bok choy into the serving plates.

Nutrition Values: calories 117, fat 9.4, fiber 2.9, carbs 6.3, protein 5.4

321. Vegan Moussaka

Preparation time: 15 minutes
Cooking time: 35 minutes
Servings:88
Ingredients:
- 2 eggplants, trimmed
- 1 white onion, chopped
- 1 garlic clove, diced
- ¼ cup tomatoes, crushed
- ½ teaspoon ground cinnamon
- 1 teaspoon salt
- 1 teaspoon ground black pepper
- 1 teaspoon ground paprika
- 2 tablespoons coconut oil
- 2 tablespoons ricotta cheese

- 1 oz Cheddar cheese, shredded
- 1 tablespoon heavy cream

Directions:
1. Place the coconut oil in the saucepan and melt it.
2. Meanwhile, chop the eggplants.
3. Place the eggplants and onion in the hot coconut oil. Add diced garlic.
4. Mix up the vegetables and cook them for 10 minutes or until they start to be soft.
5. Meanwhile, mix up together heavy cream, ricotta cheese, and shredded Cheddar cheese.
6. Transfer the roasted vegetables in the blender and blend for 3 minutes or until they are smooth.
7. After this, add all spices and crushed tomatoes, Blend the mixture 1 minute more.
8. Transfer the eggplant mixture in the casserole dish and flatten it well with the help of the spatula.
9. Place ricotta mixture over the eggplant mixture.
10. Bake moussaka for 20 minutes at the preheated to the 360F oven.
11. Chill the cooked meal for 10 minutes before serving.

Nutrition Values: calories 99, fat 5.9, fiber 5.5, carbs 10.4, protein 3

322. Cumin Fennel

Preparation time: 10 minutes
Cooking time: 15 minutes
Servings:6
Ingredients:
- 1-pound fennel bulb
- 2 tablespoons butter, softened
- 1 tablespoon ground cumin
- 1 teaspoon salt
- ¼ teaspoon garlic powder

Directions:
1. Slice fennel bulb into the medium slices.
2. Line the baking tray with the baking paper.
3. Churn butter with the ground cumin, salt, and garlic powder.
4. Arrange the sliced fennel on the tray and spread it with the churned butter mixture.
5. Bake the fennel for 15 minutes at 360F.
6. When the fennel is cooked, it has a tender taste.

Nutrition Values: calories 62, fat 4.2, fiber 2.5, carbs 6, protein 1.2

323. Mushroom Tart

Preparation time: 15 minutes
Cooking time: 40 minutes
Servings:8
Ingredients:
- 1 teaspoon baking powder
- ½ teaspoon salt
- 1 small egg, beaten

- 1 tablespoon coconut oil
- ½ cup almond flour
- 1 cup mushroom caps
- 1 tablespoon fresh dill, chopped
- 1 tablespoon butter
- 1 teaspoon ground turmeric
- 1 teaspoon ground paprika
- 2 oz Parmesan, grated
- ¼ cup heavy cream

Directions:
1. Make the tart dough: mix up together salt, egg baking powder, coconut oil, and almond flour. Knead the dough and roll it up into the pie crust.
2. Place the dough into the pie form.
3. Then arrange the mushrooms caps inside the pie form.
4. Sprinkle them with chopped dill, ground turmeric, paprika, and butter.
5. Then add Parmesan and pour it over with the heavy cream.
6. Transfer the tart in the oven.
7. Cook the mushroom tart for 40 minutes at 360F.
8. Chill the cooked tart till them room temperature and after this cut it into the servings.

Nutrition Values: calories 85, fat 7.5, fiber 0.5, carbs 1.9, protein 3.8

324. Cauliflower Cheese

Preparation time: 10 minutes
Cooking time: 25 minutes
Servings:5
Ingredients:
- 2 cups cauliflower florets
- 1 cup organic almond milk
- ½ cup heavy cream
- 2 tablespoons coconut flour
- 1 teaspoon salt
- 6 oz Cheddar cheese, shredded
- 2 cups of water

Directions:
1. Bring water to boil, add cauliflower florets and boil them for 10 minutes.
2. Then drain water and transfer cauliflower florets in the baking dish.
3. Pour almond milk and heavy cream in the saucepan. Bring the liquid to boil.
4. Add salt and coconut flour.
5. Whisk the liquid very fast for 1 minute.
6. Then switch off the heat and add shredded cheese.
7. Leave the liquid until cheese is melted. Mix it up.
8. Pour cheese over the cauliflower florets.
9. Bake the cauliflower cheese for 15 minutes at 375F or until it starts bubbling.

Nutrition Values: calories 225, fat 17.1, fiber 3, carbs 7.7, protein 10.5

325. Spinach&Kale Salad

Preparation time: 10 minutes
Servings:4
Ingredients:
- 2 cups fresh spinach
- 1 cucumber, chopped
- 1 cup kale
- ¼ teaspoon salt
- ½ teaspoon ground black pepper
- 1 teaspoon flax seeds
- 1 bell pepper
- 2 tablespoons sesame oil
- 2 tablespoons lemon juice
- ½ cup lettuce

Directions:
1. Remove stems from kale.
2. Roughly chop kale, spinach, and lettuce and transfer greens in the salad bowl.
3. Slice bell pepper.
4. Add sliced bell pepper and chopped cucumber in the salad bowl too.
5. Then sprinkle the meal with salt, ground black pepper, lemon juice, and sesame oil.
6. Mix up a salad with the help of 2 forks.
Nutrition Values: calories 99, fat 7.3, fiber 1.7, carbs 8, protein 2

326. Cauliflower Anti Pasto

Preparation time: 10 minutes
Cooking time: 20 minutes
Servings:4
Ingredients:
- 1 cup mushrooms, marinated, chopped
- 1 cup cauliflower
- 2 oz Swiss cheese, chopped
- 1 bell pepper, chopped
- 1 teaspoon dried oregano
- 1 tablespoon lemon juice
- 1 tablespoon olive oil
- ½ teaspoon dried cilantro
- 1 cup water, for the steamer

Directions:
1. Pour water in the steamer and insert trivet.
2. Place the cauliflower in the trivet and close the lid.
3. Steam the vegetable for 10 minutes totally - including preheating.
4. Preheat oven to 375F.
5. Place bell peppers in the tray and transfer in the oven.
6. Bake it for 5 minutes from each side.
7. Remove the cooked bell pepper from the oven, chill little and peel.
8. Then chop it roughly and put in the big bowl.
9. Remove the cauliflower from the steamer and cut it into the small florets.
10. Transfer the cauliflower in the zip log bag.
11. Add dried oregano, lemon juice, olive oil, and dried cilantro.

12. Shake the mixture well.
13. Remove the cauliflower from the zip log into the bowl with the bell pepper.
14. Add chopped Swiss cheese and marinated mushrooms.
15. Mix up antipasto well.
Nutrition Values: calories 105, fat 7.7, fiber 1.4, carbs 5.2, protein 5.2

327. Sour Sweet Bok Choy

Preparation time: 7 minutes
Cooking time: 12 minutes
Servings:1
Ingredients:
- 6 oz bok choy, sliced
- 1 teaspoon Erythritol
- 1 teaspoon lime juice
- ¼ teaspoon ground paprika
- 1 tablespoon water
- 1 teaspoon apple cider vinegar
- 1 tablespoon almond butter

Directions:
1. Put almond butter in the skillet and melt it.
2. Add sliced bok choy and roast it for 3 minutes from each side.
3. Meanwhile, whisk together Erythritol, lime juice, ground paprika, water, and apple cider vinegar.
4. When the bok choy is roasted from both sides sprinkle it with Erythritol mixture and mix up with the help of a spatula.
5. Bring to boil the meal and switch off the heat.
6. Let bok choy rest for 5 minutes.
Nutrition Values: calories 124, fat 9.4, fiber 3.5, carbs 7.4, protein 6

328. Celery Rosti

Preparation time: 10 minutes
Cooking time: 10 minutes
Servings:4
Ingredients:
- 8 oz celery root, peeled
- 1/3 onion, diced
- 1 teaspoon olive oil
- ½ teaspoon ground black pepper
- 2 oz Parmesan, grated
- ¼ teaspoon ground turmeric

Directions:
1. Put the diced onion in the skillet. Add olive oil and cook it until translucent.
2. Meanwhile, grated celery root and mix it up with ground black pepper, ground turmeric, and Parmesan.
3. When the mixture is homogenous, add it in the skillet.
4. Mix up well.
5. Then press the celery root mixture with the help of the spatula to get the shape of the pancake.
6. Close the lid and cook celery rosti for 6 minutes or until it is light brown.

Nutrition Values: calories 84, fat 4.4, fiber 1.3, carbs 6.9, protein 5.5

329. Garlic Snap Peas

Preparation time: 5 minutes
Cooking time: 10 minutes
Servings: 3
Ingredients:
- 1 cup snap peas
- 1 teaspoon Erythritol
- 1 teaspoon avocado oil
- ¼ teaspoon cayenne pepper
- ½ teaspoon garlic powder
- ¾ teaspoon garlic, diced

Directions:
1. Pour avocado oil in the skillet.
2. Add diced garlic and cook it for 1 minute over the medium heat.
3. Sprinkle it with garlic powder, cayenne pepper, and Erythritol.
4. Then add snap peas and mix up well.
5. Cook the snap peas for 9 minutes. Stir it all the time.
6. The cooked snap peas should be tender and crispy.

Nutrition Values: calories 44, fat 0.4, fiber 2.6, carbs 7.7, protein 2.8

320. Sheet Pan Rosemary Mushrooms

Preparation time: 10 minutes
Cooking time: 15 minutes
Servings: 2
Ingredients:
- 1 cup mushrooms
- 1 teaspoon minced rosemary
- ½ teaspoon of sea salt
- 1 tablespoon sesame oil

Directions:
- Line the baking tray with baking paper.
- Slice the mushrooms roughly and put them in the baking tray.
- Sprinkle mushrooms with minced rosemary, sea salt, and sesame oil.
- Mix up the vegetables well with the help of the hand palms.
- Preheat the oven to 360F.
- Cook mushrooms for 15 minutes.

Nutrition Values: calories 70, fat 7, fiber 0.6, carbs 1.5, protein 1.1

331. Buttered Sprouts

Preparation time: 7 minutes
Cooking time: 20 minutes
Servings: 4
Ingredients:
- 10 oz Brussel sprouts
- 2 oz prosciutto
- 3 teaspoons butter
- 1 cup of water
- 1 teaspoon salt

Directions:
1. Chop prosciutto and place in the saucepan.
2. Roast it until it starts to be crispy.
3. Then add water and Brussel sprouts.
4. Bring the mixture to boil and close the lid.
5. Boil the vegetables for 15 minutes.
6. After this, drain ½ part of all liquid and add butter.
7. Mix it up until the butter is melted and bring the meal to boil one more time in the butter liquid.
8. Serve buttered sprouts with the butter liquid.

Nutrition Values: calories 76, fat 3.9, fiber 2.7, carbs 6.7, protein 5.4

332. Bacon Cabbage Slices

Preparation time: 10 minutes
Cooking time: 15 minutes
Servings: 4
Ingredients:
- 10 oz white cabbage
- 4 oz bacon, sliced
- ½ teaspoon ground black pepper
- 1 teaspoon butter
- ½ teaspoon salt

Directions:
1. Slice the cabbage into medium slices and rub with butter.
2. Sprinkle the bacon slices with ground black pepper and salt.
3. Wrap every cabbage slice into the bacon and transfer in the tray.
4. Cook the cabbage slices in the oven at 370F for 15 minutes. You can flip the cabbage slices onto another side during cooking.

Nutrition Values: calories 180, fat 12.9, fiber 1.8, carbs 4.7, protein 11.5

333. Lemon Onion Mash

Preparation time: 15 minutes
Cooking time: 15 minutes
Servings: 4
Ingredients:
- 2 white onions
- 4 oz cauliflower
- ¼ cup heavy cream
- 4 oz Cheddar cheese, shredded
- ½ teaspoon Pink salt
- 1 teaspoon white pepper
- ½ teaspoon lemon zest
- 1 teaspoon lemon juice
- 1 teaspoon butter

Directions:
1. Peel the onion and grind it.
2. Put grinded onion and butter in the saucepan.
3. Blend cauliflower until you get cauliflower rice.
4. Add cauliflower rice in the saucepan too.

5. Add Pink salt, white pepper, lemon zest, and lemon juice. Stir it.
6. Close the lid and cook the mass for 5 minutes over the medium heat.
7. Then add shredded Cheddar cheese and heavy cream.
8. Mix up well and stir it until cheese is melted.
9. Close the lid and simmer mash for 5 minutes more over the low heat.
10. Switch off the heat and close the lid.
11. Let the lemon onion mash chill for 10 minutes.
Nutrition Values: calories 179, fat 13.3, fiber 2.1, carbs 7.6, protein 8.5

334. Chopped Ragu

Preparation time: 10 minutes
Cooking time: 25 minutes
Servings:5
Ingredients:
- 1 bell pepper, chopped
- 2 oz green beans, chopped
- 1 oz bok choy, chopped
- 2 oz collard greens, chopped
- ½ white onion, chopped
- 3 oz kale, chopped
- 2 oz jicama, chopped
- 3 oz asparagus
- ½ cup of coconut milk
- 1/3 cup water
- 1 teaspoon salt
- ½ teaspoon ground black pepper
- ½ teaspoon cayenne pepper
- 1 teaspoon marinara sauce

Directions:
1. Take the big pan and add water inside.
2. Bring water to boil and add chopped bell pepper, green beans, bok choy, collard greens, onion, kale, jicama, and asparagus.
3. Then add salt, ground black pepper, cayenne pepper, and marinara sauce.
4. Add coconut milk and carefully stir the vegetable ragu.
5. Preheat the oven to 365F.
6. Close the lid of the pan.
7. Transfer the pan in the preheated oven and bake ragu for 25 minutes.
8. When the ragu is cooked, remove it from the oven and remove the lid.
9. Don't stir ragu anymore!
10. If ragu will chill for 10-15 minutes, you will get the most delicious taste of ragu.
Nutrition Values: calories 93, fat 6, fiber 3.2, carbs 9.5, protein 2.5

EGGS AND DAIRY RECIPES

335. Eggtastic Smoothie

Servings: 1
Preparation time: 10 mins
Ingredients

- 2 tablespoons cream cheese
- 2 raw eggs
- 1 tablespoon vanilla extract
- ¼ cup heavy cream
- 3 ice cubes

Directions
1. Put all the ingredients in a blender and blend until smooth.
2. Pour into 1 glass and immediately serve.
Nutrition Values:
Calories 337
Total Fat 26.8g
Saturated Fat 14g
Cholesterol 390mg 1
Sodium 195mg
Total Carbohydrate 3.7g
Dietary Fiber 0g
Total Sugars 2.4g
Protein 13.2g

336. Eggs and Bacon

Servings: 12
Preparation time: 35 mins
Ingredients
- ½ teaspoon dried organic thyme
- 7 oz full fat cream cheese
- ½ cup parmesan cheese, shredded
- 24 organic bacon slices
- 12 hard cooked organic large eggs, peeled, yolks removed and sliced lengthwise

Directions
1. Preheat the oven to 3900F and lightly grease a baking dish.
2. Mix together thyme and cream cheese in a bowl.
3. Fill the egg white halves with the thyme mixture and close with the other egg white halves.
4. Wrap each egg tightly with 2 bacon slices and arrange on the baking dish.
5. Transfer to the oven and bake for about 25 minutes.
6. Remove from the oven to serve warm.
Nutrition Values:
Calories 340
Total Fat 25.9g
Saturated Fat 10.5g
Cholesterol 239mg
Sodium 1219mg
Total Carbohydrate 2.1g
Dietary Fiber 0.3g
Total Sugars 1.2g
Protein 23.9g

337. Cheesy Ham Souffle

Servings: 4
Preparation time: 30 mins
Ingredients
- ½ cup heavy cream
- 1 cup cheddar cheese, shredded
- 6 large eggs

- Salt and black pepper, to taste
- 6 ounces ham, diced

Directions
1.   Preheat the oven to 3750F and lightly grease ramekins.
2.   Whisk together ham with all other ingredients in a bowl.
3.   Mix well and pour the mixture into the ramekins.
4.   Transfer to the oven and bake for about 20 minutes.
5.   Remove from the oven and slightly cool before serving.

Nutrition Values:
Calories 342
Total Fat 26g
Saturated Fat 13g
Cholesterol 353mg 1
Sodium 841mg
Total Carbohydrate 3g
Dietary Fiber 0.6g
Total Sugars 0.8g
Protein 23.8g

338. Mushroom and Cheese Scrambled Eggs

Servings: 4
Preparation time: 20 mins
Ingredients
- 8 eggs
- 4 tablespoons butter
- 4 tablespoons parmesan cheese, shredded
- 1 cup fresh mushrooms, finely chopped
- Salt and black pepper, to taste

Directions
1.   Whisk together eggs with salt and black pepper in a bowl until well combined.
2.   Heat butter in a nonstick pan and stir in the whisked eggs.
3.   Cook for about 4 minutes and add mushrooms and parmesan cheese.
4.   Cook for about 6 minutes, occasionally stirring and dish out to serve.

Nutrition Values:
Calories 265
Total Fat 22.6g
Saturated Fat 11.5g
Cholesterol 365mg 1
Sodium 304mg
Total Carbohydrate 1.7g
Dietary Fiber 0.2g
Total Sugars 1g
Protein 15.1g

339. Red Pepper Frittata

Servings: 3
Preparation time: 15 mins
Ingredients
- 6 large eggs
- 2 red peppers, chopped

- Salt and black pepper, to taste
- 1¼ cups mozzarella cheese, shredded
- 3 tablespoons olive oil

Directions
1.   Whisk together the eggs in a medium bowl and add red peppers, mozzarella cheese, salt and black pepper.
2.   Heat olive oil over medium high heat in an ovenproof skillet and pour in the egg mixture.
3.   Lift the mixture with a spatula to let the eggs run under.
4.   Cook for about 5 minutes, stirring well and dish out onto a platter to serve.

Nutrition Values:
Calories 308
Total Fat 26.2g
Saturated Fat 6.4g
Cholesterol 378mg 1
Sodium 214mg
Total Carbohydrate 3.9g
Dietary Fiber 0.5g
Total Sugars 2.4g
Protein 16.5g

340. Cream Cheese Pancakes

Servings: 4
Preparation time: 25 mins
Ingredients
- ½ cup almond flour
- 2 scoops Stevia
- ½ teaspoon cinnamon
- 2 eggs
- 2 oz cream cheese

Directions
1.   Put all the ingredients in a blender and blend until smooth.
2.   Dish out the mixture to a medium bowl and set aside.
3.   Heat butter in a skillet over medium heat and add one quarter of the mixture.
4.   Spread the mixture and cook for about 4 minutes on both sides until golden brown.
5.   Repeat with rest of the mixture in batches and serve warm.

Nutrition Values:
Calories 166
Total Fat 13.8g
Saturated Fat 4.3g
Cholesterol 97mg
Sodium 78mg
Total Carbohydrate 3.8g
Dietary Fiber 1.7g
Total Sugars 0.2g
Protein 6.9g

341. Spicy Chorizo Baked Eggs

Servings: 4
Preparation time: 40 mins
Ingredients
- 5 large eggs

- 3 ounces ground chorizo sausage
- ¾ cup pepper jack cheese, shredded
- Salt and paprika, to taste
- 1 small avocado, chopped

Directions

Preheat the oven to 4000F.
1. Heat a nonstick oven safe skillet and add chorizo.
2. Cook for about 8 minutes and dish into a bowl.
3. Break the eggs in the skillet and season with salt and paprika.
4. Add cooked chorizo and avocado and cook for about 2 minutes.
5. Top with pepper jack cheese and transfer to the oven.
6. Bake for about 20 minutes and remove from the oven to serve.

Nutrition Values:

Calories 334
Total Fat 28.3g
Saturated Fat 10.3g
Cholesterol 269mg
Sodium 400mg
Total Carbohydrate 5.7g
Dietary Fiber 3.6g
Total Sugars 0.8g
Protein 16.9g

342. Cheesy Taco Pie

Servings: 6
Preparation time: 45 mins

Ingredients

- 1 tablespoon garlic powder
- 1 pound ground beef
- 6 large eggs
- Salt and chili powder, to taste
- 1 cup cheddar cheese, shredded

Directions

1. Preheat the oven to 3500F and lightly grease a pie plate.
2. Heat a large nonstick skillet and add beef, garlic powder, salt and chili powder.
3. Cook for about 6 minutes over medium low heat and transfer to the pie plate.
4. Top with cheddar cheese and transfer to the oven.
5. Bake for about 30 minutes and remove from the oven to serve hot.

Nutrition Values:

Calories 294
Total Fat 16g
Saturated Fat 7.3g
Cholesterol 273mg
Sodium 241mg
Total Carbohydrate 1.9g
Dietary Fiber 0.3g
Total Sugars 0.9g
Protein 34.2g

343. Sausage Egg Casserole

Servings: 8
Preparation time: 40 mins

Ingredients

- 1 cup almond milk, unsweetened
- 6 large eggs
- Salt and black pepper, to taste
- 2 cups cheddar cheese, shredded
- 1 pound ground pork sausage, cooked

Directions

1. Preheat the oven to 3500F and lightly grease a casserole dish.
2. Whisk together eggs with almond milk, salt and black pepper in a bowl.
3. Put the cooked sausages in the casserole dish and top with the egg mixture and cheddar cheese.
4. Transfer to the oven and bake for about 30 minutes.
5. Remove from the oven and serve hot.

Nutrition Values:

Calories 429
Total Fat 36.3g
Saturated Fat 18.6g
Cholesterol 217mg
Sodium 657mg
Total Carbohydrate 2.3g
Dietary Fiber 0.7g
Total Sugars 1.4g
Protein 23.5g

344. Egg Bites

Servings: 8
Preparation time: 25 mins

Ingredients

- 12 large eggs
- 1 -8 ouncepackage cream cheese, softened
- 8 slices bacon, cooked and crumbled
- 1 cup gruyere cheese, shredded
- Salt and paprika, to taste

Directions

1. Put eggs, cream cheese, salt and paprika in a blender and blend until smooth.
2. Grease 8 egg poaching cups lightly with cooking spray and put half the gruyere cheese, bacon and egg mixture in them.
3. Put the cups in a large saucepan with boiling water and cover the lid.
4. Lower the heat and cook for about 10 minutes.
5. Dish out the eggs into a serving dish and slice to serve.

Nutrition Values:

Calories 365
Total Fat 29.7g
Saturated Fat 13.7g
Cholesterol 346mg 1
Sodium 673mg
Total Carbohydrate 1.7g

Dietary Fiber 0g
Total Sugars 0.7g
Protein 22.6g

345. Chorizo and Eggs

Servings: 2
Preparation time: 20 mins
Ingredients
- ½ small yellow onion, chopped
- 1 teaspoon olive oil
- 2 -3 ouncechorizo sausages
- Salt and black pepper, to taste
- 4 eggs

Directions
1. Open the sausage casings and dish the meat into a bowl.
2. Heat olive oil over medium high heat in a large skillet and add onions.
3. Sauté for about 3 minutes and stir in the chorizo sausage.
4. Cook for about 4 minutes and add eggs, salt and black pepper.
5. Whisk well and cook for about 3 minutes.
6. Dish into a bowl and serve warm.

Nutrition Values:
Calories 270
Total Fat 21.8g
Saturated Fat 7.6g
Cholesterol 201mg
Sodium 587mg
Total Carbohydrate 2g
Dietary Fiber 0.2g
Total Sugars 0.7g
Protein 15.9g

346. Egg in the Avocado

Servings: 6
Preparation time: 25 mins
Ingredients
- 3 medium avocados, cut in half, pitted, skin on
- 1 teaspoon garlic powder
- ¼ cup parmesan cheese, grated
- 6 medium eggs
- Sea salt and black pepper, to taste

Directions
1. Preheat the oven to 3500F and grease 6 muffin tins.
2. Put the avocado half in each muffin tin and season with garlic powder, sea salt, and black pepper.
3. Break 1 egg into each avocado and top with the parmesan cheese.
4. Transfer into the oven and bake for about 15 minutes.
5. Remove from the oven and serve warm.

Nutrition Values:
Calories 107
Total Fat 7.9g
Saturated Fat 2.5g
Cholesterol 167mg

Sodium 105mg
Total Carbohydrate 2.4g
Dietary Fiber 1.6g
Total Sugars 0.5g
Protein 7.6g

347. Egg, Bacon and Cheese Cups

Servings: 6
Preparation time: 30 mins
Ingredients
- ¼ cup frozen spinach, thawed and drained
- 6 large eggs
- 6 strips bacon
- Salt and black pepper, to taste
- ¼ cup sharp cheddar cheese

Directions
1. Preheat the oven to 4000and grease 6 muffin cups.
2. Whisk together eggs, spinach, salt and black pepper in a bowl.
3. Put the bacon slices in the muffin cups and pour in the egg spinach mixture.
4. Top with sharp cheddar cheese and transfer to the oven.
5. Bake for 15 minutes and remove from the oven to serve warm.

Nutrition Values:
Calories 194
Total Fat 14.5g
Saturated Fat 5.2g
Cholesterol 212mg
Sodium 539mg
Total Carbohydrate 0.8g
Dietary Fiber 0g
Total Sugars 0.4g
Protein 14.5g

348. Steak and Eggs

Servings: 4
Preparation time: 25 mins
Ingredients
- 6 eggs
- 2 tablespoons butter
- 8 oz. sirloin steak
- Salt and black pepper, to taste
- ½ avocado, sliced

Directions
1. Heat butter in a pan on medium heat and fry the eggs.
2. Season with salt and black pepper and dish out onto a plate.
3. Cook the sirloin steak in another pan until desired doneness and slice into bite sized strips.
4. Season with salt and black pepper and dish out alongside the eggs.
5. Put the avocados with the eggs and steaks and serve.

Nutrition Values:
Calories 302
Total Fat 20.8g

Saturated Fat 8.1g
Cholesterol 311mg 1
Sodium 172mg
Total Carbohydrate 2.7g
Dietary Fiber 1.7g
Total Sugars 0.6g
Protein 26g

349. Butter Coffee

Servings: 4
Preparation time: 20 mins
Ingredients
- ½ cup coconut milk
- ½ cup water
- 2 tablespoons coffee
- 1 tablespoon coconut oil
- 1 tablespoon grass fed butter

Directions
1. Heat water in a saucepan and add coffee.
2. Simmer for about 3 minutes and add coconut milk.
3. Simmer for another 3 minutes and allow to cool down.
4. Transfer to a blender along with coconut oil and butter.
5. Pour into a mug and serve immediately.

Nutrition Values:
Calories 111
Total Fat 11.9g
Saturated Fat 10.3g
Cholesterol 4mg
Sodium 18mg
Total Carbohydrate 1.7g
Dietary Fiber 0.7g
Total Sugars 1g
Protein 0.7g

350. California Chicken Omelet

Servings: 1
Preparation time: 20 mins
Ingredients
- 2 bacon slices, cooked and chopped
- 2 eggs
- 1 oz. deli cut chicken
- 3 tablespoons avocado mayonnaise
- 1 Campari tomato

Directions
1. Whisk together eggs in a bowl and pour into a nonstick pan.
2. Season with salt and black pepper and cook for about 5 minutes.
3. Add chicken, bacon, tomato and avocado mayonnaise and cover with lid.
4. Cook for 5 more minutes on medium low heat and dish out to serve hot.

Nutrition Values:
Calories 208
Total Fat 15g
Saturated Fat 4.5g
Cholesterol 189mg

Sodium 658mg
Total Carbohydrate 3g
Dietary Fiber 1.1g
Total Sugars 0.9g
Protein 15.3g

351. Eggs Oopsie Rolls

Servings: 3
Preparation time: 25 mins
Ingredients
- 3 oz cream cheese
- 3 large eggs, separated
- 1/8 teaspoon cream of tartar
- 1 scoop stevia
- 1/8 teaspoon salt

Directions
1. Preheat oven to 3000F and line a cookie sheet with parchment paper.
2. Beat the egg whites with cream of tartar until soft peaks form.
3. Mix together egg yolks, salt and cream cheese in a bowl.
4. Combine the egg yolk and egg white mixtures and spoon them onto the cookie sheet.
5. Transfer to the oven and bake for about 40 minutes.
6. Remove from the oven and serve warm.

Nutrition Values:
Calories 171
Total Fat 14.9g
Saturated Fat 7.8g
Cholesterol 217mg
Sodium 251mg
Total Carbohydrate 1.2g
Dietary Fiber 0g
Total Sugars 0.5g
Protein 8.4g

352. Easy Blender Pancakes

Servings: 2
Preparation time: 25 mins
Ingredients
- 2 eggs
- 2 oz. cream cheese
- 1 scoop Isopure Protein Powder
- 1 pinch salt
- 1 dash cinnamon

Directions
1. Mix together eggs with cream cheese, protein powder, salt and cinnamon in a bowl.
2. Transfer to a blender and blend until smooth.
3. Heat a nonstick pan and pour quarter of the mixture.
4. Cook for about 2 minutes on each side and dish out.
5. Repeat with the remaining mixture and dish out in a platter to serve warm.

Nutrition Values:
Calories 215

Total Fat 14.5g
Saturated Fat 7.7g
Cholesterol 196mg
Sodium 308mg
Total Carbohydrate 1.2g
Dietary Fiber 0.1g
Total Sugars 0.4g
Protein 20.2g

353. Shakshuka

Servings: 2
Preparation time: 25 mins
Ingredients
- 1 chili pepper, chopped
- 1 cup marinara sauce
- 4 eggs
- Salt and black pepper, to taste
- 1 oz. feta cheese

Directions
1. Preheat the oven to 3900F.
2. Heat a small oven proof skillet on medium heat and add marinara sauce and chili pepper.
3. Cook for about 5 minutes and stir in the eggs.
4. Season with salt and black pepper and top with feta cheese.
5. Transfer into the oven and bake for about 10 minutes.
6. Remove from the oven and serve hot shakshuka.

Nutrition Values:
Calories 273
Total Fat 15.1g
Saturated Fat 5.7g
Cholesterol 342mg 1
Sodium 794mg
Total Carbohydrate 18.7g
Dietary Fiber 3.3g
Total Sugars 12.4g
Protein 15.4g

354. Rooibos Tea Latte

Servings: 1
Preparation time: 20 mins
Ingredients
- 2 bags rooibos tea
- 1 cup water
- 1 tablespoon grass fed butter
- 1 scoop collagen peptides
- ¼ cup full fat canned coconut milk

Directions
1. Put the tea bags in boiling water and steep for about 5 minutes.
2. Discard the tea bags and stir in butter and coconut milk.
3. Pour this mixture into a blender and blend until smooth.
4. Add collagen to the blender and blend on low speed until incorporated.

5. Pour into a mug to serve hot or chilled as desired.
Nutrition Values:
Calories 283
Total Fat 23.5g
Saturated Fat 18.3g
Cholesterol 31mg
Sodium 21mg
Total Carbohydrate 3.4g
Dietary Fiber 0g
Total Sugars 2.4g
Protein 15g

355. Feta and Pesto Omelet

Servings: 3
Preparation time: 10 mins
Ingredients
- 3 eggs
- 2 tablespoons butter
- 1 oz. feta cheese
- Salt and black pepper, to taste
- 1 tablespoon pesto

Directions
1. Heat butter in a pan and allow it to melt.
2. Whisk together eggs in a bowl and pour into the pan.
3. Cook for about 3 minutes until done and add feta cheese and pesto.
4. Season with salt and black pepper and fold it over.
5. Cook for another 5 minutes until the feta cheese is melted and dish out onto a platter to serve.

Nutrition Values:
Calories 178
Total Fat 16.2g
Saturated Fat 8.1g
Cholesterol 194mg
Sodium 253mg
Total Carbohydrate 1.1g
Dietary Fiber 0.1g
Total Sugars 1.1g
Protein 7.5g

356.Eggs Benedict

Servings: 2
Preparation time: 25 mins
Ingredients
- 4 oopsie rolls
- 4 eggs
- 4 Canadian bacon slices, cooked and crisped
- 1 tablespoon white vinegar
- 1 teaspoon chives

Directions
1. Boil water with vinegar and create a whirlpool in it with a wooden spoon.
2. Break an egg in a cup and place in the boiling water for about 3 minutes.
3. Repeat with rest of the eggs and dish out onto a platter.

4. Place oopsie rolls on the plates and top with bacon slices.
5. Put the poached eggs onto bacon slices and garnish with chives to serve.
Nutrition Values:
Calories 190
Total Fat 13.5g
Saturated Fat 5.8g
Cholesterol 275mg
Sodium 587mg
Total Carbohydrate 1.5g
Dietary Fiber 0g
Total Sugars 0.6g
Protein 15.3g

357. Egg Clouds

Servings: 2
Preparation time: 25 mins
Ingredients
- 6 strips bacon
- ¼ teaspoon cayenne pepper
- 2 eggs, separated
- Salt and black pepper, to taste
- ½ teaspoon garlic powder

Directions
1. Preheat oven to 3500F and grease a baking sheet lightly.
2. Whisk the egg whites in a bowl until fluffy and add garlic powder and salt.
3. Make 2 bacon weaves and spoon the egg white mixture on to it to form a cloud.
4. Make a hole in the egg cloud and put the egg yolks in it.
5. Season with cayenne pepper and black pepper and transfer to the oven.
6. Bake for about 10 minutes and dish out on a platter to serve.
Nutrition Values:
Calories 374
Total Fat 28.2g
Saturated Fat 9.2g
Cholesterol 226mg
Sodium 1379mg
Total Carbohydrate 1.8g
Dietary Fiber 0.1g
Total Sugars 0.5g
Protein 26.8g

358. Spicy Shrimp Omelet

Servings: 6
Preparation time: 15 mins
Ingredients
- 6 eggs
- 10 large shrimp, boiled
- 4 grape tomatoes
- Sriracha salt and cayenne pepper, to taste
- 1 handful spinach

Directions
1. Whisk together eggs with all other ingredients in a bowl.

2. Heat a nonstick pan and pour the mixture in it.
3. Cook for about 5 minutes on medium low heat and flip the side.
4. Cook for another 5 minutes and dish out onto a platter to serve.
Nutrition Values:
Calories 90
Total Fat 4.7g
Saturated Fat 1.4g
Cholesterol 183mg
Sodium 93mg
Total Carbohydrate 3.9g
Dietary Fiber 1.1g
Total Sugars 2.5g
Protein 8.5g

359. Egg Pizza Crust

Servings: 4
Preparation time: 25 mins
Ingredients
- 4 eggs
- 2 tablespoons coconut flour
- 2 cups cauliflower, grated
- ½ teaspoon salt
- 1 tablespoon psyllium husk powder

Directions
1. Preheat the oven to 3600F and lightly grease a pizza tray.
2. Mix together all the ingredients in a bowl until well combined and set aside for about 10 minutes.
3. Pour this mixture into the pizza tray and place in the oven.
4. Bake for about 15 minutes until golden brown and remove from the oven.
5. Add your favorite toppings and serve.
Nutrition Values:
Calories 98
Total Fat 4.8g
Saturated Fat 1. 6g
Cholesterol 164mg
Sodium 367mg
Total Carbohydrate 7.5g
Dietary Fiber 4.5g
Total Sugars 1.5g
Protein 7g

360. Coffee Egg Latte

Servings: 2
Preparation time: 15 mins
Ingredients
- 8 ounces black coffee
- 2 tablespoons grass fed butter
- 2 pasture raised eggs
- 1 scoop vanilla collagen protein
- ¼ teaspoon Ceylon cinnamon

Directions
1. Put eggs, butter and coffee in a blender.

2.	Blend until smooth and stir in the collagen protein.
3.	Blend on low and pour into 2 mugs.
4.	Sprinkle with cinnamon and serve hot or chilled as desired.
Nutrition Values:
Calories 189
Total Fat 16g
Saturated Fat 8.8g
Cholesterol 246mg
Sodium 94mg
Total Carbohydrate 1.3g
Dietary Fiber 0.2g
Total Sugars 0g
Protein 10.3g

361. Buttery Egg Waffles

Servings: 4
Preparation time: 30 mins
Ingredients
- 4 tablespoons coconut flour
- 5 eggs, whites separated
- 4 scoops Stevia
- 1 teaspoon baking powder
- ½ cup butter, melted

Directions
1.	Mix together coconut flour, egg yolks, Stevia and baking powder in a bowl.
2.	Add butter and mix well to form a smooth batter.
3.	Whisk egg whites in another bowl until fluffy and pour into the flour mixture.
4.	Put this mixture into a waffle maker and cook until golden in color.
5.	Dish out on plates to serve.
Nutrition Values:
Calories 313
Total Fat 29.3g
Saturated Fat 16.8g
Cholesterol 266mg
Sodium 242mg
Total Carbohydrate 6g
Dietary Fiber 3g
Total Sugars 0.4g
Protein 8.2g

362. Egg and Bacon Breakfast Muffins

Servings: 4
Preparation time: 40 mins
Ingredients
- 4 large eggs
- 4 bacon slices, cooked and crisped
- 1/3 cup green onions, chopped green stem only
- Salt and black pepper, to taste
- ¼ teaspoon paprika

Directions
1.	Preheat the oven to 3500F and lightlygrease muffin tin cavities.

2.	Whisk together eggs in a bowl and add green onions, bacon, paprika, salt and black pepper.
3.	Pour this mixture into the muffin tin cavities and transfer to the oven.
4.	Bake for about 25 minutes and remove from oven to serve.
Nutrition Values:
Calories 177
Total Fat 13g
Saturated Fat 4.2g
Cholesterol 207mg
Sodium 510mg
Total Carbohydrate 1.4g
Dietary Fiber 0.3g
Total Sugars 0.6g
Protein 13.5g

363. Egg Bacon Fat Bombs

Servings: 6
Preparation time: 15 mins
Ingredients
- ¼ cup butter, softened
- 4 large slices bacon, baked
- 2 large eggs, boiled
- 2 tablespoons mayonnaise
- Salt and black pepper, to taste

Directions
1.	Preheat the oven to 3750F and lightly grease a baking tray.
2.	Put the bacon on the baking tray and bake for about 15 minutes.
3.	Remove from the oven, crumble it and set aside.
4.	Mash together boiled eggs with butter, mayonnaise, salt and black pepper with a fork.
5.	Refrigerate for about 1 hour and then form small balls out of this mixture.
6.	Roll the balls into the bacon crumbles and refrigerate for an hour to serve.
Nutrition Values:
Calories 180
Total Fat 16.2g
Saturated Fat 7.4g
Cholesterol 98mg
Sodium 406mg
Total Carbohydrate 1.5g
Dietary Fiber 0g
Total Sugars 0.5g

364. Soft Boiled Eggs with Butter and Thyme

Servings: 3
Preparation time: 20 mins
Ingredients
- 2 tablespoons butter, melted
- 3 large eggs
- ½ teaspoon black pepper
- 2 tablespoons thyme leaves
- ½ teaspoon Himalayan pink salt

Directions

1. Boil eggs in water for about 6 minutes and then put under cold water.
2. Peel the eggs and dip in the melted butter.
3. Top with thyme leaves and season with salt and black pepper to serve.

Nutrition Values:
Calories 145
Total Fat 12.8g
Saturated Fat 6.5g
Cholesterol 206mg
Sodium 631mg
Total Carbohydrate 1.8g
Dietary Fiber 0.8g
Total Sugars 0.4g
Protein 6.6g

SALADS & SOUPS

365. Easy Shrimp Salad

Preparation time: 10 mins
Servings: 6
Ingredients:
For the shrimp:
- 2 minced garlic cloves
- 1 lb. shrimp
- 1 tsp. Cajun spice
- 2 tbsps. olive oil
- For the salad:
- 6 c. lettuce leaves
- 4 chopped tomatoes
- 1 chopped yellow onion
- 1 sliced cucumber
- 2 chopped avocados
- 1 c. corn
- 1 lemon
- ½ bunch chopped parsley
- 2 tbsps. olive oil
- Black pepper

Directions:
1. In a bowl, combine the shrimp with Cajun spice and garlic and toss.
2. Heat up a pan with 2 tablespoons oil over medium-high heat, add shrimp, cook each side for 2 minutes and set to a bowl.
3. Add lettuce, tomatoes, onion, cucumber, avocado, corn and a pinch of pepper and toss.
4. In a small bowl, mix 2 tablespoons oil with parsley and lemon juice, whisk well, pour over the salad, toss and serve for lunch.

Nutrition Values:
Calories: 210 Fat 4g, Carbs 28g, protein 14g.

366. Easy Veggie Soup

Preparation time: 10 mins
Servings: 6
Ingredients:
- 1 tbsp. olive oil
- 1 chopped yellow onion
- 2 chopped celery ribs
- 2 chopped carrots
- 2 c. mixed zucchini and cauliflower florets
- black pepper
- 1 tsp. dried thyme
- ½ tsp. garlic powder
- 1 tsp. dried oregano
- 8 c. veggie stock
- 1 bay leaf
- 14 oz. chopped canned tomatoes

Directions:
1. Add oil in a pot and heat over medium-high heat, add onion, celery and carrots, stir and sauté them for 4 minutes.
2. Add zucchini, cauliflower, black pepper, thyme, garlic powder, oregano, bay leaf, tomatoes and stock, stir, bring to a simmer and cook for 16 minutes.
3. Stir the soup one more time, ladle it into bowls and serve for a dash diet lunch. Enjoy!

Nutrition Values:
Calories: 180 Fat 2g, Carbs 28g, protein 8g .

367. Seafood Salad

Preparation time: 15 mins
Servings: 4
Ingredients:
- 1 big octopus
- 1 lb. mussels
- 2 lbs. clams
- 1 big squid
- 3 chopped garlic cloves
- 1 celery rib
- ½ c. sliced celery rib
- 1 carrot
- 1 chopped white onion
- 1 bay leaf
- ¾ c. veggie stock
- 2 c. sliced radicchio
- 1 sliced red onion
- 1 c. chopped parsley
- 1 c. olive oil
- 1 c. red wine vinegar
- Black pepper

Directions:
1. Place the octopus in a large pot with celery rib cut into thirds, garlic, carrot, bay leaf, white onion and stock. Add water to cover the octopus, cover the pot, bring to a boil over high heat, and reduce temperature to low, simmer for 1 hour and 30 minutes. Drain octopus, reserve boiling liquid and leave it aside to cool down.
2. Put ¼ cup octopus cooking liquid in another pot, add mussels, heat up over medium-high heat, cook until they open, transfer to a bowl and leave aside.
3. Add clams to the pan, cover, cook over medium-high heat until they open as well, transfer to the bowl with mussels and leave aside.

4.   Add squid to the pan, cover and cook over medium-high heat for 3 minutes, transfer to the bowl with mussels and clams.
5.   Meanwhile, slice octopus into small pieces and mix with the rest of the seafood.
6.   Add sliced celery, radicchio, red onion, vinegar, olive oil, parsley, salt and pepper, toss and leave aside in the fridge for 2 hours before serving. Enjoy!

Nutrition Values:
Calories: 200 Fat 8g, carbs 28g, protein 4g

368. Caesar Salad

Preparation time: 10 mins
Servings: 4
Ingredients:
- 1 lb. chicken breast
- Cooking spray
- Black pepper
- ½ c. cubed feta cheese
- 2 tbsps. lemon juice
- 1½ tsps. Dijon mustard
- 1 tbsp. olive oil
- 1½ tsps. red wine vinegar
- ¾ tsp. minced garlic
- 1 tbsp. water
- 1 tsp. Worcestershire sauce
- 8 c. lettuce leaves
- 4 tbsps. grated parmesan
- 1¼ whole wheat croutons

Directions:
1.   Spray chicken breasts with some cooking spray and season black pepper to the taste.
2.   Heat up your kitchen grill over medium-high heat, add chicken breasts, cook for 6 minutes on each side, transfer to a cutting board, cool down for a few minutes, cut in small pieces, transfer to a salad bowl, add lettuce and croutons and leave aside.
3.   In your blender, mix feta with lemon juice, olive oil, mustard, vinegar, Worcestershire sauce and garlic and pulse well.
4.   Add the water and half of the parmesan and blend some more.
5.   Add this to your salad, toss to coat, sprinkle the rest of the parmesan and serve.

Nutrition Values:
Calories: 200 Fat 10g, Carbs 18g, protein 10g.

369. Greek Chicken Salad

Preparation time: 10 minutes
Servings: 4
Ingredients:
- 15 oz. canned chickpeas
- 9 oz. chicken breast
- 1 chopped cucumber
- 4 chopped green onions
- Black pepper
- ½ c. yoghurt
- ¼ c. chopped mint

- 2 c. baby spinach
- 2 minced garlic cloves
- 1/3 c. feta cheese
- 4 lemon wedges

Directions:
1.   In a salad bowl, mix chicken meat with chickpeas, cucumber, onions, mint, garlic, salt and pepper.
2.   Add yogurt, spinach and feta and toss to coat.
3.   Serve with lemon wedges on the side.
4.   Enjoy!

Nutrition Values:
Calories: 180 Fat 10g, Carbs 16g, protein 10g.

370. Chicken Soup

Preparation time: 10 mins
Servings: 6
Ingredients:
- 1 whole chicken
- 6 chopped celery stalks
- 6 sliced carrots
- 1 onion
- 1 bunch parsley springs
- 1 bunch dill springs
- 2 tbsps. chopped dill
- 3 garlic cloves
- 2 tbsps. black peppercorns
- black pepper
- 2 bay leaves
- ¼ tsp. saffron threads

Directions:
1.   Put chicken pieces in a pot, add water to cover, bring to a boil over medium-high heat, cook for 15 minutes and skim foam.
2.   Add celery, onion, carrots, parsley springs, dill springs, whole cloves, bay leaves, peppercorns and some black pepper, stir, cover pot, reduce heat to medium-low and simmer for 1 hour and 30 minutes.
3.   Take chicken pieces out and leave them aside to cool down.
4.   Strain soup into another pot, reserve carrots and celery but discard herbs and spices.
5.   Discard bones from the chicken, cut meat into strips and return to pot.
6.   Heat up the soup with reserved veggies, add chicken pieces, crushed saffron and chopped dill and stir.
7.   Ladle soup into bowls and serve. Enjoy!

Nutrition Values:
Calories: 200 Fat 10g, Carbs 16g, protein 12g.

371. Pumpkin Soup

Preparation time: 10 mins
Servings: 4
Ingredients:
- 1 chopped yellow onion
- ¾ c. water
- 15 oz. pumpkin puree

- 2 c. veggie stock
- ½ tsp. cinnamon powder
- ¼ tsp. ground nutmeg
- 1 c. fat-free milk
- Black pepper
- 1 chopped green onion

Directions:
1.	Put the water in a pot, bring to a simmer over medium heat, add onion, stock and pumpkin puree and stir.
2.	Add cinnamon, nutmeg, milk and black pepper, stir, cook for 10 minutes, ladle into bowls, sprinkle green onion on top and serve.
3.	Enjoy!

Nutrition Values:
Calories: 180 Fat 10g, Carbs 22g, protein 14g.

372. Spicy Black Bean Soup

Preparation time: 10 mins
Servings: 8
Ingredients:
- 1 lb. black beans
- 2 chopped yellow onions
- 2 quarts low-sodium veggie stock
- 2 tbsps. olive oil
- 6 minced garlic cloves
- 2 chopped tomatoes
- 2 chopped jalapenos
- ½ tsp. dried oregano
- 1 tsp. ground cumin
- 1 tsp. grated ginger
- 2 bay leaves
- 1 tbsp. chili powder
- 3 tbsps. balsamic vinegar
- Black pepper
- ½ c. chopped scallions

Directions:
1.	Put the stock in a pot, bring to a simmer over medium heat, add beans, cover and cook for 45 minutes.
2.	Meanwhile, heat up a pan with the oil over medium-high heat, add ginger, garlic and onion, stir and cook for 5 minutes.
3.	Add tomatoes, cumin, jalapeno, oregano and chili powder, stir, cook for 3 minutes more and transfer to the pot with the beans.
4.	Add bay leaves, and cook the soup for 40 minutes more while the pot is covered.
5.	Add vinegar, stir, cook the soup for 15 minutes more, discard bay leaves, blend the soup using an immersion blender, ladle into bowls and serve with scallions on top. Enjoy!

Nutrition Values:
Calories: 220, fat 10, carbs 34, protein 14

373. Shrimp Soup

Preparation time: 10 mins
Servings: 6
Ingredients:

- 8 oz. shrimp
- 1 stalk lemongrass
- 2 grated ginger
- 6 c. low-sodium chicken stock
- 2 chopped jalapenos
- 4 lime leaves
- 1½ c. chopped pineapple
- 1 c. chopped shiitake mushroom caps
- 1 chopped tomato
- ½ cubed bell pepper
- 1 tsp. stevia
- ¼ c. lime juice
- 1/3 c. chopped cilantro
- 2 sliced scallions

Directions:
1.	In a pot, mix ginger with lemongrass, stock, jalapenos and lime leaves, stir, bring to a boil over medium heat, cover, cook for 15 minutes, strain liquid in a bowl and discard solids.
2.	Return soup to the pot again, add pineapple, tomato, mushrooms, bell pepper, sugar and fish sauce, stir, bring to a boil over medium heat, cook for 5 minutes, add shrimp and cook for 3 more minutes.
3.	Add lime juice, cilantro and scallions, stir, ladle into soup bowls and serve.
4.	Enjoy!

Nutrition Values:
Calories: 190 Fat 8g, Carbs 30g, protein 6g.

374. Mayo-less Tuna Salad

Preparation time: 5 mins
Servings: 2
Ingredients:
- 5 oz. Tuna
- 1 tbsp. extra virgin Olive oil
- 1 tbsp. Red wine vinegar
- ¼ c. chopped green onion
- 2 c. Arugula
- 1 c. cooked Pasta
- 1 tbsp. Parmesan cheese
- Black pepper

Directions:
1.	Combine all your ingredients into a medium bowl.
2.	Split mixture between two plates.
3.	Serve, and enjoy.

Nutrition Values:
Calories: 213.2 Protein 22.7g, Carbs 20.3g, Fat 6.2g,

375. Chestnut Soup

Preparation time: 10 mins
Servings: 3
Ingredients:
- 30 oz. whole roasted chestnuts
- 1 chopped shallot
- ½ c. heavy cream
- ½ c. chicken stock
- 1 chopped leek
- 2 tbsps. butter

- 1 sprig thyme
- 1 bay leaf
- 1 chopped celery stalk
- ½ tsp. nutmeg
- Salt
- pepper

Directions:
1. Add butter, carrot, leek, shallot, and celery in a saucepan over medium heat. Cook for 6-7 minutes or until the vegetables are tender.
2. Add stock, thyme, bay leaf, chestnuts and bring to boil. Reduce heat and simmer for 25 minutes.
3. Remove from the heat and discard the thyme and bay leaf.
4. Allow to cool slightly and puree using an immersion blender.
5. Heat the soup again as you stir in the cream, nutmeg and season to taste.
6. Cook for 5 minutes more.
7. Serve while still hot.

Nutrition Values:
Calories: 191 Protein 6g, Carbs 25g, Fat 18g.

376. Pepper Pot Soup

Preparation time: 10 mins
Servings: 6
- **Ingredients:**
- 4 quarts chicken stock
- 3 tbsps. butter
- 2 diced potatoes
- ½ diced breadfruit
- 1 lb. diced yam
- ½ lb. diced cocoa
- 2 crushed garlic cloves
- 2 sprigs thyme
- 1 scotch bonnet
- 3 chopped green onion
- ½ c. Coconut Milk
- 10 pimento berries
- 2 chopped callaloo

Directions:
1. In a reasonable size soup pot, boil 4 quarts of stock.
2. Add garlic, potato, breadfruit, yam, cocoa, and stir.
3. Bring soup to a boil add thyme, green onion, pimento, callaloo, coconut milk, and pepper.
4. Stir, and cook until done.

Nutrition Values:
Calories: 250.3 Protein 15.5g, Carbs 22.8g, Fat 11.3g.

377. Quinoa & Avocado Salad

Preparation time: 10 mins
Servings: 2
Ingredients:
- 1½ c. Cooked Quinoa
- 4 oz. julienned Cucumber
- 4 oz. julienned Carrots
- ½ diced Avocado

- ½ c. Brussels Sprouts

Directions:
1. Split your Quinoa into 2 medium bowls.
2. Mix in your minced nori.
3. Top with your cucumber, avocado, and carrot.
4. Add blanched Brussel Sprouts.
5. Serve and enjoy!

Nutrition Values:
Calories: 472 Protein 11.2g, Carbs 50.6g, Fat 27.4g.

378. Kale Salad with Mixed Vegetables

Preparation time: 10 mins
Servings: 4
Ingredients:
- 1 bunch chopped Premier kale
- 1 c. fresh peas
- 2 chopped carrots
- 1 c. boiled potatoes
- 1 c. sliced cabbage
- 2 tbsps. apple cider vinegar
- 1 tsp. chili powder
- ½ tsp. salt
- 2 tbsps. coconut oil
- 1 tsp. coconut powder

Directions:
1. Combine all vegetables with kale.
2. Drizzle vinegar and coconut oil.
3. Season with salt and chili powder.
4. Sprinkle coconut powder and toss to combine.
5. Add to a serving dish and serve. Enjoy.

Nutrition Values:
Calories: 240 Protein 9g, Carbs 36g, Fat 9g.

379. Cream of Corn Soup

Preparation time: 15 mins
Servings: 4
Ingredients:
- 0.5 lb. Corn puree
- 0.5 lb. carrots
- 2 c. vegetable stock
- ½ c. chopped onion
- ½ tsp. Salt
- ¼ tsp. Pepper
- 1 tsp. dried thyme
- 2 oz. chopped celery
- ½ tbsp. olive oil
- 1 anise star

Directions:
1. Heat olive oil in medium pot and add onion; add celery, carrots and sauté for 15 minutes, until onion is caramelized.
2. Add corn and stir until corn is tender.
3. Add thyme and stir well.
4. Transfer the vegetables in a blender, add pumpkin puree, vegetable stock, and pulse until smooth.

5. Transfer the mixture into sauce pan and simmer, add anise star and simmer over medium-high heat for 5-8 minutes or until heated through.
6. Remove the anise star and discard.
7. Serve immediately.
Nutrition Values:
Calories: 223 Protein 7.84g, Carbs 23.98g, Fat 11.51g.

380. Clam Soup

Preparation time: 15 mins
Servings: 4
Ingredients:
- 1½ c. Water
- ½ fresh ginger
- 1 lb. Manila clams
- 1 tbsp. Chinese rice white wine
- ¼ tsp. Salt
- ¼ tsp. White Pepper

Directions:
1. In a large pot, boil water and add clams and ginger.
2. Cook until clams open then add wine.
3. Add pepper and salt and serve hot.
Nutrition Values:
Calories: 80 Protein 3g, Carbs 16g, Fat 0.5g.

381. Apple & Peach Salad

Preparation time: 3 mins
Servings: 3
Ingredients:
- 2 chopped apples
- 1 c. peach
- 1 c. blackberries
- 1 tbsp. lime juice
- 1 tbsp. honey
- ¼ tsp. dried thyme
- ¼ tsp. sugar
- 1 tsp. salt

Directions:
1. Toss all ingredients together and put into serving dish.
2. Serve and enjoy.
Nutrition Values:
Calories: 528 Protein 34g, Carbs 13g, Fat 37g.

382. Chicken, Apple & Basil Salad

Preparation time: 6 mins
Servings: 4
Ingredients:
- 4 c. Basil
- 2 c. chopped Apple
- 2 c. chopped Chicken Breast
- ½ c. sliced Red Onion
- ¼ c. chopped Pecans
- ¾ c. Acai Dressing

Directions:
1. Set 4 salad bowls on the table and add basil to each.
2. Add each of your remaining ingredients as layers on top of the greens.

3. Once satisfied, drizzle each bowl of salad with 3 tablespoons of dressing.
Nutrition Values:
Calories: 269 Protein 34g, Carbs 20g, Fat 8g.

383. Curried Quinoa Sweet Potato Salad

Preparation time: 12 mins
Servings: 6
Ingredients:
- 1 c. Curried Quinoa
- 6 chopped Sweet Potatoes
- 1 c. Water
- ¼ c. chopped Onion
- 1 chopped Celery
- Salt
- Pepper
- 3 boiled Eggs
- 1 tbsp. chopped Dill
- ½ c. Mayonnaise
- 1 tsp. Yellow Mustard
- 1 tsp. Vinegar

Directions:
1. Pour in your potatoes and water into the cooker.
2. Securely close the lid and allow to rise to high pressure over a high flame. Cook for about 3 minutes.
3. Remove the cooker from the flame and cool under cold running water.
4. Proceed to peel and dice potatoes then layer them alternately with celery and onion.
5. Season with salt and pepper then add your dill and chopped eggs.
6. In a separate bowl combine the mustard, mayonnaise, and vinegar then fold the mixture gently into the potatoes.
7. Stir in your cooked quinoa.
8. Chill, serve and enjoy!
Nutrition Values:
Calories: 335.3 Protein 5.5g, Carbs 55.2g, Fat 9g.

384. Banana Salad

Preparation time: 5 mins
Servings: 3
Ingredients:
- 4 sliced bananas
- ¼ c. pineapple sauce
- ¼ sliced onion
- 1 tbsp. lime juice
- ¼ tsp. cinnamon powder
- ¼ tsp. chili flakes

Directions:
1. In a bowl add bananas, pineapple sauce, lemon juice, ad mix.
2. Now season with cinnamon and chili flakes.
3. Serve and enjoy.
Nutrition Values:
Calories: 221 Protein 1.1g, Carbs 57.5g, Fat 0.3g.

385. Ranch Dressing

Servings: 12
Preparation time: 10 minutes
Ingredients
- 1 cup mayonnaise
- ½ cup sour cream
- ¼ cup unsweetened almond milk
- 2 teaspoons fresh lemon juice
- 2 teaspoons dried parsley
- 1 teaspoon dried chives
- 1 teaspoon dried dill
- ½ teaspoon garlic powder
- ½ teaspoon onion powder
- Salt and ground black pepper, as required

Directions:
1. Add all the ingredients in a large bowl and beat until well combined.
2. Refrigerate to chill before serving.

Nutrition Values:
Calories: 99
Net Carbs: 5.3g
Carbohydrate: 5.4g
Fiber: 0.1g
Protein: 0.6g
Fat: 8.6g
Sugar: 1.4g
Sodium: 60mg

386. French Dressing

Servings: 20
Preparation time: 10 minutes
Ingredients
- 1 small yellow onion, roughly chopped
- 1½ cups olive oil
- 1 cup sugar-free ketchup
- ¾ cup Erythritol
- ½ cup balsamic vinegar
- 1 teaspoon fresh lemon juice
- 1 teaspoon paprika
- ½ teaspoon salt

Directions:
1. Add all the ingredients in a blender and pulse until smooth.
2. Serve immediately.

Nutrition Values:
Calories: 144
Net Carbs: 3.3g
Carbohydrate: 3.5g
Fiber: 0.2g
Protein: 0.3g
Fat: 15.2g
Sugar: 2.9g
Sodium: 61mg

387. Caesar Dressing

Servings: 16
Preparation time: 10 minutes
Ingredients
- 1 organic egg yolk
- 2 tablespoons fresh lemon juice
- 1 tablespoon anchovy paste
- 2 teaspoons Dijon mustard
- 2 garlic cloves, peeled
- 1 tablespoon fresh oregano
- Salt and ground black pepper, as required
- ½ cup olive oil
- ½ cup Parmesan cheese, shredded

Directions:
1. Place all the ingredients except oil and Parmesan in a blender and pulse until smooth.
2. While the motor is running gradually, add the oil and pulse until smooth.
3. Add the Parmesan cheese and pulse for about 20 seconds.
4. Serve immediately.

Nutrition Values:
Calories: 72
Net Carbs: 0.3g
Carbohydrate: 0.5g
Fiber: 0.2g
Protein: 1.3g
Fat: 8.7g
Sugar: 0.1g
Sodium: 121mg

388. Yogurt Dressing

Servings: 8
Preparation time: 10 minutes
Ingredients
- 1 -8-ouncescontainer plain Greek yogurt
- 2 teaspoons fresh lemon juice
- 1 teaspoon fresh chives, chopped
- 1 teaspoon fresh parsley, chopped
- 1 teaspoon Dijon mustard

Directions:
1. Place the yogurt and lemon juice in a bowl and beat until well combined and smooth.
2. Now, place the remaining ingredients and stir until well combined.
3. Refrigerate before serving.

Nutrition Values:
Calories: 21
Net Carbs: 2.1g
Carbohydrate: 2.1g
Fiber: 0g
Protein: 1.7g
Fat: 0.4g
Sugar: 2g
Sodium: 27mg

389. Blue Cheese Dressing

Servings: 24
Preparation time: 10 minutes
Ingredients
- 1 cup blue cheese, crumbled
- 1 cup sour cream
- 1 cup mayonnaise
- 2-4 drops liquid stevia

- 2 teaspoons fresh lemon juice
- 2 teaspoons Worcestershire sauce
- 1 teaspoon hot pepper sauce
- 2 tablespoons fresh parsley, chopped
- Salt and ground black pepper, as required

Directions:
1. Add all the ingredients in a large bowl and beat until well combined.
2. Refrigerate to chill before serving.

Nutrition Values:
Calories: 101
Net Carbs: 0.7g
Carbohydrate: 0.7g
Fiber: 0g
Protein: 1.5g
Fat: 10.3g
Sugar: 0.1g
Sodium: 156mg

390. Olives & Feta Dressing

Servings: 16
Preparation time: 10 minutes
Ingredients
- 3 tablespoons feta cheese, crumbled
- 3 tablespoons kalamata olives, pitted and chopped
- 2 tablespoons yellow onion, chopped
- 1 garlic clove, chopped
- 6-8 drops liquid stevia
- 1 tablespoon Dijon mustard
- 3 tablespoons fresh lemon juice
- 3 tablespoons olive oil
- 1 teaspoon dried oregano, crushed
- Salt and ground black pepper, as required

Directions:
1. Add all the ingredients in a blender and pulse until smooth.
2. Serve immediately.

Nutrition Values:
Calories: 31
Net Carbs: 0.3g
Carbohydrate: 0.5g
Fiber: 0.2g
Protein: 0.4g
Fat: 3.2g
Sugar: 0.2g
Sodium: 57mg

391. Creamy Mustard Dressing

Servings: 8
Preparation time: 10 minutes
Ingredients
- ½ cup sour cream
- ¼ cup water
- ¼ cup Dijon mustard
- 1 tablespoon organic apple cider vinegar
- 1 tablespoon granulated Erythritol

Directions:

Add all the ingredients in a large bowl and beat until well combined.
Serve immediately.
Nutrition Values:
Calories: 36
Net Carbs: 0.8g
Carbohydrate: 1.1g
Fiber: 0.3g
Protein: 0.8g
Fat: 3.3g
Sugar: 0.1g
Sodium: 97mg

392. Sunflower Seeds Dressing

Servings: 5
Preparation time: 1 minutes
Ingredients
- ½ cup sunflower seeds
- 1/3 cup organic apple cider vinegar
- ½ cup water
- 1 tablespoon Dijon mustard
- 1 teaspoon ground turmeric
- Salt and ground black pepper, as required
- ¼ cup olive oil

Directions:
1. Add all the ingredients except oil in a blender and pulse until smooth.
2. While the motor is running gradually, add the oil and pulse until smooth.
3. Serve immediately.

Nutrition Values:
Calories: 120
Net Carbs: 0.9g
Carbohydrate: 1.5g
Fiber: 0.6g
Protein: 1.1g
Fat: 12.6g
Sugar: 0.2g
Sodium: 69mg

393. Italian Dressing

Servings: 12
Preparation time: 10 minutes
Ingredients
- 1 cup olive oil
- ½ cup balsamic vinegar
- 1 teaspoon dried basil
- ½ teaspoon dried oregano
- 1/8 teaspoon dried marjoram
- Salt and ground black pepper, as required
- 2 tablespoons Pecorino Romano cheese, grated finely
- 1 tablespoon garlic, minced

Directions:
1. Place the oil, vinegar, dried herbs, salt, and black pepper in a blender and pulse until well combined.
2. Place the dressing into a bowl and stir in the cheese and garlic.
3. Serve.

Nutrition Values:
Calories: 152
Net Carbs: 0.4g
Carbohydrate: 0.4g
Fiber: 0g
Protein: 0.4g
Fat: 17.1g
Sugar: 0.1g
Sodium: 36mg

394. Raspberry Dressing

Servings: 10
Preparation time: 10 minutes
Ingredients
- ½ cup olive oil
- ¼ cup MCT oil
- ¼ cup organic apple cider vinegar
- 2 tablespoons Dijon mustard
- 1½ teaspoons fresh tarragon leaves, chopped
- ¼ teaspoon Erythritol
- Pinch of salt
- ½ cup fresh raspberries, mashed

Directions:
1. Place all the ingredients except raspberries in a bowl and beat until smooth.
2. Transfer the mixture into a bowl.
3. Now, add the mashed raspberries and stir to combine well.
4. Serve immediately.

Nutrition Values:
Calories: 133
Net Carbs: 0.5g
Carbohydrate: 1g
Fiber: 0.5g
Protein: 0.2g
Fat: 15.9g
Sugar: 0.2g
Sodium: 51mg

395. Cranberry Sauce

Servings: 6
Preparation time: 10 minutes
Cooking Time: 15 minutes
Ingredients
- 12 ounces fresh cranberries
- 1 cup powdered Erythritol
- ¾ cup water
- 1 teaspoon fresh lemon zest, grated
- ½ teaspoon organic vanilla extract

Directions:
1. Place the cranberries, water, Erythritol and lemon zest in a medium pan and mix well.
2. Place the pan over medium heat and bring to a boil.
3. Adjust the heat to low and simmer for about 12-15 minutes, stirring frequently.
4. Remove the pan from heat and mix in the vanilla extract.

5. Set aside at room temperature to cool completely.
6. Transfer the sauce into a bowl and refrigerate to chill before serving.

Nutrition Values:
Calories: 32
Net Carbs: 3.1g
Carbohydrate: 5.2g
Fiber: 2.1g
Protein: 0g
Fat: 0g
Sugar: 2.1g
Sodium: 160mg

396. Ketchup

Servings: 12
Preparation time: 10 minutes
Cooking Time: 30 minutes
Ingredients
- 6 ounces sugar-free tomato paste
- 1 cup water
- ¼ cup powdered Erythritol
- 3 tablespoons balsamic vinegar
- ½ teaspoon garlic powder
- ½ teaspoon onion powder
- ¼ teaspoon paprika
- 1/8 teaspoon ground cloves
- 1/8 tsp mustard powder
- Salt, as required

Directions:
1. Add all the ingredients in a small pan and beat until smooth.
2. Now, place the pan over medium heat and bring to a gentle simmer, stirring continuously.
3. Adjust the heat to low and simmer, covered for about 30 minutes or until desired thickness, stirring occasionally.
4. Remove the pan from heat and let it cool completely before serving.
5. You can preserve this ketchup in the refrigerator by placing in an airtight container.

Nutrition Values:
Calories: 13
Net Carbs: 2.3g
Carbohydrate: 2.9g
Fiber: 0.6g
Protein: 0.7g
Fat: 0.1g
Sugar: 1.8g
Sodium: 26mg
-Note: For the best consistency, puree the ketchup in a high-speed blender until smooth.

397. Cilantro Sauce

Servings: 6
Preparation time: 10 minutes
Ingredients
- ½ cup plain Greek yogurt
- ½ cup fresh cilantro, chopped
- 6 garlic cloves, peeled

- 1 jalapeño pepper, chopped
- Salt, as required
- ¼ cup water

Directions:
1. Add all the ingredients in a blender and pulse until smooth.
2. Transfer the sauce into a bowl and set aside for about 15-20 minutes before serving.

Nutrition Values:
Calories: 20
Net Carbs: 2.4g
Carbohydrate: 2.6g
Fiber: 0.2g
Protein: 1.4g
Fat: 0.3g
Sugar: 1.6g
Sodium: 43mg

398. Avocado Sauce

Servings: 8
Preparation time: 15 minutes
Ingredients
1. 2 avocados, peeled, pitted and chopped
2. ½ cup yellow onion, chopped
3. 1 cup fresh cilantro leaves
4. 2 garlic cloves, chopped
5. 1 jalapeño pepper, chopped
6. 1 cup homemade vegetable broth
7. 2 tablespoons fresh lemon juice
8. 2 teaspoons balsamic vinegar
9. 1 teaspoon ground cumin
10. Pinch of cayenne pepper
11. Salt, as required

Directions:
1. Add all the ingredients in a blender and pulse until smooth.
2. Serve immediately.

Nutrition Values:
Calories: 115
Net Carbs: 2.1g
Carbohydrate: 5.8g
Fiber: 3.7g
Protein: 1.8g
Fat: 10.1g
Sugar: 0.8g
Sodium: 120mg

398. Herbed Capers Sauce

Servings: 4
Preparation time: 10 minutes
Ingredients
- ½ cup fresh parsley, finely chopped
- 3 tablespoons fresh basil, finely chopped
- 2 garlic cloves, crushed
- 1 tablespoon fresh lemon juice
- 2 tablespoons small capers
- ¾ cup olive oil
- Salt and ground black pepper, as required

Directions:

1. Add all the ingredients into a shallow bowl and with an immersion blender, blend until the desired consistency is achieved.
2. Serve immediately.

Nutrition Values:
Calories: 331
Net Carbs: 0.8g
Carbohydrate: 1.3g
Fiber: 0.5g
Protein: 0.5g
Fat: 38g
Sugar: 0.2g
Sodium: 172mg

400. Basil Pesto

Servings: 6
Preparation time: 10 minutes
Ingredients
- 2 cups fresh basil
- 4 garlic cloves, peeled
- 2/3 cup Parmesan cheese, grated
- 1/3 cup pine nuts
- ½ cup olive oil
- Salt and ground black pepper, as required

Directions:
1. Place the basil, garlic, Parmesan cheese and pine nuts in a food processor and pulse until a chunky mixture is formed.
2. While the motor is running gradually, add the oil and pulse until smooth.
3. Now, add the salt, and black pepper and pulse until well combined.
4. Serve immediately.

Nutrition Values:
Calories: 232
Net Carbs: 1.4g
Carbohydrate: 1.9g
Fiber: 0.5g
Protein: 5g
Fat: 24.2g
Sugar: 0.3g
Sodium: 104mg

401. Veggie Hummus

Servings: 8
Preparation time: 10 minutes
Ingredients
- 2½ tablespoons olive oil, divided
- 1 cup zucchini, peeled and chopped
- ¾ cup pumpkin puree
- ¼ cup tahini
- 2 tablespoons fresh lemon juice
- 1 teaspoon ground cumin
- 1 teaspoon garlic powder
- ½ teaspoon smoked paprika
- Salt, as required

Directions:
1. Place 2 tablespoons of oil and the remaining ingredients in a blender and pulse until smooth.

2.   Place the hummus into a bowl and drizzle with remaining oil.
3.   Serve immediately.

Nutrition Values:
Calories: 96
Net Carbs: 2.7g
Carbohydrate: 4.4g
Fiber: 1.7g
Protein: 1.9g
Fat: 8.6g
Sugar: 1.2g
Sodium: 32mg

402. Tzatziki

Servings: 12
Preparation time: 10 minutes

Ingredients
- 1 large English cucumber, peeled and grated
- Salt, as required
- 2 cups plain Greek yogurt
- 1 tablespoon fresh lemon juice
- 4 garlic cloves, minced
- 1 tablespoon fresh mint leaves, chopped
- 2 tablespoons fresh dill, chopped
- Pinch of cayenne pepper
- Freshly ground black pepper, as required

Directions:
1.   Arrange a colander in the sink.
2.   Place the cucumber into colander and sprinkle with salt.
3.   Let it drain for about 10-15 minutes.
4.   With your hands, squeeze the cucumber well.
5.   Place the cucumber and remaining ingredients in a large bowl and stir to combine.
6.   Cover the bowl and refrigerate to chill for at least 4-8 hours before serving.

Nutrition Values:
Calories: 36
Net Carbs: 4.2g
Carbohydrate: 4.5g
Fiber: 0.3g
Protein: 2.7g
Fat: 0.6g
Sugar: 3.3g
Sodium: 42mg

403. Baba Ghanoush

Servings: 8
Preparation time: 15 minutes
Cooking Time: 35 minutes

Ingredients
- 2 large eggplants
- 3 teaspoons olive oil
- 2 garlic cloves, chopped
- 2 tablespoons tahini
- 2 tablespoons fresh lemon juice
- 1 teaspoon ground cumin
- Salt and ground black pepper, as required

- 1 tablespoon fresh parsley leaves

Directions:
1.   Preheat the oven to 400 degrees F. Grease a baking dish.
2.   Arrange the eggplants into prepared baking dish in a single layer.
3.   Bake for about 35 minutes.
4.   Remove the eggplants from oven and immediately, place into a bowl of cold water to cool slightly.
5.   Now, peel off the skin of eggplants.
6.   Place the eggplants, 2 teaspoons of oil and remaining ingredients except parsley and pulse until smooth.
7.   Place the mixture into a serving bowl and refrigerate to chill before serving.
8.   Drizzle with the remaining oil and serve with garnishing of fresh parsley.

Nutrition Values:
Calories: 75
Net Carbs: 4g
Carbohydrate: 9.3g
Fiber: 5.3g
Protein: 2.1g
Fat: 4.1g
Sugar: 4.2g
Sodium: 28mg

404. Salsa Verde

Servings: 10
Preparation time: 15 minutes
Cooking Time: 40 minutes

Ingredients
- 2 pounds medium tomatillos, husks removed and halved
- 2 large yellow onions, roughly chopped
- 6 garlic cloves, peeled and halved
- 2 Serrano peppers, seeded and chopped
- ¼ cup olive oil
- 1/3-½ cup water
- ½ cup fresh cilantro, chopped
- 2 tablespoons fresh lime juice
- Pinch of salt

Directions:
1.   Preheat the oven to 425 degrees F.
2.   In a large bowl, add the tomatillos, onions, garlic, peppers, and oil and toss to coat well.
3.   Place the mixture onto 2 -15x10x1-inchbaking sheets and spread in an even layer.
4.   Roast for about 35-40 minutes, stirring occasionally.
5.   Remove both baking sheets from the oven and set aside to cool slightly.
6.   Place the tomatillo mixture and enough water in a food processor and pulse until smooth.
7.   Now, add the remaining ingredients and pulse until just combined.
8.   Transfer the mixture into a bowl and refrigerate to chill before serving.

Nutrition Values:

Calories: 84
Net Carbs: 5.8g
Carbohydrate: 8.1g
Fiber: 2.3g
Protein: 1.3g
Fat: 6g
Sugar: 1g
Sodium: 18mg

405. Pizza Sauce

Servings: 8
Preparation time: 15 minutes
Cooking Time: 45 minutes
Ingredients
- 2 tablespoons olive oil
- 2 anchovy fillets
- 2 tablespoons fresh oregano leaves, finely chopped
- 3 garlic cloves, minced
- ½ teaspoon dried oregano, crushed
- ½ teaspoon red pepper flakes, crushed
- 1 -28-ouncescan whole peeled tomatoes, crushed
- ½ teaspoon Erythritol
- Salt, as required
- Pinch of freshly ground black pepper
- Pinch of organic baking powder

Directions:
1. Heat the olive oil in a medium pan over medium-low heat and cook the anchovy fillets for about 1 minute, stirring occasionally.
2. Stir in the fresh oregano, garlic, dried oregano, and red pepper flakes and sauté for about 2-3 minutes.
3. Add the remaining ingredients except baking powder and bring to a gentle simmer.
4. Reduce the heat to low and simmer for about 35-40 minutes, stirring occasionally.
5. Stir in the baking powder and remove from heat.
6. Set aside at room temperature to cool completely before serving.
7. You can preserve this sauce in refrigerator by placing into an airtight container.

Nutrition Values:
Calories: 56
Net Carbs: 3.4g
Carbohydrate: 5.1g
Fiber: 1.7g
Protein: 1.4g
Fat: 4g
Sugar: 2.7g
Sodium: 61mg

406. Marinara Sauce

Servings: 12
Preparation time: 10 minutes / Total Cooking Time: 5 minutes
Ingredients
- 2 tablespoons olive oil

- 1 garlic clove
- 2 teaspoons onion flakes
- 2 teaspoons fresh thyme, finely chopped
- 2 teaspoons fresh oregano, finely chopped
- 24 ounces tomato puree
- 1 tablespoon balsamic vinegar
- 2 teaspoons Erythritol
- Salt and ground black pepper, as required
- 2 tablespoons fresh parsley, finely chopped

Directions:
1. Heat the olive oil in a medium pan over medium-low heat and sauté the garlic, onion flakes, thyme and oregano for about 3 minutes.
2. Stir in the tomato puree, vinegar, Erythritol, salt, and black pepper and bring to a gentle simmer.
3. Remove the pan of sauce from heat and stir in the parsley.
4. Set aside at room temperature to cool completely before serving.
5. You can preserve this sauce in refrigerator by placing into an airtight container.

Nutrition Values:
Calories: 36
Net Carbs: 3.6g
Carbohydrate: 4.7g
Fiber: 1.1g
Protein: 0.9g
Fat: 2g
Sugar: 2.3g
Sodium: 168mg

407. BBQ Sauce

Servings: 20
Preparation time: 15 minutes
Cooking Time: 20 minutes
Ingredients
- 2½ -6-ouncescans tomato paste
- ½ cup organic apple cider vinegar
- 1/3 cup powdered Erythritol
- 2 tablespoons Worcestershire sauce
- 1 tablespoon liquid hickory smoke
- 2 teaspoons smoked paprika
- 1 teaspoon garlic powder
- ½ teaspoon onion powder
- Salt, as required
- ¼ teaspoon red chili powder
- ¼ teaspoon cayenne pepper
- 1½ cups water

Directions:
1. Add all the ingredients except water in a pan and beat until well combined.
2. Add 1 cup of water and beat until combined.
3. Add the remaining water and beat until well combined.
4. Place the pan over medium-high heat and bring to a gentle boil.
5. Adjust the heat to medium-low and simmer, uncovered for about 20 minutes, stirring frequently.

6.　　　Remove from the heat and set aside to cool slightly before serving.
7.　　　You can preserve this sauce in refrigerator by placing into an airtight container.
Nutrition Values:
Calories: 22
Net Carbs: 3.7g
Carbohydrate: 4.7g
Fiber: 1g
Protein: 1g
Fat: 0.1g
Sugar: 3g
Sodium: 85mg

408. Enchilada Sauce

Servings: 6
Preparation time: 10 minutes / Total Cooking Time: 10 minutes
Ingredients
- 3 ounces salted butter
- 1½ tablespoons Erythritol
- 2 teaspoons dried oregano
- 3 teaspoons ground cumin
- 2 teaspoons ground coriander
- 2 teaspoons onion powder
- ¼ teaspoon cayenne pepper
- Salt and ground black pepper, as required
- 12 ounces tomato puree

Directions:
1.　　　Melt the butter in a medium pan over medium heat and sauté all the ingredients except tomato puree for about 3 minutes.
2.　　　Add the tomato puree and simmer for about 5 minutes.
3.　　　Remove the pan from heat and let it cool slightly before serving.
4.　　　You can preserve this sauce in the refrigerator by placing into an airtight container.
Nutrition Values:
Calories: 132
Net Carbs: 5.1g
Carbohydrate: 6.6g
Fiber: 1.5g
Protein: 1.4g
Fat: 11.9g
Sugar: 3.1g
Sodium: 127mg
-**Note:** You can add a little water, if you prefer a thinner sauce.

409. Teriyaki Sauce

Servings: 8
Preparation time: 10 minutes / Total Cooking Time: 15 minutes
Ingredients
- ½ cup low-sodium soy sauce
- 1 cup water
- 2 tablespoons organic apple cider vinegar
- ¼ cup Erythritol
- 1 tablespoon sesame oil

- ½ teaspoon ginger powder
- 2 teaspoons garlic powder
- ½ teaspoon xanthan gum
- 2 teaspoons sesame seeds

Directions:
1.　　　Place all the ingredient except xanthan gum and sesame seeds in a small pan and mix well.
2.　　　Now, place the pan over medium heat and bring to a boil.
3.　　　Sprinkle with the xanthan gum and beat until well combined.
4.　　　Cook for about 8-10 minutes or until the sauce becomes thick.
5.　　　Remove the pan from heat and mix in the sesame seeds.
6.　　　Serve hot.
7.　　　You can preserve this cooled sauce in the refrigerator by placing into an airtight container.
Nutrition Values:
Calories: 29
Net Carbs: 1.6g
Carbohydrate: 2g
Fiber: 0.4g
Protein: 1.3g
Fat: 2.1g
Sugar: 1.2g
Sodium: 886mg

410. Hoisin Sauce

Servings: 8
Preparation time: 10 minutes
Ingredients
- 4 tablespoons low-sodium soy sauce
- 2 tablespoons natural peanut butter
- 1 tablespoon Erythritol
- 2 teaspoons balsamic vinegar
- 2 teaspoons sesame oil
- 1 teaspoon Sriracha
- 1 garlic clove, peeled
- Ground black pepper, as required

Directions:
1.　　　Add all the ingredients in a food processor and pulse until smooth.
2.　　　You can preserve this sauce in the refrigerator by placing into an airtight container.
Nutrition Values:
Calories: 39
Net Carbs: 1.2g
Carbohydrate: 1.5g
Fiber: 0.3g
Protein: 1.8g
Fat: 3.1g
Sugar: 0.8g
Sodium: 445mg

411. Hot Sauce

Servings: 40
Preparation time: 15 minutes
Cooking Time: 15 minutes
Ingredients

- 1 tablespoon olive oil
- 1 cup carrot, peeled and chopped
- ½ cup yellow onion, chopped
- 5 garlic cloves, minced
- 6 habanero peppers, stemmed
- 1 tomato, chopped
- 1 tablespoon fresh lemon zest
- ¼ cup fresh lemon juice
- ¼ cup balsamic vinegar
- ¼ cup water
- Salt and ground black pepper, as required

Directions:

1. Heat the oil in a large pan over medium heat and cook the carrot, onion and garlic for about 8-10 minutes, stirring frequently.
2. Remove the pan from heat and let it cool slightly.
3. Place the onion mixture and remaining ingredients in a food processor and pulse until smooth.
4. Return the mixture into the same pan over medium-low heat and simmer for about 3-5 minutes, stirring occasionally.
5. Remove the pan from heat and let it cool completely.
6. You can preserve this sauce in the refrigerator by placing into an airtight container.

Nutrition Values:
Calories: 9
Net Carbs: 1g
Carbohydrate: 1.3g
Fiber: 0.3g
Protein: 0.2g
Fat: 0.4g
Sugar: 0.7g
Sodium: 7mg

412. Worcestershire Sauce

Servings: 10
Preparation time: 5 minutes / Total Cooking Time: 5 minutes

Ingredients

- ½ cup organic apple cider vinegar
- 2 tablespoons low-sodium soy sauce
- 2 tablespoons water
- ¼ teaspoon ground mustard
- ¼ teaspoon ground ginger
- ¼ teaspoon garlic powder
- ¼ teaspoon onion powder
- 1/8 teaspoon ground cinnamon
- 1/8 teaspoon ground black pepper

Directions:

1. Add all the ingredients in a small pan and mix well.
2. Now, place the pan over medium heat and bring to a boil.
3. Adjust the heat to low and simmer for about 1-2 minutes.

4. Remove the pan from heat and let it cool completely.
5. You can preserve this sauce in refrigerator by placing into an airtight container.

Nutrition Values:
Calories: 5
Net Carbs: 0.4g
Carbohydrate: 0.5g
Fiber: 0.1g
Protein: 0.2g
Fat: 0g
Sugar: 0.3g
Sodium: 177mg

413. Almond Butter

Servings: 6
Preparation time: 15 minutes
Cooking Time: 15 minutes

Ingredients

- 2¼ cups raw almonds
- 1 tablespoon coconut oil
- ¾ teaspoon salt
- 4-6 drops liquid stevia
- ½ teaspoon ground cinnamon

Directions:

1. Preheat the oven to 325 degrees F.
2. Arrange the almonds onto a rimmed baking sheet in an even layer.
3. Bake for about 12-15 minutes.
4. Remove the almonds from oven and let them cool completely.
5. In a food processor, fitted with metal blade, place the almonds and pulse until a fine meal forms.
6. Add the coconut oil, and salt and pulse for about 6-9 minutes.
7. Add the stevia, and cinnamon and pulse for about 1-2 minutes.
8. You can preserve this almond butter in refrigerator by placing into an airtight container.

Nutrition Values:
Calories: 226
Net Carbs: 3.2g
Carbohydrate: 7.8g
Fiber: 4.6g
Protein: 7.6g
Fat: 20.1g
Sugar: 1.5g
Sodium: 291mg

414. Mayonnaise

Servings: 10
Preparation time: 10 minutes

Ingredients

- 2 organic egg yolks
- 3 teaspoons fresh lemon juice, divided
- 1 teaspoon mustard
- ½ cup coconut oil, melted
- ½ cup olive oil
- Salt and ground black pepper, as required - optional

Directions:

1.   Place the egg yolks, 1 teaspoon of lemon juice, and mustard in a blender and pulse until combined.

2.   While the motor is running gradually, add both oils and pulse until a thick mixture forms.

3.   Add the remaining lemon juice, salt, and black pepper and pulse until well combined.

4.   You can preserve this mayonnaise in refrigerator by placing into an airtight container.

Nutrition Values:
Calories: 193
Net Carbs: 0.2g
Carbohydrate: 0.3g
Fiber: 0.1g
Protein: 0.6g
Fat: 22g
Sugar: 0.1g
Sodium: 17mg
-**Note:** If the mayonnaise seems too thin, slowly add more oils while the motor is running until thick.

415. Seasoned Salt

Servings: 18
Preparation time: 5 minutes
Ingredients
- ¼ cup kosher salt
- ½ teaspoon onion powder
- 1 teaspoon garlic powder
- 1 teaspoon paprika
- ½ teaspoon ground red pepper
- 4 teaspoons freshly ground black pepper

Directions:
- Add all the ingredients in a bowl and stir to combine.
- Transfer into an airtight jar to preserve.

Nutrition Values:
Calories: 2
Net Carbs: 0.4g
Carbohydrate: 0.6g
Fiber: 0.2g
Protein: 0.1g
Fat: 0.1g
Sugar: 0.1g
Sodium: 1500mg

416. Poultry Seasoning

Servings: 10
Preparation time: 5 minutes
Ingredients
- 2 teaspoons dried sage, crushed finely
- 1 teaspoon dried marjoram, crushed finely
- ¾ teaspoon dried rosemary, crushed finely
- 1½ teaspoons dried thyme, crushed finely
- ½ teaspoon ground nutmeg
- ½ teaspoon ground black pepper

Directions:
1.   Add all the ingredients in a bowl and stir to combine.
2.   Transfer into an airtight jar to preserve.

Nutrition Values:
Calories: 2
Net Carbs: 0.2g
Carbohydrate: 0.4g
Fiber: 0.2g
Protein: 0.1g
Fat: 0.1g
Sugar: 0g
Sodium: 0mg

417. Taco Seasoning

Servings: 12
Preparation time: 5 minutes
Ingredients
- ½ teaspoon dried oregano, crushed
- ½ teaspoon ground cumin
- 2 teaspoons hot chili powder
- 1½ teaspoons paprika
- Pinch of red pepper flakes, crushed
- Pinch of cayenne pepper
- ¼ teaspoon ground black pepper
- 1 teaspoon onion powder
- ½ teaspoon garlic powder
- ½ teaspoon sea salt

Directions:
1.   Add all the ingredients in a bowl and stir to combine.
2.   Transfer into an airtight jar to preserve.

Nutrition Values:
Calories: 4
Net Carbs: 0.5g
Carbohydrate: 0.8g
Fiber: 0.3g
Protein: 0.2g
Fat: 0.1g
Sugar: 0.2g
Sodium: 83mg
Pumpkin Pie Spice
Servings: 3
Preparation time: 5 minutes
Ingredients
- 1 teaspoon ground cinnamon
- ¼ teaspoon ground ginger
- ¼ teaspoon ground nutmeg
- 1/8 teaspoon ground cloves

Directions:
1.   Add all the ingredients in a bowl and stir to combine.
2.   Transfer into an airtight jar to preserve.

Nutrition Values:
Calories: 4
Net Carbs: 0.4g
Carbohydrate: 0.9g
Fiber: 0.5g
Protein: 0.1g
Fat: 0.1g
Sugar: 0.1g
Sodium: 0mg

418. Curry Powder

Servings: 20
Preparation time: 10 minutes
Cooking Time: 10 minutes

Ingredients

- ¼ cup coriander seeds
- 2 tablespoons mustard seeds
- 2 tablespoons cumin seeds
- 2 tablespoons anise seeds
- 1 tablespoon whole allspice berries
- 1 tablespoon fenugreek seeds
- 5 tablespoons ground turmeric

Directions:

1.   In a large nonstick frying pan, place all the spices except turmeric over medium heat and cook for about 9-10 minutes or until toasted completely, stirring continuously.
2.   Remove the frying pan from heat and set aside to cool.
3.   In a spice grinder, add the toasted spices, and turmeric and grind until a fine powder forms.
4.   Transfer into an airtight jar to preserve.

Nutrition Values:

Calories: 19
Net Carbs: 0.6g
Carbohydrate: 2.4g
Fiber: 1.8g
Protein: 0.8g
Fat: 0.8g
Sugar: 0.1g
Sodium: 2mg

SNACKS

419. Chickpeas And Pepper Hummus

Preparation time: 10 minutes
Cooking time: 0 minutes
Servings: 4
Ingredients:
- 14 ounces canned chickpeas, no-salt-added, drained and rinsed
- 1 tablespoon sesame paste
- 2 roasted red peppers, chopped
- Juice of ½ lemon
- 4 walnuts, chopped

Directions:
1. In your blender, combine the chickpeas with the sesame paste, red peppers, lemon juice and walnuts, pulse well, divide into bowls and serve as a snack.
2. Enjoy!
Nutrition Values: calories 231, fat 12, fiber 6, carbs 15, protein 14

420. Lemony Chickpeas Dip

Preparation time: 10 minutes
Cooking time: 0 minutes
Servings: 4
Ingredients:
- 14 ounces canned chickpeas, drained, no-salt-added, rinsed
- Zest of 1 lemon, grated
- Juice of 1 lemon
- 1 tablespoon olive oil
- 4 tablespoons pine nuts
- ½ cup coriander, chopped

Directions:
1. In a blender, combine the chickpeas with lemon zest, lemon juice, coriander and oil, pulse well, divide into small bowls, sprinkle pine nuts on top and serve as a party dip.
2. Enjoy!
Nutrition Values: calories 200, fat 12, fiber 4, carbs 9, protein 7

421. Chili Nuts

Preparation time: 10 minutes
Cooking time: 10 minutes
Servings: 4
Ingredients:
- ½ teaspoon chili flakes
- 1 egg white
- ½ teaspoon curry powder
- ½ teaspoon ginger powder
- 4 tablespoons coconut sugar
- A pinch of cayenne pepper
- 14 ounces mixed nuts

Directions:
1. In a bowl, combine the egg white with the chili flakes, curry powder, curry powder, ginger powder, coconut sugar and cayenne and whisk well.

2. Add the nuts, toss well, spread them on a lined baking sheet, introduce in the oven and bake at 400 degrees F for 10 minutes.
3. Divide the nuts into bowls and serve as a snack.
4. Enjoy!
Nutrition Values: calories 234, fat 12, fiber 5, carbs 14, protein 7

422. Protein Bars

Preparation time: 10 minutes
Cooking time: 0 minutes
Servings: 4
Ingredients:
- 4 ounces apricots, dried
- 2 ounces water
- 2 tablespoons rolled oats
- 1 tablespoon sunflower seeds
- 2 tablespoons coconut, shredded
- 1 tablespoon sesame seeds
- 1 tablespoon cranberries
- 3 tablespoons hemp seeds
- 1 tablespoon chia seeds

Directions:
1. In your food processor, combine the apricots with the water and the oats, pulse well, transfer to a bowl, add coconut, sunflower seeds, sesame seeds, cranberries, hemp and chia seeds and stir until you obtain a paste.
2. Roll this into a log, wrap, cool in the fridge, slice and serve as a snack.
3. Enjoy!
Nutrition Values: calories 100, fat 3, fiber 4, carbs 8, protein 5

423. Red Pepper Muffins

Preparation time: 10 minutes
Cooking time: 30 minutes
Servings: 12
Ingredients:
- 1 and ¾ cups whole wheat flour
- 2 teaspoons baking powder
- 2 tablespoons coconut sugar
- A pinch of black pepper
- 1 egg
- ¾ cup almond milk
- 2/3 cup roasted red pepper, chopped
- ½ cup low-fat mozzarella, shredded

Directions:
1. In a bowl, combine the flour with baking powder, coconut sugar, black pepper, egg, milk, red pepper and mozzarella, stir well, divide into a lined muffin tray, introduce in the oven and bake at 400 degrees F for 30 minutes.
2. Serve as a snack.
3. Enjoy!
Nutrition Values: calories 149, fat 4, fiber 2, carbs 14, protein 5

424. Nuts And Seeds Mix

Preparation time: 10 minutes
Cooking time: 0 minutes
Servings: 6
Ingredients:
- 1 cup pecans
- 1 cup hazelnuts
- 1 cup almonds
- ¼ cup coconut, shredded
- 1 cup walnuts
- ½ cup papaya pieces, dried
- ½ cup dates, dried, pitted and chopped
- ½ cup sunflower seeds
- ½ cup pumpkin seeds
- 1 cup raisins

Directions:
1. In a bowl, combine the pecans with the hazelnuts, almonds, coconut, walnuts, papaya, dates, sunflower seeds, pumpkin seeds and raisins, toss and serve as a snack.
2. Enjoy!
Nutrition Values: calories 188, fat 4, fiber 6, carbs 8, protein 6

425. Tortilla Chips

Preparation time: 10 minutes
Cooking time: 25 minutes
Servings: 6
Ingredients:
- 12 whole wheat tortillas, cut into 6 wedges each
- 2 tablespoons olive oil
- 1 tablespoon chili powder
- A pinch of cayenne pepper

Directions:
1. Spread the tortillas on a lined baking sheet, add the oil, chili powder and cayenne, toss, introduce in the oven and bake at 350 degrees F for 25 minutes.
2. Divide into bowls and serve as a side dish.
3. Enjoy!
Nutrition Values: calories 199, fat 3, fiber 4, carbs 12, protein 5

426. Kale Chips

Preparation time: 10 minutes
Cooking time: 15 minutes
Servings: 8
Ingredients:
- 1 bunch kale leaves
- 1 tablespoon olive oil
- 1 teaspoon smoked paprika
- A pinch of black pepper

Directions:
1. Spread the kale leaves on a baking sheet, add black pepper, oil and paprika, toss, introduce in the oven and bake at 350 degrees F for 15 minutes.
2. Divide into bowls and serve as a snack.
3. Enjoy!

Nutrition Values: calories 177, fat 2, fiber 4, carbs 13, protein 6

427. Potato Chips

Preparation time: 10 minutes
Cooking time: 30 minutes
Servings: 6
Ingredients:
- 2 gold potatoes, cut into thin rounds
- 1 tablespoon olive oil
- 2 teaspoons garlic, minced

Directions:
1. In a bowl, combine the potato chips with the oil and the garlic, toss, spread on a lined baking sheet, introduce in the oven and bake at 400 degrees F for 30 minutes.
2. Divide into bowls and serve.
3. Enjoy!
Nutrition Values: calories 200, fat 3, fiber 5, carbs 13, protein 6

428. Peach Dip

Preparation time: 10 minutes
Cooking time: 0 minutes
Servings: 2
Ingredients:
- ½ cup nonfat yogurt
- 1 cup peaches, chopped
- A pinch of cinnamon powder
- A pinch of nutmeg, ground

Directions:
1. In a bowl, combine the yogurt with the peaches, cinnamon and nutmeg, whisk, divide into small bowls and serve as a snack.
2. Enjoy!
Nutrition Values: calories 165, fat 2, fiber 3, carbs 14, protein 13

429. Cereal Mix

Preparation time: 10 minutes
Cooking time: 40 minutes
Servings: 6
Ingredients:
- 3 tablespoons olive oil
- 1 teaspoon hot sauce
- ½ teaspoon garlic powder
- ½ teaspoon onion powder
- ½ teaspoon cumin, ground
- A pinch of cayenne pepper
- 3 cups rice cereal squares
- 1 cup cornflakes
- ½ cup pepitas

Directions:
1. In a bowl, combine the oil with the hot sauce, garlic powder, onion powder, cumin, cayenne, rice cereal, cornflakes and pepitas, toss, spread on a lined baking sheet, introduce in the oven and bake at 350 degrees F for 40 minutes.
2. Divide into bowls and serve as a snack.
3. Enjoy!

Nutrition Values: calories 199, fat 3, fiber 4, carbs 12, protein 5

430. Goji Berry Mix

Preparation time: 10 minutes
Cooking time: 0 minutes
Servings: 4
Ingredients:
- 1 cup almonds
- 1 cup goji berries
- ½ cup sunflower seeds
- ½ cup pumpkin seeds
- ½ cup walnuts, halved
- 12 apricots, dried and quartered

Directions:
1. In a bowl, combine the almond with the goji berries, sunflower seeds, pumpkin seeds, walnuts and apricots, toss, divide into bowls and serve.
2. Enjoy!

Nutrition Values: calories 187, fat 2, fiber 5, carbs 12, protein 6

431. Artichoke Spread

Preparation time: 10 minutes
Cooking time: 15 minutes
Servings: 4
Ingredients:
- 10 ounces spinach, chopped
- 12 ounces canned artichoke hearts, no-salt-added, drained and chopped
- 1 cup coconut cream
- 1 cup low-fat cheddar, shredded
- A pinch of black pepper

Directions:
1. In a bowl, combine the spinach with the artichokes, cream, cheese and black pepper, stir well, transfer to a baking dish, introduce in the oven and bake at 400 degrees F for 15 minutes.
2. Divide into bowls and serve.
3. Enjoy!

Nutrition Values: calories 200, fat 4, fiber 6, carbs 14, protein 8

432. Avocado Salsa

Preparation time: 10 minutes
Cooking time: 0 minutes
Servings: 4
Ingredients:
- 1 small yellow onion, minced
- 1 jalapeno, minced
- ¼ cup cilantro, chopped
- A pinch of black pepper
- 2 avocados, peeled, pitted and cubed
- 2 tablespoons lime juice

Directions:
1. In a bowl, combine the onion with the jalapeno, cilantro, black pepper, avocado and lime juice, toss and serve.
2. Enjoy!

Nutrition Values: calories 198, fat 2, fiber 5, carbs 14, protein 7

433. Onion Spread

Preparation time: 10 minutes
Cooking time: 35 minutes
Servings: 4
Ingredients:
- 2 tablespoons olive oil
- 2 yellow onions, sliced
- A pinch of black pepper
- 8 ounces low-fat cream cheese
- 1 cup coconut cream
- 2 tablespoons chives, chopped

Directions:
1. Heat up a pan with the oil over low heat, add the onions and the black pepper, stir and cook for 35 minutes.
2. In a bowl, combine the onions with the cream cheese, coconut cream and chives, stir well and serve as a party spread.
3. Enjoy!

Nutrition Values: calories 212, fat 3, fiber 5, carbs 14, protein 8

434. Eggplant Salsa

Preparation time: 10 minutes
Cooking time: 7 hours
Servings: 4
Ingredients:
- 1 and ½ cups tomatoes, chopped
- 3 cups eggplant, cubed
- 6 ounces green olives, pitted and sliced
- 4 garlic cloves, minced
- 2 teaspoons balsamic vinegar
- 1 tablespoon oregano, chopped
- Black pepper to the taste

Directions:
1. In your slow cooker, mix tomatoes with eggplant, green olives, garlic, vinegar, oregano and pepper, toss, cover, cook on Low for 7 hours, divide into small bowls and serve as an appetizer.
2. Enjoy!

Nutrition Values: calories 190, fat 6, fiber 5, carbs 12, protein 2

435. Artichoke and Beans Spread

Preparation time: 10 minutes
Cooking time: 30 minutes
Servings: 8
Ingredients:
- 4 cups spinach, chopped
- 2 cups artichoke hearts
- Black pepper to the taste
- 1 teaspoon thyme, chopped
- 2 garlic cloves, minced
- 1 cup white beans, already cooked
- 1 tablespoon parsley, chopped
- 2 tablespoons low-fat parmesan, grated

- ½ cup low-fat sour cream

Directions:
1. In your slow cooker, mix artichokes with spinach, black pepper, thyme, garlic, beans, parmesan, parsley and sour cream, stir, cover and cook on Low for 5 hours.
2. Transfer to your blender, pulse well divide into bowls and serve.
3. Enjoy!

Nutrition Values: calories 180, fat 2, fiber 6, carbs 11, protein 5

436. Stuffed White Mushrooms

Preparation time: 10 minutes
Cooking time: 5 hours
Servings: 20

Ingredients:
- 20 mushrooms, stems removed
- ¼ cup low-fat butter, melted
- 1 and ½ cups whole wheat breadcrumbs
- 2 tablespoons parsley, chopped
- 2 cups basil, chopped
- 1 cup tomato sauce, no-salt-added
- ¼ cup low-fat parmesan, grated
- 1 tablespoon garlic, minced
- 2 teaspoons lemon juice
- 1 tablespoon olive oil

Directions:
1. In a bowl, mix butter with breadcrumbs and parsley, stir well and leave aside.
2. In your blender, mix basil with oil, parmesan, garlic and lemon juice and pulse really well.
3. Stuff mushrooms with this mix, pour the tomato sauce on top, sprinkle breadcrumbs mix at the end, cover and cook on Low for 5 hours.
4. Arrange mushrooms on a platter and serve.
5. Enjoy!

Nutrition Values: calories 170, fat 1, fiber 3, carbs 14, protein 4

437. Italian Tomato Appetizer

Preparation time: 10 minutes
Cooking time: 2 hours
Servings: 4

Ingredients:
- 2 teaspoons olive oil
- 8 tomatoes, chopped
- ¼ cup basil, chopped
- 3 tablespoons low-sodium veggie stock
- 1 garlic clove, minced
- 4 Italian whole wheat bread slices, toasted
- Black pepper to the taste

Directions:
1. In your slow cooker, mix tomatoes with basil, garlic, oil, stock and black pepper, stir, cover, cook on High for 2 hours and then leave aside to cool down.
2. Divide this mix on the toasted bread and serve as an appetizer.

3. Enjoy!

Nutrition Values: calories 174, fat 2, fiber 1, carbs 10, protein 4

438. Sweet Pineapple Snack

Preparation time: 10 minutes
Cooking time: 2 hours
Servings: 8

Ingredients:
- 1 tablespoon lime juice
- 2 tablespoons stevia
- 1 tablespoon olive oil
- 1 teaspoon cinnamon powder
- 1 pineapple, peeled and cut into medium sticks
- ¼ teaspoon cloves, ground
- 1 tablespoon lime zest, grated

Directions:
1. In a bowl, mix lime juice with stevia, oil, cinnamon and cloves and whisk well.
2. Add the pineapple sticks to your slow cooker, add lime mix, toss, cover and cook on High for 2 hours.
3. Serve the pineapple sticks as a snack with lime zest sprinkled on top.
4. Enjoy!

Nutrition Values: calories 130, fat 4, fiber 1, carbs 10, protein 3

439. Chickpeas Hummus

Preparation time: 10 minutes
Cooking time: 5 hours
Servings: 6

Ingredients:
- 1 cup chickpeas, soaked overnight and drained
- 2 garlic cloves
- 3 cups water
- 1 tablespoon olive oil
- 2 tablespoons sherry vinegar
- ¾ cup green onions, chopped
- 1 teaspoon cumin, ground
- 3 tablespoons cilantro, chopped

Directions:
1. Put the water in your slow cooker, add chickpeas and garlic, cover and cook on Low for 5 hours.
2. Drain chickpeas, transfer them to your blender, add ½ cup of the cooking liquid, green onions, vinegar, oil, cilantro and cumin, blend well, divide into bowls and serve.
3. Enjoy!

Nutrition Values: calories 133, fat 1, fiber 3, carbs 10, protein 3

440. Asparagus Snack

Preparation time: 4 weeks
Cooking time: 2 hours
Servings: 6

Ingredients:

118

- 3 cups asparagus spears, halved
- ¼ cup apple cider vinegar
- 1 tablespoon dill
- ¼ cup white wine vinegar
- 2 cloves
- 1 cup water
- 3 garlic cloves, sliced
- ¼ teaspoon red pepper flakes
- 8 black peppercorns
- 1 teaspoon coriander seeds

Directions:

1.   In your slow cooker, mix the asparagus with the cider vinegar, white vinegar, dill, cloves, water, garlic, pepper flakes, peppercorns and coriander, cover and cook on High for 2 hours.
2.   Drain asparagus, transfer it to bowls and serve as a snack.
3.   Enjoy!

Nutrition Values: calories 90, fat 1, fiber 2, carbs 7, protein 2

441. Shrimp and Beans Appetizer Salad

Preparation time: 10 minutes
Cooking time: 5 hours and 30 minutes.
Servings: 8
Ingredients:

- ¼ pound shrimp, peeled, deveined and chopped
- Zest and juice of 2 limes
- Zest and juice of 2 lemons
- 2 teaspoons cumin, ground
- 2 tablespoons olive oil
- 1 cup tomato, chopped
- ½ cup red onion, chopped
- 2 tablespoons garlic, minced
- 1 cup canned black beans, no-salt-added, drained and rinsed
- 1 cup cucumber, chopped
- ¼ cup cilantro, chopped

Directions:

1.   In a bowl, mix lime juice and lemon juice with shrimp and toss.
2.   Grease the slow cooker with the oil, add black beans, tomato, onion, garlic and cumin, cover and cook on Low for 5 hours.
3.   Add shrimp, cover, cook on Low for 30 minutes, more, transfer everything to a bowl, add cucumber and cilantro, toss, leave aside to cool down, divide between small bowls and serve as an appetizer.
4.   Enjoy!

Nutrition Values: calories 200, fat 3, fiber 2, carbs 15, protein 5

442. Pepper and Chickpeas Dip

Preparation time: 10 minutes
Cooking time: 2 hours
Servings: 12
Ingredients:

- 1 cup red bell pepper, sliced
- 1 tablespoon olive oil
- 2 tablespoons white sesame seeds
- 2 cups canned chickpeas, no-salt-added, drained and rinsed
- 1 tablespoon lemon juice
- 1 teaspoon garlic powder
- 1 teaspoon onion powder
- A pinch of cayenne pepper
- 1 and ¼ teaspoons cumin, ground

Directions:

1.   In your slow cooker, mix red bell pepper with oil, sesame seeds, chickpeas, lemon juice, garlic and onion powder, cayenne pepper and cumin, cover and cook on High for 2 hours.
2.   Transfer this mix to your blender, pulse well, divide into serving bowls and serve cold.
3.   Enjoy!

Nutrition Values: calories 180, fat 2, fiber 2, carbs 15, protein 3

443. White Bean Spread

Preparation time: 10 minutes
Cooking time: 6 hours
Servings: 8
Ingredients:

- 15 ounces canned white beans, no-salt-added, drained and rinsed
- 1 cup low-sodium veggie stock
- 2 tablespoons olive oil
- 8 garlic cloves, roasted
- 2 tablespoons lemon juice

Directions:

1.   In your blender, mix beans with oil, stock, garlic and lemon juice, cover, cook on Low for 6 hours, transfer to your blender, pulse well, divide into bowls and serve as a snack.
2.   Enjoy!

Nutrition Values: calories 159, fat 4, fiber 3, carbs 14, protein 2

444. Minty Spinach Dip

Preparation time: 20 minutes
Cooking time: 2 hours
Servings: 4
Ingredients:

- 1 bunch spinach leaves, roughly chopped
- 1 scallion, sliced
- 2 tablespoons mint leaves, chopped
- ¾ cup low-fat sour cream
- Black pepper to the taste

Directions:

1.   In your slow cooker, mix the spinach with the scallion, mint, cream and black pepper, cover, cook on High for 2 hours, stir well, divide into bowls and serve.
2.   Enjoy!

Nutrition Values: calories 160, fat 3, fiber 3, carbs 12, protein 5

445. Turnips and Cauliflower Spread

Preparation time: 10 minutes
Cooking time: 7 hours
Servings: 4
Ingredients:
- 2 cups cauliflower florets
- 1/3 cup cashews, chopped
- 1 cup turnips, chopped
- 2 and ½ cups water
- 1 cup coconut milk
- 1 teaspoon garlic powder
- ¼ teaspoon smoked paprika
- ¼ teaspoon mustard powder

Directions:
1.   In your slow cooker, mix cauliflower with cashews, turnips and water, stir, cover, cook on Low for 7 hours, drain, transfer to a blender, add milk, garlic powder, paprika and mustard powder, blend well, divide into bowls and serve as a snack
2.   Enjoy!
Nutrition Values: calories 221, fat 7, fiber 4, carbs 14, protein 3

446. Italian Veggie Dip

Preparation time: 10 minutes
Cooking time: 5 hours
Servings: 7
Ingredients:
- ½ cauliflower head, riced
- 54 ounces canned tomatoes, no-salt-added and crushed
- 10 ounces white mushrooms, chopped
- 3 cups eggplant, cubed
- 6 garlic cloves, minced
- 2 tablespoons stevia
- 2 tablespoons balsamic vinegar
- 2 tablespoons tomato paste, no-salt-added
- 1 tablespoon basil, chopped
- 1 and ½ tablespoons oregano, chopped
- A pinch of black pepper

Directions:
1.   In your slow cooker, mix cauliflower with tomatoes, mushrooms, eggplant, garlic, stevia, vinegar, tomato paste and pepper, stir, cover and cook on High for 5 hours.
2.   Add basil and oregano, stir, mash a bit with a potato masher, divide into bowls and serve as a dip.
3.   Enjoy!
Nutrition Values: calories 261, fat 7, fiber 6, carbs 11, protein 6

447. Cajun Peas Spread

Preparation time: 10 minutes
Cooking time: 5 hours
Servings: 5
Ingredients:
- 1 and ½ cups black-eyed peas
- 3 cups water
- 1 teaspoon Cajun seasoning
- ½ cup pecans, toasted
- ½ teaspoon garlic powder
- ½ teaspoon chili powder
- A pinch of black pepper
- ½ teaspoon cayenne powder

Directions:
1.   In your slow cooker, mix the peas with Cajun seasoning, pepper and water, stir, cover and cook on High for 5 hours.
2.   Drain, transfer to a blender, add pecans, garlic powder, chili powder and cayenne powder, pulse well, divide into bowls and serve as a snack
3.   Enjoy!
Nutrition Values: calories 241, fat 4, fiber 7, carbs 12, protein 4

448. Cashew Spread

Preparation time: 10 minutes
Cooking time: 3 hours
Servings: 10
Ingredients:
- 1 cup water
- 1 cup cashews
- 10 ounces hummus, no-salt-added
- ¼ teaspoon garlic powder
- ¼ teaspoon onion powder
- A pinch of black pepper
- 1 teaspoon apple cider vinegar

Directions:
1.   In your slow cooker, mix water with cashews and pepper, stir, cover, cook on High for 3 hours, transfer to your blender, add hummus, garlic powder, onion powder and vinegar, pulse well, divide into bowls and serve.
2.   Enjoy!
Nutrition Values: calories 212, fat 7, fiber 7, carbs 15, protein 4

449. Coconut Spinach Dip

Preparation time: 10 minutes
Cooking time: 1 hour
Servings: 4
Ingredients:
- 1 cup coconut cream
- 10 ounces spinach leaves
- 8 ounces water chestnuts, chopped
- 1 garlic clove, minced
- Black pepper to the taste

Directions:
1.   In your slow cooker, mix coconut cream with spinach, chestnuts, black pepper and garlic, stir, cover, cook on High for 1 hour, blend with an immersion blender, divide into bowls and serve as a dip
2.   Enjoy!
Nutrition Values: calories 192, fat 5, fiber 7, carbs 12, protein 5

450. Black Bean Salsa

Preparation time: 10 minutes

Cooking time: 4 hours
Servings: 7
Ingredients:
- 1 tablespoon low sodium soy sauce
- ½ teaspoon cumin, ground
- 1 cup canned black beans, no-salt-added, drained and rinsed
- 1 cup chunky salsa, salt-free
- 6 cups romaine lettuce, torn
- ½ cup avocado, peeled, pitted and mashed

Directions:
1. In your slow cooker, mix the beans with salsa, cumin and soy sauce, stir, cover and cook on Low for 4 hours.
2. In a salad bowl, mix lettuce leaves with black beans mix and mashed avocado, toss, divide into small bowls and serve.
3. Enjoy!

Nutrition Values: calories 199, fat 4, fiber 7, carbs 14, protein 4

Chili Coconut Corn Spread

Preparation time: 10 minutes
Cooking time: 2 hours
Servings: 8
Ingredients:
- 30 ounces canned corn, no-salt-added, drained
- 2 green onions, chopped
- ½ cup coconut cream
- 8 ounces low-fat cream cheese
- 1 jalapeno, chopped
- ½ teaspoon chili powder

Directions:
1. In your slow cooker, mix corn with green onions, coconut cream, cream cheese, chili powder and jalapeno, cover, cook on Low for 2 hours, whisk well, divide into bowls and serve as a dip.
2. Enjoy!

Nutrition Values: calories 302, fat 5, fiber 7, carbs 12, protein 4

452. Artichoke and Spinach Dip

Preparation time: 10 minutes
Cooking time: 2 hours
Servings: 8
Ingredients:
- 28 ounces canned artichokes, no-salt-added, drained and chopped
- 10 ounces spinach
- 8 ounces coconut cream
- 1 yellow onion, chopped
- 2 garlic cloves, minced
- ¾ cup coconut milk
- 3 tablespoons avocado mayonnaise
- 1 tablespoon red vinegar
- A pinch of black pepper

Directions:

1. In your slow cooker, mix artichokes with spinach, cream, onion, garlic, milk, mayo, vinegar and pepper, stir, cover, cook on Low for 2 hours, divide into bowls and serve as a snack.
2. Enjoy!

Nutrition Values: calories 255, fat 7, fiber 4, carbs 20, protein 13

453. Mushroom and Bell Pepper Dip

Preparation time: 10 minutes
Cooking time: 4 hours
Servings: 6
Ingredients:
- 3 cups green bell peppers, chopped
- 1 red onion, chopped
- 3 garlic cloves, minced
- 1 pound mushrooms, chopped
- 28 ounces tomato sauce, no-salt-added
- ½ cup low-fat cheddar, grated
- Black pepper to the taste

Directions:
1. In your slow cooker, mix bell peppers with mushrooms, onion, garlic, tomato sauce, cheese and pepper, stir, cover, cook on Low for 4 hours, divide into bowls and serve.
2. Enjoy!

Nutrition Values: calories 253, fat 4, fiber 7, carbs 15, protein 3

454. Warm French Veggie Salad

Preparation time: 10 minutes
Cooking time: 9 hours
Servings: 6
Ingredients:
- 2 yellow onions, chopped
- 1 eggplant, sliced
- 4 zucchinis, sliced
- 2 garlic cloves, minced
- 2 green bell peppers, cut into medium strips
- 6 ounces canned tomato paste, no-salt-added
- 2 tomatoes, cut into medium wedges
- 1 teaspoon oregano, dried
- 1 tablespoon basil, chopped
- 2 tablespoons parsley, chopped
- 3 tablespoons olive oil
- A pinch of black pepper

Directions:
1. In your slow cooker, mix oil with onions, eggplant, zucchinis, garlic, bell peppers, tomato paste, tomatoes, basil, oregano and pepper, cover and cook on Low for 9 hours.
2. Add parsley, toss, divide into small bowls and serve warm as an appetizer.
3. Enjoy!

Nutrition Values: calories 219, fat 7, fiber 6, carbs 18, protein 4

455. Bulgur and Beans Salad

Preparation time: 10 minutes
Cooking time: 8 hours
Servings: 4
Ingredients:
- 2 cups white mushrooms, sliced
- ¾ cup bulgur, soaked and drained
- 2 cups yellow onion, chopped
- ½ cup red bell pepper, chopped
- 1 cup low sodium veggie stock
- 2 garlic cloves, minced
- 1 cup strong coffee
- 14 ounces canned kidney beans, no-salt-added, drained
- 14 ounces canned pinto beans, no-salt-added, drained
- 2 tablespoons stevia
- 2 tablespoons chili powder
- 1 tablespoon cocoa powder
- 1 teaspoon oregano, dried
- 2 teaspoons cumin, ground
- Black pepper to the taste

Directions:
1. In your slow cooker, mix mushrooms with bulgur, onion, bell pepper, stock, garlic, coffee, kidney and pinto beans, stevia, chili powder, cocoa, oregano, cumin and pepper, stir gently, cover and cook on Low for 12 hours.
2. Divide the mix into small bowls and serve cold as an appetizer.
3. Enjoy!

456. Cheese Sticks

Preparation Time: 1 hour 30 minutes
Servings: 16
Ingredients:
- 2 eggs, whisked
- 8 mozzarella cheese strings, cut in halves
- 1/2 cup olive oil
- 1 garlic clove, minced
- 1 cup parmesan, grated
- 1 tablespoon Italian seasoning
- Salt and black pepper to the taste.

Directions:
1. In a bowl, mix parmesan with salt, pepper, Italian seasoning and garlic and stir well.
2. Put whisked eggs in another bowl.
3. Dip mozzarella sticks in egg mixture, then in the cheese mix.
4. Dip them again in egg and in parm mix and keep them in the freezer for 1 hour.
5. Heat up a pan with the oil over medium high heat; add cheese sticks, fry them until they are golden on one side, flip and cook them the same way on the other side
6. Arrange them on a platter and serve
Nutrition Values: Calories: 140; Fat : 5; Fiber : 1; Carbs : 3; Protein : 4

457. Fried Queso Snack

Preparation Time: 20 minutes
Servings: 6
Ingredients:
- 5 ounces queso Blanco, cubed and freeze for a couple of minutes
- 1 ½ tablespoons olive oil
- 2 ounces olives, pitted and chopped.
- A pinch of red pepper flakes

Directions:
1. Heat up a pan with the oil over medium high heat; add queso cubes and cook until the bottom melts a bit.
2. Flip cubes with a spatula and sprinkle black olives on top.
3. Leave cubes to cook a bit more, flip and sprinkle red pepper flakes and cook until they are crispy.
4. Flip, cook on the other side until it's crispy as well, transfer to a cutting board, cut into small blocks and then serve as a snack.
Nutrition Values: Calories: 500; Fat : 43; Fiber : 4; Carbs : 2; Protein : 30

458. Halloumi Cheese Fries

Preparation Time: 15 minutes
Servings: 4
Ingredients:
- 1 cup marinara sauce
- 2 ounces tallow
- 8 ounces halloumi cheese, pat dried and sliced into fries

Directions:
1. Heat up a pan with the tallow over medium high heat.
2. Add halloumi pieces, cover, cook for 2 minutes on each side and transfer to paper towels
3. Drain excess grease, transfer them to a bowl and serve with marinara sauce on the side
Nutrition Values: Calories: 200; Fat : 16; Fiber : 1; Carbs : 1; Protein : 13

459. Artichoke Dip

Preparation Time: 25 minutes
Servings: 16
Ingredients:
- 28 ounces canned artichoke hearts, chopped.
- 1/4 cup sour cream
- 1/4 cup heavy cream
- 1/4 cup mayonnaise
- 1/4 cup shallot, chopped.
- 1/2 cup parmesan cheese, grated
- 1 cup mozzarella cheese, shredded
- 4 ounces feta cheese, crumbled
- 1 tablespoon balsamic vinegar
- 10 ounces spinach, chopped.
- 1 tablespoon olive oil
- 2 garlic cloves, minced
- 4 ounces cream cheese

- Salt and black pepper to the taste.

Directions:

1. Heat up a pan with the oil over medium heat; add shallot and garlic; stir and cook for 3 minutes
2. Add heavy cream and cream cheese and stir.
3. Also add sour cream, parmesan, mayo, feta cheese and mozzarella cheese; stir and reduce heat.
4. Add artichoke, spinach, salt, pepper and vinegar; stir well, take off heat and transfer to a bowl.
5. Serve as a tastydip.

Nutrition Values: Calories: 144; Fat : 12; Fiber : 2; Carbs : 5; Protein : 5

460. Maple And Pecan Bars

Preparation Time: 35 minutes
Servings: 12
Ingredients:

- 2 cups pecans, toasted and crushed.
- 1 cup almond flour
- 1/4 teaspoon stevia
- 1/2 cup coconut, shredded
- 1/2 cup coconut oil
- 1/2 cup flaxseed meal
- 1/4 cup "maple syrup"
- For the maple syrup:
- 2 teaspoons maple extract
- 1/2 teaspoon vanilla extract
- 1 tablespoon ghee
- ¾ cup water
- 1/4 teaspoon xanthan gum
- 1/4 cup erythritol
- 2 ¼ teaspoons coconut oil

Directions:

1. In a heatproof bowl, mix ghee with 2¼ teaspoons coconut oil and xanthan gum; stir, introduce in your microwave and heat up for 1 minute
2. Add erythritol, water, maple and vanilla extract; stir well and heat up in the microwave for 1 minute more
3. In a bowl, mix flaxseed meal with coconut and almond flour and stir.
4. Add pecans and stir again.
5. Add 1/4 cup "maple syrup", stevia and 1/2 cup coconut oil and stir well.
6. Spread this in a baking dish, press well, introduce in the oven at 350 degrees F and bake for 25 minutes
7. Leave aside to cool down, cut into 12 bars and serve as asnack.
8. Nutrition Values: Calories: 300; Fat : 30; Fiber : 12; Carbs : 2; Protein : 5

461. Muffins Snack

Preparation Time: 25 minutes
Servings: 20
Ingredients:

- 3 hot dogs, cut into 20 pieces
- 1/2 cup flaxseed meal
- 1/2 cup almond flour
- 1/4 cup coconut milk
- 1/3 cup sour cream
- 3 tablespoons swerve
- 1 tablespoon psyllium powder
- 1/4 teaspoon baking powder
- 1 egg
- Cooking spray
- A pinch of salt

Directions:

1. In a bowl, mix flaxseed meal with flour, psyllium powder, swerve, salt and baking powder and stir.
2. Add egg, sour cream and coconut milk and whisk well.
3. Grease a muffin tray with cooking oil, divide the batter you've just make, stick a hot dog piece in the middle of each muffin, introduce in the oven at 350 degrees F and bake for 12 minutes
4. Broil in preheated broil for 3 minutes more, divide on a platter and serve

Nutrition Values: Calories: 80; Fat : 6; Fiber : 1; Carbs : 1; Protein : 3

462. Chia Seeds Snack

Preparation Time: 45 minutes
Servings: 36
Ingredients:

- 1/2 cup chia seeds, ground
- 1/4 teaspoon oregano, dried
- 1/4 teaspoon garlic powder
- 1/4 teaspoon sweet paprika
- 3 ounces cheddar, cheese, grated
- 1/4 teaspoon xanthan gum
- 1/4 teaspoon onion powder
- 1¼ cup ice water
- 2 tablespoons olive oil
- 2 tablespoons psyllium husk powder
- Salt and black pepper to the taste.

Directions:

1. In a bowl, mix chia seeds with xanthan gum, psyllium powder, oregano, garlic and onion powder, paprika, salt and pepper and stir.
2. Add oil and stir well.
3. Add ice water and stir until you obtain a firm dough.
4. Spread this on a baking sheet, introduce in the oven at 350 degrees F and bake for 35 minutes
5. Leave aside to cool down, cut into 36 crackers and serve them as asnack.

Nutrition Values: Calories: 50; Fat : 3; Fiber : 1; Carbs : 0.1; Protein : 2

463. Taco Cups

Preparation Time: 50 minutes
Servings: 30
Ingredients:

- 1 pound beef, ground
- 2 cups cheddar cheese, shredded

- 2 tablespoons cumin
- 2 tablespoons chili powder
- 1/4 cup water
- Pico de gallo for serving
- Salt and black pepper to the taste.

Directions:

1. Divide spoonful of parmesan on a lined baking sheet, introduce in the oven at 350 degrees F and bake for 7 minutes
2. Leave cheese to cool down for 1 minute, transfer them to mini cupcake molds and shape them into cups
3. Meanwhile; heat up a pan over medium high heat; add beef; stir and cook until it browns
4. Add the water, salt, pepper, cumin and chili powder; stir and cook for 5 minutes more
5. Divide into cheese cups, top with pico de gallo, transfer them all to a platter and serve

Nutrition Values: Calories: 140; Fat : 6; Fiber : 0; Carbs : 6; Protein : 15

464. Jalapeno Balls

Preparation Time: 20 minutes
Servings: 3
Ingredients:

- 3 bacon slices
- 3 ounces cream cheese
- 1/2 teaspoon parsley, dried
- 1/4 teaspoon garlic powder
- 1/4 teaspoon onion powder
- 1 jalapeno pepper, chopped.
- Salt and black pepper to the taste.

Directions:

1. Heat up a pan over medium high heat; add bacon, cook until it's crispy, transfer to paper towels, drain grease and crumble
2. Reserve bacon fat from the pan.
3. In a bowl, mix cream cheese with jalapeno pepper, onion and garlic powder, parsley, salt and pepper and stir well.
4. Add bacon fat and bacon crumbles; stir gently, shape balls from this mix and serve

Nutrition Values: Calories: 200; Fat : 18; Fiber : 1; Carbs : 2; Protein : 5

465. Pumpkin Muffins

Preparation Time: 25 minutes
Servings: 18
Ingredients:

- 1/4 cup sunflower seed butter
- 3/4 cup pumpkin puree
- 1/2 teaspoon nutmeg, ground
- 1/2 teaspoon baking soda
- 1 egg
- 1/2 teaspoon baking powder
- 1 teaspoon cinnamon, ground
- 2 tablespoons flaxseed meal
- 1/4 cup coconut flour
- 1/2 cup erythritol

- A pinch of salt

Directions:

1. In a bowl, mix butter with pumpkin puree and egg and blend well.
2. Add flaxseed meal, coconut flour, erythritol, baking soda, baking powder, nutmeg, cinnamon and a pinch of salt and stir well.
3. Spoon this into a greased muffin pan, introduce in the oven at 350 degrees F and bake for 15 minutes
4. Leave muffins to cool down and serve them as a snack.

Nutrition Values: Calories: 50; Fat : 3; Fiber : 1; Carbs : 2; Protein : 2

466. Pepper Nachos

Preparation Time: 30 minutes
Servings: 6
Ingredients:

- 1 pound mini bell peppers, cut in halves
- 1 pound beef meat, ground
- 1 teaspoon cumin, ground
- 1/2 cup tomato, chopped.
- 1 teaspoon garlic powder
- 1 teaspoon sweet paprika
- 1/2 teaspoon oregano, dried
- 1/4 teaspoon red pepper flakes
- 1½ cups cheddar cheese, shredded
- 1 tablespoons chili powder
- Sour cream for serving
- Salt and black pepper to the taste.

Directions:

1. In a bowl, mix chili powder with paprika, salt, pepper, cumin, oregano, pepper flakes and garlic powder and stir.
2. Heat up a pan over medium heat; add beef; stir and brown for 10 minutes
3. Add chili powder mix; stir and take off heat.
4. Arrange pepper halves on a lined baking sheet, stuff them with the beef mix, sprinkle cheese, introduce in the oven at 400 degrees F and bake for 10 minutes
5. Take peppers out of the oven, sprinkle tomatoes and divide between plates and serve with sour cream on top.

Nutrition Values: Calories: 350; Fat : 22; Fiber : 3; Carbs : 6; Protein : 27

467. Yummy Spinach Balls

Preparation Time: 22 minutes
Servings: 30
Ingredients:

- 4 tablespoons melted ghee
- 2 eggs
- 1 cup almond flour
- 16 ounces spinach
- 1/3 cup feta cheese, crumbled
- 1/4 teaspoon nutmeg, ground
- 1/3 cup parmesan, grated

- 1 tablespoon onion powder
- 3 tablespoons whipping cream
- 1 teaspoon garlic powder
- Salt and black pepper to the taste.

Directions:

1. In your blender, mix spinach with ghee, eggs, almond flour, feta cheese, parmesan, nutmeg, whipping cream, salt, pepper, onion and garlic pepper and blend very well.
2. Transfer to a bowl and keep in the freezer for 10 minutes
3. Shape 30 spinach balls, arrange on a lined baking sheet, introduce in the oven at 350 degrees F and bake for 12 minutes
4. Leave spinach balls to cool down and serve as a party appetizer.

Nutrition Values: Calories: 60; Fat : 5; Fiber : 1; Carbs : 0.7; Protein : 2

468. Tortilla Chips

Preparation Time: 24 minutes
Servings: 6
Ingredients:
For the tortillas:
- 2 teaspoons olive oil
- 2 tablespoons psyllium husk powder
- 1/4 teaspoon xanthan gum
- 1/2 teaspoon curry powder
- 3 teaspoons coconut flour
- 1 cup flax seed meal
- 1 cup water

For the chips:
- 6 flaxseed tortillas
- 3 tablespoons vegetable oil
- Fresh salsa for serving
- Sour cream for serving
- Salt and black pepper to the taste.

Directions:

1. In a bowl, mix flaxseed meal with psyllium powder, olive oil, xanthan gum, water and curry powder and mix until you obtain an elastic dough.
2. Spread coconut flour on a working surface
3. Divide dough into 6 pieces, place each piece on the working surface and roll into a circle and cut each into 6 pieces
4. Heat up a pan with the vegetable oil over medium high heat; add tortilla chips, cook for 2 minutes on each side and transfer to paper towels
5. Put tortilla chips in a bowl, season with salt and pepper and serve with some fresh salsa and sour cream on the side

Nutrition Values: Calories: 30; Fat : 3; Fiber : 1. 2; Carbs : 0.5; Protein : 1

469. Onion And Cauliflower Dip

Preparation Time: 40 minutes
Servings: 24
Ingredients:
- 1 cauliflower head, florets separated
- 1½ cups chicken stock

- 1/2 teaspoon chili powder
- 1/2 teaspoon garlic powder
- 1/4 cup mayonnaise
- 1/2 cup yellow onion, chopped.
- 1/2 teaspoon cumin, ground
- ¾ cup cream cheese
- Salt and black pepper to the taste.

Directions:

1. Put the stock in a pot, add cauliflower and onion, heat up over medium heat and cook for 30 minutes
2. Add chili powder, salt, pepper, cumin and garlic powder and stir.
3. Also add cream cheese and stir a bit until it melts
4. Blend using an immersion blender and mix with the mayo.
5. Transfer to a bowl and keep in the fridge for 2 hours before you serve it.

Nutrition Values: Calories: 60; Fat : 4; Fiber : 1; Carbs : 1; Protein : 1

470. Delightful Bombs

Preparation Time: 10 minutes
Servings: 6
Ingredients:
- 8 black olives, pitted and chopped.
- 4 ounces cream cheese
- 1 tablespoons basil, chopped.
- 2 tablespoons sun-dried tomato pesto
- 14 pepperoni slices, chopped.
- Salt and black pepper to the taste.

Directions:

1. In a bowl, mix cream cheese with salt, pepper, pepperoni, basil, sun dried tomato pesto and black olives and stir well.
2. Shape balls from this mix, arrange on a platter and serve

Nutrition Values: Calories: 110; Fat : 10; Fiber : 0; Carbs : 1. 4; Protein : 3

471. Pesto Crackers

Preparation Time: 27 minutes
Servings: 6
Ingredients:
- 1/2 teaspoon baking powder
- 1/4 teaspoon basil, dried
- 1¼ cups almond flour
- 1 garlic clove, minced
- 2 tablespoons basil pesto
- A pinch of cayenne pepper
- 3 tablespoons ghee
- Salt and black pepper to the taste.

Directions:

1. In a bowl, mix salt, pepper, baking powder and almond flour.
2. Add garlic, cayenne and basil and stir.
3. Add pesto and whisk.

4. Also add ghee and mix your dough with your finger.
5. Spread this dough on a lined baking sheet, introduce in the oven at 325 degrees F and bake for 17 minutes
6. Leave aside to cool down, cut your crackers and serve them as a snack.
Nutrition Values: Calories: 200; Fat : 20; Fiber : 1; Carbs : 4; Protein : 7

Zucchini Chips
Preparation Time: 3 hours 10 minutes
Servings: 8
Ingredients:
- 3 zucchinis, very thinly sliced
- 2 tablespoons balsamic vinegar
- 2 tablespoons olive oil
- Salt and black pepper to the taste.

Directions:
1. In a bowl, mix oil with vinegar, salt and pepper and whisk well.
2. Add zucchini slices, toss to coat well and spread on a lined baking sheet, introduce in the oven at 200 degrees F and bake for 3 hours
3. Leave chips to cool down and serve them as asnack.
Nutrition Values: Calories: 40; Fat : 3; Fiber : 7; Carbs : 3; Protein : 7

472. Avocado Dip

Preparation Time: 3 hours 20 minutes
Servings: 4
Ingredients:
- 2 avocados, pitted, peeled and cut into slices
- 1/2 cup cilantro, chopped.
- 1 cup coconut milk
- 1/4 cup erythritol powder
- 1/4 teaspoon stevia
- Juice and zest of 2 limes

Directions:
1. Place avocado slices on a lined baking sheet, squeeze half of the lime juice over them and keep in your freezer for 3 hours
2. Heat up the coconut milk in a pan over medium heat.
3. Add lime zest; stir and bring to a boil.
4. Add erythritol powder; stir, take off heat and leave aside to cool down a bit.
5. Transfer avocado to your food processor, add the rest of the lime juice and the cilantro and pulse well.
6. Add coconut milk mix and stevia and blend well.
7. Transfer to a bowl and serve right away.
Nutrition Values: Calories: 150; Fat : 14; Fiber : 2; Carbs : 4; Protein : 2

473. Broccoli And Cheddar Biscuits

Preparation Time: 35 minutes
Servings: 12

Ingredients:
- 4 cups broccoli florets
- 1½ cup almond flour
- 2 eggs
- 1/2 teaspoon apple cider vinegar
- 1/2 teaspoon baking soda
- 1 teaspoon paprika
- 1/4 cup coconut oil
- 2 cups cheddar cheese, grated
- 1 teaspoon garlic powder
- Salt and black pepper to the taste.

Directions:
1. Put broccoli florets in your food processor, add some salt and pepper and blend well.
2. In a bowl, mix almond flour with salt, pepper, paprika, garlic powder and baking soda and stir.
3. Add cheddar cheese, coconut oil, eggs and vinegar and stir everything.
4. Add broccoli and stir again.
5. Shape 12 patties, arrange on a baking sheet, introduce in the oven at 375 degrees F and bake for 20 minutes
6. Turn the oven to broiler and broil your biscuits for 5 minutes more
7. Arrange on a platter and serve
Nutrition Values: Calories: 163; Fat : 12; Fiber : 2; Carbs : 2; Protein : 7

474. Celery Sticks

Preparation Time: 10 minutes
Servings: 12
Ingredients:
- 2 cups rotisserie chicken, shredded
- 6 celery sticks cut in halves
- 3 tablespoons hot tomato sauce
- 1/4 cup mayonnaise
- 1/2 teaspoon garlic powder
- Some chopped chives for serving
- Salt and black pepper to the taste.

Directions:
1. In a bowl, mix chicken with salt, pepper, garlic powder, mayo and tomato sauce and stir well.
2. Arrange celery pieces on a platter, spread chicken mix over them, sprinkle some chives and serve
Nutrition Values: Calories: 100; Fat : 2; Fiber : 3; Carbs : 1; Protein : 6

475. Delightful Cucumber Cups

Preparation Time: 10 minutes
Servings: 24
Ingredients:
- 2 cucumbers, peeled, cut into ¾ inch slices and some of the seeds scooped out
- 1/2 cup sour cream
- 2 teaspoons lime juice
- 1 tablespoon lime zest
- 6 ounces smoked salmon, flaked

- 1/3 cup cilantro, chopped.
- A pinch of cayenne pepper
- Salt and white pepper to the taste.

Directions:
1. In a bowl mix salmon with salt, pepper, cayenne, sour cream, lime juice and zest and cilantro and stir well.
2. Fill each cucumber cup with this salmon mix, arrange on a platter and serve as aappetizer.

Nutrition Values: Calories: 30; Fat : 11; Fiber : 1; Carbs : 1; Protein : 2

476. Egg Chips

Preparation Time: 15 minutes
Servings: 2
Ingredients:
- 4 eggs whites
- 2 tablespoons parmesan, shredded
- 1/2 tablespoon water
- Salt and black pepper to the taste.

Directions:
1. In a bowl, mix egg whites with salt, pepper and water and whisk well.
2. Spoon this into a muffin pan, sprinkle cheese on top, introduce in the oven at 400 degrees F and bake for 15 minutes
3. Transfer egg white chips to a platter and serve with adip on the side

Nutrition Values: Calories: 120; Fat : 2; Fiber : 1; Carbs : 2; Protein : 7

477. Cheese Burger Muffins

Preparation Time: 40 minutes
Servings: 9
Ingredients:
- 1/2 cup flaxseed meal
- 1 teaspoon baking powder
- 1/4 cups sour cream
- 1/2 cup almond flour
- 2 eggs
- Salt and black pepper to the taste.

For the filling:
- 1/2 teaspoon onion powder
- 2 tablespoons tomato paste
- 1/2 teaspoon garlic powder
- 1/2 cup cheddar cheese, grated
- 16 ounces beef, ground
- 2 tablespoons mustard
- Salt and black pepper to the taste.

Directions:
1. In a bowl, mix almond flour with flaxseed meal, salt, pepper and baking powder and whisk.
2. Add eggs and sour cream and stir very well.
3. Divide this into a greased muffin pan and press well using your fingers
4. Heat up a pan over medium high heat; add beef; stir and brown for a few minutes
5. Add salt, pepper, onion powder, garlic powder and tomato paste and stir well.

6. Cook for 5 minutes more and take off heat.
7. Fill cupcakes crusts with this mix, introduce in the oven at 350 degrees F and bake for 15 minutes
8. Spread cheese on top, introduce in the oven again and bake muffins for 5 minutes more
9. Serve with mustard and your favorite toppings on top.

Nutrition Values: Calories: 245; Fat : 16; Fiber : 6; Carbs : 2; Protein : 14

478. Tomato Tarts

Preparation Time: 1 hour 20 minutes
Servings: 12
Ingredients:
- 2 tomatoes, sliced
- 1/4 cup olive oil
- Salt and black pepper to the taste.
- For the base:
- 5 tablespoons ghee
- 1 tablespoon psyllium husk
- 1/2 cup almond flour
- 2 tablespoons coconut flour
- A pinch of salt
- For the filling:
- 3 ounces goat cheese, crumbled
- 1 small onion, thinly sliced
- 3 teaspoons thyme, chopped.
- 2 tablespoons olive oil
- 2 teaspoons garlic, minced

Directions:
1. Spread tomato slices on a lined baking sheet, season with salt and pepper, drizzle 1/4 cup olive oil, introduce in the oven at 425 degrees F and bake for 40 minutes
2. Meanwhile; in your food processor mix almond flour with psyllium husk, coconut flour, salt, pepper and cold butter and stir until you obtain a dough.
3. Divide this dough into silicone cupcake molds, press well, introduce in the oven at 350 degrees F and bake for 20 minutes
4. Take cupcakes out of the oven and leave aside
5. Also take tomato slices out of the oven and cool them down a bit.
6. Divide tomato slices on top of cupcakes
7. Heat up a pan with 2 tablespoons olive oil over medium high heat; add onion; stir and cook for 4 minutes
8. Add garlic and thyme; stir, cook for 1 minute more and take off heat.
9. Spread this mix on top of tomato slices
10. Sprinkle goat cheese, introduce in the oven again and cook at 350 degrees F for 5 minutes more
11. Arrange on a platter and serve

Nutrition Values: Calories: 163; Fat : 13; Fiber : 1; Carbs : 3; Protein : 3

479. Pizza Dip

Preparation Time: 30 minutes

Servings: 4

Ingredients:

- 4 ounces cream cheese, soft
- 1/2 cup tomato sauce
- 1/4 cup mayonnaise
- 1/2 cup mozzarella cheese
- 6 pepperoni slices, chopped.
- 1/2 teaspoon Italian seasoning
- 1/4 cup sour cream
- 1/4 cup parmesan cheese, grated
- 1 tablespoon green bell pepper, chopped.
- 4 black olives, pitted and chopped.
- Salt and black pepper to the taste.

Directions:

1. In a bowl, mix cream cheese with mozzarella, sour cream, mayo, salt and pepper and stir well.
2. Spread this into 4 ramekins, add a layer of tomato sauce, then layer parmesan cheese, top with bell pepper, pepperoni, Italian seasoning and black olives
3. Introduce in the oven at 350 degrees F and bake for 20 minutes Serve warm.

Nutrition Values: Calories: 400; Fat : 34; Fiber : 4; Carbs : 4; Protein : 15

480. Prosciutto And Shrimp Appetizer

Preparation Time: 30 minutes

Servings: 16

Ingredients:

- 11 prosciutto sliced
- 10 ounces already cooked shrimp, peeled and deveined
- 2 tablespoons olive oil
- 1/3 cup blackberries, ground
- 1/3 cup red wine
- 1 tablespoons mint, chopped.
- 2 tablespoons erythritol

Directions:

1. Wrap each shrimp in prosciutto slices, arrange on a lined baking sheet, drizzle the olive oil over them, introduce in the oven at 425 degrees F and bake for 15 minutes
2. Heat up a pan with ground blackberries over medium heat; add mint, wine and erythritol; stir, cook for 3 minutes and take off heat.
3. Arrange shrimp on a platter, drizzle blackberries sauce over them and serve

Nutrition Values: Calories: 245; Fat : 12; Fiber : 2; Carbs : 1; Protein : 14

481. Parmesan Wings

Preparation Time: 34 minutes

Servings: 6

Ingredients:

- 6-pound chicken wings, cut in halves
- 1/2 teaspoon Italian seasoning
- 2 tablespoons ghee
- 1/2 cup parmesan cheese, grated
- 1 teaspoon garlic powder
- 1 egg
- A pinch of red pepper flakes, crushed.
- Salt and black pepper to the taste.

Directions:

1. Arrange chicken wings on a lined baking sheet, introduce in the oven at 425 degrees F and bake for 17 minutes
2. Meanwhile; in your blender, mix ghee with cheese, egg, salt, pepper, pepper flakes, garlic powder and Italian seasoning and blend very well.
3. Take chicken wings out of the oven, flip them, turn oven to broil and broil them for 5 minutes more
4. Take chicken pieces out of the oven again, pour sauce over them, toss to coat well and broil for 1 minute more
5. Serve them as a quickappetizer.

Nutrition Values: Calories: 134; Fat : 8; Fiber : 1; Carbs : 0.5; Protein : 14

DESURTS

482. Chocolate Pudding

Preparation time: 10 minutes
Cooking time: 10 minutes
Servings:2
Ingredients:
- ½ cup heavy cream
- 2 eggs, beaten
- 1 teaspoon almond flour
- 2 tablespoons monk fruit
- ¼ oz dark chocolate

Directions:
1. Place heavy cream in the saucepan and start to preheat it.
2. Add eggs and whisk it very carefully.
3. Keep whisking and add almond flour, monk fruit, and dark chocolate.
4. Start to stir the liquid with the help of a spatula.
5. When the liquid starts to be thick, remove it from the heat and chill well.
6. The chilled pudding will be thick and soft. Transfer it into the serving pudding glasses.
Nutrition Values: calories 266, fat 23.7, fiber 1.8, carbs 6.2, protein 9.3

483. Bacon Cookies

Preparation time: 15 minutes
Cooking time: 20 minutes
Servings:6
Ingredients:
- 2 oz bacon, chopped
- 1 tablespoon ghee
- 1 tablespoon butter
- 1 cup almond flour
- 2 tablespoons monk fruit
- 1 teaspoon vanilla extract
- 1 oz dark chocolate sugar-free, chopped
- ½ teaspoon baking powder
- 1 teaspoon apple cider vinegar

Directions:
1. Roast the bacon in the skillet for 5-7 minutes or until it is crunchy.
2. Then chill it.
3. After this, make the cookies dough: mix up together ghee, butter, almond flour, monk fruit, vanilla extract, baking powder, and apple cider vinegar.
4. Add bacon and chocolate.
5. Mix up the mixture little and them knead the dough.
6. Make 6 dough balls.
7. Line the baking tray with baking paper.
8. Place the dough balls in the tray. Press them little.
9. Preheat the oven to 360F and bake the cookies for 15 minutes.

10. Then chill the cookies and store them in the paper bags or glass jar with the closed lid.
Nutrition Values: calories 119, fat 10.4, fiber 0.6, carbs 2.2, protein 4.6

484. Nut Cookies

Preparation time: 15 minutes
Cooking time: 10 minutes
Servings:12
Ingredients:
- 2 tablespoons peanuts
- ¼ cup of coconut milk
- 1 teaspoon baking powder
- 1 cup almond flour
- ½ cup of rice flour
- 2 tablespoons Erythritol
- ½ teaspoon vanilla extract

Directions:
1. Chop the peanuts.
2. Mix up together coconut milk, baking powder, almond flour, and rice flour.
3. Stir gently and add Erythritol and vanilla extract.
4. Knead the dough.
5. Add peanuts and knead the dough again with the help of the hand palms.
6. Then cut the dough into 12 pieces.
7. Roll the small balls and press them gently with the help of hand. The nut cookies are prepared.
8. Line the baking tray with parchment.
9. Put the nut cookies on the tray and transfer the tray in the preheated to 360F oven.
10. Bake the cookies for 10 minutes.
11. Remove the cooked cookies from the oven and chill them well.
Nutrition Values: calories 58, fat 3.2, fiber 0.7, carbs 6.6, protein 1.3

485. Vanilla Mug Cake

Preparation time: 7 minutes
Cooking time: 2 minutes
Servings:4
Ingredients:
- 4 teaspoons almond flour
- 4 teaspoons rice flour
- 2 eggs, beaten
- ½ teaspoon baking powder
- ½ teaspoon lemon juice
- 1 teaspoon vanilla extract
- 3 teaspoons butter, softened
- 1 tablespoon monk fruit
- 1 tablespoon cream cheese

Directions:
1. Mix up together cream cheese with butter and stir gently.
2. Preheat the mixture in the microwave oven for 30 seconds.

3. Then add almond flour and rice flour in the mixture.
4. Stir it.
5. Add baking powder, lemon juice, vanilla extract, egg, and monk fruit.
6. Stir well until homogenous.
7. Pour the mixture into 4 small mugs and flatten the surface.
8. Then place the mugs in the microwave oven and cook for 1 minute.
9. After this, cook for 30 seconds more.
Nutrition Values: calories 241, fat 20, fiber 3.1, carbs 9.3, protein 9.2

486. Blackberry Muffins

Preparation time: 10 minutes
Cooking time: 12 minutes
Servings:6
Ingredients:
- 1/3 cup butter, softened
- 1 teaspoon vanilla extract
- ¾ cup monk fruit
- 1 cup almond flour
- ¾ cup blackberries
- 1 egg, whisked
- 1 teaspoon baking powder
- ½ teaspoon lemon juice

Directions:
1. In the mixing bowl, mix up together butter, vanilla extract, monk fruit, almond flour, egg, baking powder, and lemon juice.
2. When the mixture is smooth, add blackberries and mix up.
3. Then pour the mixture in the muffin molds.
4. Preheat the oven to 365F.
5. Transfer the muffins in the oven and bake them for 12 minutes.
6. Chill the cooked muffins well and discard from the molds.
Nutrition Values: calories 205, fat 12.4, fiber 1.5, carbs 3.1, protein 20.9

487. Avocado Sheet Cake

Preparation time: 10 minutes
Cooking time: 40 minutes
Servings:6
Ingredients:
- 1 tablespoon cocoa powder
- 1 avocado, peeled
- ¾ teaspoon salt
- 4 tablespoons monk fruit
- ½ cup heavy cream
- 1 cup almond flour
- 1 teaspoon ground cinnamon
- 1 tablespoon butter, melted
- 1 egg, beaten

Directions:
1. Line the baking tray with the baking paper.
2. Preheat the oven to 360F.

3. In the mixing bowl, combine together all the ingredients except avocado.
4. Whisk the mixture with the help of the hand blender for 5 minutes. The batter is cooked.
5. After this, chop the avocado and put it in the blender. Blend it until smooth.
6. Add avocado mash in the batter and whisk for 2 minutes more.
7. After this, pour the batter in the prepared baking tray and flatten the surface with the help of the spatula.
8. Transfer the tray with cake in the oven and cook for 40 minutes.
9. When the time is over, check if the cake is cooked with the help of the wooden toothpick: pin the cake, if it is clean, the cake is cooked.
10. Chill the cooked cake to the room temperature and slice into servings.
Nutrition Values: calories 160, fat 15.3, fiber 3.2, carbs 5, protein 3

488. Mint Bars

Preparation time: 15 minutes
Cooking time: 30 minutes
Servings:4
Ingredients:
- 1 teaspoon dried mint
- 1 egg, whisked
- 1 tablespoon coconut oil
- ½ teaspoon peppermint extract
- ½ cup almond flour
- 1 tablespoon Truvia
- ¾ cup of coconut milk
- Cooking spray

Directions:
1. Place whisked egg, coconut oil, and coconut milk in the mixing bowl.
2. Blend the mixture until homogenous.
3. Then add peppermint extract, almond flour, Truvia, and dried mint.
4. Stir the mass until you get a smooth batter.
5. Spray the springform pan with the cooking spray.
6. Pour the mint butter in the pan and flatten its surface with the spatula.
7. Preheat the oven to 360F.
8. Transfer the springform pan in the oven and bake it for 30 minutes.
9. Then switch off the oven and let the dessert rest for 10 minutes.
10. Remove the pan with dessert from the oven, cut it into bars and transfer in the serving plate.
Nutrition Values: calories 170, fat 17, fiber 1.4, carbs 4.6, protein 3.2

489. Matcha-Coconut Muffins

Preparation time: 10 minutes
Cooking time: 12 minutes
Servings:4
Ingredients:

- ½ teaspoon matcha tea
- 2 tablespoons coconut flakes
- 1 cup coconut flour
- ½ teaspoon baking powder
- ½ teaspoon apple cider vinegar
- 1 tablespoon liquid stevia
- ¼ cup organic almond milk
- ½ teaspoon ground ginger
- 1teaspoon butter, melted

Directions:
1. Put all ingredients in the big bowl.
2. Then use the hand blender and blend the mixture until homogenous.
3. With the help of the spoon put the blended mixture in the muffin molds.
4. Flatten the surface of the muffins if needed.
5. Let the muffins rest for 10 minutes.
6. Meanwhile, preheat the oven to 360F.
7. Transfer the muffins in the oven and cook them for 12 minutes.
8. When the muffins are cooked, remove them from the oven and chill for 5-10 minutes.
9. After this, discard them from the muffin molds.

Nutrition Values: calories 44, fat 3.1, fiber 1.8, carbs 3.5, protein 0.9

490. Cake Shake

Preparation time: 5 minutes
Cooking time: 8 minutes
Servings:3
Ingredients:
- 1 ½ cup heavy cream
- ½ cup of coconut milk
- 1 tablespoon cocoa powder
- 2 tablespoons monk fruit
- ½ teaspoon vanilla extract
- ½ oz dark chocolate, melted

Directions:
1. Blend the heavy cream until soft peaks.
2. Then keep whisking and add coconut milk, cocoa powder, monk fruit, vanilla extract, and melted chocolate.
3. Blend the mixture for 3 minutes at maximum speed.
4. Pour the cooked cake shake in the glasses.

Nutrition Values: calories 330, fat 33.4, fiber 1.6, carbs 7.8, protein 2.8

491. Hazelnut Biscotti

Preparation time: 10 minutes
Cooking time: 45 minutes
Servings:7
Ingredients:
- 1 cup almond flour
- 1 teaspoon baking powder
- 1 tablespoon Psyllium Husk
- 1/3 teaspoon ground cinnamon
- 1 teaspoon vanilla extract

- 2 tablespoons butter, softened
- 1 egg, beaten
- 1 tablespoon monk fruit
- ¼ cup hazelnuts, chopped

Directions:
1. Make the biscotti dough: in the mixing bowl mix up together almond flour, baking powder Psyllium husk, ground cinnamon, vanilla extract, and softened butter.
2. Then add egg and monk fruit.
3. Mix up the mixture well, add chopped hazelnuts, and knead the dough.
4. Line the baking tray with baking paper and place the dough on it.
5. Flatten the dough with the help of the fingertips.
6. Bake the dough for 35 minutes at 350F.
7. When the time is over, remove the baked dough from the oven and slice it into the biscotti.
8. Then return the biscotti back in the oven and bake at 345F for 10 minutes.
9. Chill the cooked hazelnut biscotti and store in the closed glass jars.

Nutrition Values: calories 93, fat 7.6, fiber 4.8, carbs 6.7, protein 2.1

492. Sweet Zucchini Pie

Preparation time: 15 minutes
Cooking time: 50 minutes
Servings:6
Ingredients:
- 1 zucchini, grated
- 2 eggs, whisked
- ½ teaspoon baking powder
- 1 tablespoon Psyllium Husk
- ½ cup heavy cream
- 1 cup almond flour
- 2 tablespoons Erythritol
- ½ teaspoon vanilla extract
- ¾ teaspoon ground nutmeg
- 1 teaspoon ground cinnamon

Directions:
1. Mix up together whisked eggs with heavy cream and Psyllium Husk.
2. Add baking powder, grated zucchini, almond flour, Erythritol, vanilla extract, ground nutmeg, and ground cinnamon.
3. Take the spoon and mix up the mass until homogenous.
4. Line the loaf pan with the baking paper.
5. Pour the homogenous zucchini mass in the loaf pan, flatten it and cover with baking paper.
6. Bake the zucchini pie for 40 minutes at 350F.
7. Then remove the baking paper from the surface of the pie and bake it for 10 minutes more at 360F.
8. Chill the cooked pie very well and then cut into servings.

Nutrition Values: calories 105, fat 7.7, fiber 5.8, carbs 12.8, protein 3.5

493. Ginger Cookies

Preparation time: 15 minutes
Cooking time: 8 minutes
Servings:6
Ingredients:
- 1 teaspoon minced ginger
- ½ teaspoon ground ginger
- ½ teaspoon ground cinnamon
- 2 tablespoons Erythritol
- 1 tablespoon butter, softened
- ½ cup almond flour
- 3 tablespoons flax meal
- 2 tablespoons coconut oil

Directions:
1. Mix up together ground ginger, minced ginger, ground cinnamon, Erythritol, butter, flour, flax meal, and coconut oil.
2. With the help of the fingertips knead the dough and cut it into 6 pieces.
3. Make the balls from the dough.
4. Then press the center of every ball with the help of the teaspoon to make the small holes.
5. Place the cookies in the tray and transfer in the oven.
6. Bake the cookies at 360F for 8 minutes.
Nutrition Values: calories 74, fat 7.6, fiber 1.2, carbs 5, protein 1.1

494. Pumpkin Bars

Preparation time: 15 minutes
Cooking time: 15 minutes
Servings:4
Ingredients:
- 1 teaspoon pumpkin puree
- 1 egg, whisked
- ½ teaspoon vanilla extract
- ½ cup almond flour
- ¼ teaspoon ground cinnamon
- 1 tablespoon cream cheese
- ½ teaspoon turmeric
- 1 tablespoon Erythritol

Directions:
1. Mix up together pumpkin puree, whisked egg, vanilla extract, almond flour, ground cinnamon, cream cheese, turmeric, and Erythritol.
2. When you get a smooth batter, transfer it into the non-sticky square pan and flatten it with the help of a spatula.
3. After this, transfer the pan in the oven and bake it at 360F for 15 minutes.
4. The cooked pumpkin dessert will be soft and a little bit wet.
5. Chill the dessert for 10-15 minutes. Then cut it into the bars.
Nutrition Values: calories 48, fat 3.7, fiber 0.6, carbs 1.4, protein 2.4

495. Chocolate Fudge

Preparation time: 10 minutes
Cooking time: 7 minutes
Servings:2
Ingredients:
- ¼ oz dark chocolate -
- ½ teaspoon of cocoa powder
- 4 tablespoons peanut butter

Directions:
1. Put peanut butter and cocoa powder in the saucepan.
2. Churn the mixture until homogenous.
3. Then add dark chocolate and start to preheat the mixture.
4. When it is melted and smooth, switch off the heat.
5. Pour the peanut butter mixture into the silicone muffin molds and freeze until solid.
6. Remove the chocolate fudge from the freezer and transfer in the serving plate.
Nutrition Values: calories 208, fat 17.2, fiber 2.2, carbs 8.7, protein 8.4

496. Cheesecake Fat Bombs

Preparation time: 10 minutes
Cooking time: 17 minutes
Servings:5
Ingredients:
- 5 tablespoons cream cheese
- 1 teaspoon vanilla extract
- ¾ teaspoon ground cinnamon
- 2 eggs, whisked
- 2 tablespoons Erythritol
- ½ teaspoon ricotta cheese
- ¾ teaspoon lime zest, grated

Directions:
1. Whisk the cream cheese with the ricotta cheese using the hand mixer.
2. When the mixture is fluffy, add eggs and whisk until homogenous.
3. Then add ground cinnamon, vanilla extract, Erythritol, and lime zest.
4. Stir the mass and transfer into the silicone muffin molds.
5. Bake the cheesecake fat bombs for 17 minutes at 355F.
6. Chill the cooked fat bombs and remove them from the muffin molds.
Nutrition Values: calories 64, fat 5.3, fiber 0.2, carbs 0.9, protein 3

497. Cardamom Donuts

Preparation time: 10 minutes
Cooking time: 18 minutes
Servings:4
Ingredients:
- 4 tablespoons almond flour
- 2 tablespoons flax meal
- 1 teaspoon ground cardamom

- 2 tablespoons Erythritol
- 2 eggs, whisked
- 2 tablespoons coconut milk
- 1 teaspoon butter, softened

Directions:
1. In the mixing bowl, mix up together flax meal, almond flour, ground cardamom, whisked eggs coconut milk, and butter.
2. When the mixture is smooth pour it into the donut cavities. -Fill only 1/3 part of every donut cavity
3. Bake the donuts in the oven at 350F for 18 minutes or until they are light brown.
4. Then remove the cooked donuts from the donut cavities and coat into Erythritol.
5. Do it very fast until donuts are hot.
Nutrition Values: calories 234, fat 20.2, fiber 4.3, carbs 7.9, protein 9.8

498. Caramel Sauce

Preparation time: 8 minutes
Cooking time: 7 minutes
Servings:4
Ingredients:
- 4 teaspoons butter
- 1 tablespoon xylitol
- 2 tablespoons Monk fruit
- ½ cup heavy cream
- 1 teaspoon vanilla extract

Directions:
1. Toss butter in the saucepan and melt.
2. Add xylitol, Monk fruit, and vanilla extract.
3. Add heavy cream and mix up until homogenous.
4. Bring the liquid to boil.
5. Then stir it well and let caramel sauce chill to the room temperature.
6. Store the dessert in the fridge up to 2 days.
Nutrition Values: calories 91, fat 9.4, fiber 0, carbs 1.2, protein 0.4

499. Mascarpone Mousse with Blueberries

Preparation time: 10 minutes
Servings:2
Ingredients:
- 4 tablespoons mascarpone cheese
- 1 tablespoon blueberries
- 1 tablespoon coconut milk
- 1 teaspoon Erythritol
- ½ teaspoon of cocoa powder

Directions:
- Mix up together coconut milk and mascarpone cheese.
- Use the hand blender to whisk the mixture until fluffy.
- Then add Erythritol and whisk it for 10 seconds.
- After this, transfer the cooked mousse into the serving glasses and add cocoa powder.

- Stir the mixture with the help of the toothpick gently. You will need to get chocolate swirls.
- After this, top the mousse with blueberries.
Nutrition Values: calories 75, fat 5.9, fiber 0.4, carbs 4.3, protein 3.8

500. Chocolate Heaven

Preparation time: 15 minutes
Cooking time: 25 minutes
Servings:6
Ingredients:
- 1/3 cup cocoa powder
- 6 tablespoons butter, softened
- 6 tablespoons ricotta
- 1 teaspoon vanilla extract
- ¼ cup Monk fruit

Directions:
1. Blend together Monk fruit and softened butter.
2. After 3 minutes of blending, add ricotta cheese, vanilla extract, and cocoa powder.
3. Whisk the mixture with the help of the hand blender for 5 minutes or until you get the soft and fluffy texture of the chocolate mixture.
4. Then transfer the mass into the square springform pan and flatten it.
5. Make the light swirls with the help of the spoon -like clouds.
6. Transfer the pan in the fridge and freeze the dessert for 25 minutes or until it is solid.
7. Cut the chocolate into the bars.
Nutrition Values: calories 136, fat 13.4, fiber 1.4, carbs 3.5, protein 2.8

501. Meringue Clouds

Preparation time: 15 minutes
Cooking time: 60 minutes
Servings:5
Ingredients:
- 2 egg whites, from the fridge
- 5 teaspoons Erythritol
- 1 teaspoon lemon juice
- 1 tablespoon almond flour

Directions:
1. Put egg whites in the mixer bowl and start to mix them on the low heat.
2. Then gradually increase the speed till maximum.
3. When egg whites turn into the mass of the light peak, add lemon juice and Erythritol.
4. Whisk the mass for 1 minute and add the almond flour.
5. Whisk the mass until it has strong peaks - appx. 4-5 minutes on the maximum speed of mixer.
6. Meanwhile, lime the baking tray with the baking paper.
7. Transfer the egg white mass in the paper cone and make medium meringue clouds on the baking paper.

8. Bake the clouds for 60 minutes at 300F.
9. The cooked meringue clouds will be dry and very light.
Nutrition Values: calories 39, fat 2.8, fiber 0.6, carbs 6.3, protein 2.7

502. Silk Pie

Preparation time: 20 minutes
Cooking time: 10 minutes
Servings:8
Ingredients:
- ½ cup almond flour
- 1 tablespoon coconut oil
- 1 egg, beaten
- ¾ teaspoon salt
- ½ cup cream cheese
- 1 tablespoon sour cream
- ½ cup whipped cream
- 4 tablespoons Monk fruit
- 1 teaspoon vanilla extract
- 1 tablespoon cocoa powder
- 1 tablespoon butter

Directions:
1. Make the pie crust: mix up together coconut oil, almond flour, egg, and salt.
2. Knead the dough and transfer it in the springform pan.
3. Flatten the dough to make pie crust.
4. Bake it for 10 minutes at 355F or until the pie crust is golden brown.
5. Meanwhile, make the silk filling.
6. Put the cream cheese in the mixer bowl.
7. Add sour cream, Monk fruit, vanilla extract, and butter.
8. With the help of the mixer mix up it until smooth and fluffy.
9. Then add whipped cream, and carefully stir the mass with the help of the spatula.
10. Remove the pie crust from the oven and chill it till the room temperature.
11. Then place the cream cheese silk mass over the pie crust. Flatten it well.
12. Refrigerate the pie for at least 1 hour.
Nutrition Values: calories 124, fat 12.4, fiber 0.4, carbs 1.5, protein 2.5

503. Almond Bun

Preparation time: 15 minutes
Cooking time: 30 minutes
Servings:6
Ingredients:
- 3 tablespoons almond butter
- 1 cup almond flour
- ½ teaspoon ground cinnamon
- ½ teaspoon baking powder
- ½ teaspoon lemon juice
- 1 tablespoon Erythritol
- 2 tablespoons ground flax meal
- 1 tablespoon cream cheese

Directions:
1. Mix up together almond butter, cream cheese, and lemon juice.
2. When the mixture is homogenous, add almond flour, ground cinnamon, baking powder, Erythritol, and ground flax meal.
3. Stir the mass with the help of the spoon carefully.
4. Line the baking dish with the parchment.
5. Then with the help of the scopper make the buns and place them in the prepared baking dish.
6. Bake the buns for 30 minutes at 350F.
7. Then check if the buns are cooked – press them gently with the help of the fingertips, if they are too soft – cook them for an extra 10 minutes.
8. Chill the almond buns well before serving.
Nutrition Values: calories 93, fat 8.2, fiber 2.1, carbs 3.6, protein 3.3

504. Flan

Preparation time: 10 minutes
Cooking time: 35 minutes
Servings:4
Ingredients:
- 4 teaspoons Erythritol
- 1 tablespoon butter
- 4 tablespoons water
- 1 teaspoon vanilla extract
- 4 eggs, beaten
- 1 cup heavy cream
- 2 tablespoons monk Fruit

Directions:
1. Make flan caramel: in the saucepan combine together Erythritol and water.
2. When the liquid starts to boil, add butter and stir well.
3. Boil caramel for 3-4 minutes over the low heat.
4. Then pour caramel into the flan ramekins.
5. Nake flan: mix up together Monk fruit, heavy cream, and beaten eggs.
6. Whisk the liquid with the help of the hand mixer.
7. When it is homogenous, pour it into the ramekins over the caramel.
8. Place the ramekins into the casserole dish.
9. Pour hot water into the casserole dish to cover ½ part of every ramekin.
10. Bake flan for 30 minutes at 350F.
11. Chill cooked flan well and remove from the ramekins.
Nutrition Values: calories 195, fat 18.4, fiber 0, carbs 6.3, protein 6.2

505. Matcha Crepe Cake

Preparation time: 10 minutes
Cooking time:15 minutes
Servings:6
Ingredients:
- 1 tablespoon matcha tea

- 1 cup almond flour
- 1 teaspoon baking powder
- ¼ cup of coconut milk
- 1 tablespoon Erythritol
- 1 teaspoon olive oil
- 4 tablespoons cream cheese
- 1 teaspoon sour cream

Directions:
1. Make the crepe batter: mix up together almond flour, matcha tea, baking powder, coconut milk, and olive oil.
2. With the help of the hand mixer, blend the batter until smooth.
3. Preheat non-stick skillet.
4. Ladle one ladle of the batter in the skillet and flatten it in the shape of crepe.
5. Cook the crepe for 1 minute from each side.
6. Repeat the same steps with remaining batter.
7. After this, blend together Erythritol, sour cream, and cream cheese.
8. Spread the fluffy cream cheese mixture on every crepe and combine them together to make the shape of the cake.
9. Let the cooked crepe cake cool for 10 minutes in the fridge.

Nutrition Values: calories 84, fat 8, fiber 0.7, carbs 5.1, protein 1.8

506. Pumpkin Spices Mini Pies

Preparation time: 15 minutes
Cooking time: 30 minutes
Servings:7
Ingredients:
- 1 tablespoon pumpkin pie spices
- 1 tablespoon pumpkin puree
- 1 teaspoon ground turmeric
- 2 tablespoons butter
- 1 cup coconut flour
- 3 tablespoons heavy cream
- ½ teaspoon ground nutmeg
- 1 tablespoon coconut oil
- 1 teaspoon baking powder
- 3 tablespoons Truvia
- Cooking spray

Directions:
1. In the mixing bowl, mix up together pumpkin pie spices and pumpkin puree.
2. Add the ground turmeric, butter, coconut flour, heavy cream, ground nutmeg, coconut oil, baking powder, and Truvia.
3. Use the spoon to mix up the mixture until homogenous.
4. Spray the silicone molds with cooking spray.
5. Put the pumpkin spices mixture in the silicone molds.
6. Bake the pies for 30 minutes at 355F.
7. Then chill the cooked mini pies well and remove them from the molds.

Nutrition Values: calories 154, fat 10.7, fiber 7.2, carbs 13.8, protein 3.7

507. Nut Bars

Preparation time: 15 minutes
Cooking time: 20 minutes
Servings:4
Ingredients:
- 4 pecans, chopped
- 2 tablespoons walnuts, chopped
- 1 tablespoon chia seeds
- 1 tablespoons almonds, chopped
- 1 tablespoon pumpkin seeds
- 2 tablespoons coconut flakes
- 1 tablespoon Erythritol
- 3 tablespoon peanut butter

Directions:
1. Put the peanut butter and Erythritol in the bowl and stir well.
2. Then microwave the mixture for 15 seconds.
3. In the separate bowl, mix up together chopped pecans, walnuts, chis seeds, almonds, pumpkin seeds, and coconut flakes.
4. Then add melted peanut butter and mix up the mixture.
5. Line the baking tray with parchment and transfer the nut mixture in it.
6. Flatten it into the shape of a square and cut into bars.
7. Dry the nutbars in the preheated to the 300F oven for 20 minutes.
8. Then let the cooked nut bars rest for 30minutes more in a dry and warm place.

Nutrition Values: calories 233, fat 21.6, fiber 3.8, carbs 10.6, protein 6.8

508. Pound Cake

Preparation time: 15 minutes
Cooking time: 30 minutes
Servings:4
Ingredients:
- 1 teaspoon baking powder
- 1 teaspoon apple cider vinegar
- 1 cup almond flour
- 2 tablespoons butter
- 1/3 cup whipped cream
- 2 tablespoons Erythritol
- ½ teaspoon vanilla extract
- 2 egg, beaten

Directions:
1. Mix up together baking powder, apple cider vinegar, almond flour, butter, vanilla extract, and eggs.
2. When the mixture is homogenous and smooth, transfer it in the pound cake pan.
3. Flatten the surface of the cake and transfer it in the preheated to the 360F oven.
4. Cook the pound cake for 30 minutes.

5.   Check if the cake is cooked with the help of the toothpick. Pierce the cake with it; if the toothpick is dry, the cake is cooked.
6.   Stir Erythritol in the whipped cream.
7.   Chill the pound cake well and remove it from the pan.
8.   Spread the surface of the pound cake with the sweet whipped cream mixture.
9.   Slice the cake into the servings.
Nutrition Values: calories 155, fat 14.6, fiber 0.8, carbs 8.6, protein 4.6

509. Tortilla Chips with Cinnamon Recipe

Preparation Time: 10 minutes
Servings: 4
Ingredients:
- 4 flour tortillas
- 2 tbsp. vegan margarine, melted
- 1 tbsp. cinnamon
- 1 tbsp. sugar

Directions:
1.   Start by preparing all the ingredients together then slice the tortillas like a pizza into 6 slices to create tortilla chips.
2.   Drizzle each tortilla "chips" with melted margarine and then sprinkle with cinnamon and sugar.
3.   Bake the tortilla chips at 350 F for at least 10 minutes, or until desired crispy.
4.   Serve with your favourite smoothies or fruit shake.
5.   Enjoy!

510. Granola Yogurt with Berries

Preparation Time: 5 minutes
Servings: 4
Ingredients:
- 2 cups unsweetened plain yogurt
- 2 teaspoons pure vanilla extract
- ½ cup Granola, divided
- ½ cup sliced fresh strawberries
- ½ cup fresh blueberries

Directions:
1.   Start by preparing all the ingredients together then mix the yogurt and vanilla in a small bowl.
2.   Scoop ½ cup of the yogurt mixture into each of two small cups.
3.   Top each with 2 tablespoons of granola, strawberries, and blueberries.
4.   Add another ½ cup of the yogurt mixture to each cup and top with the remaining granola and fruit.
5.   Serve and enjoy!

511. Berry Sorbet

Preparation Time: 25 minutes
Servings: 4
Ingredients:
- 1 cup halved strawberries
- 1 cup blueberries
- Juice of 1 lemon
- ⅓ Cup maple syrup

Directions:
1.   Start by preparing all the ingredients together and use a blender then add the strawberries, blueberries, lemon juice, and maple syrup.
2.   Blend until the mixture has a smooth and even texture.
3.   Pour the mixture into an ice cream maker and freeze the sorbet according to the manufacturer's instructions. It takes about 25 minutes.
4.   Transfer the sorbet into an airtight, freezer-safe container and let freeze for at least 2 hours.
5.   Serve and enjoy!

512. Coconut Berry Smoothie

Preparation Time: 5 minutes
Servings: 2
Ingredients:
- ¼ cup blanched almonds
- 1 cup mixed berries
- 4 Medjool dates
- 2 cups coconut milk
- 1 tbsp. honey

Directions:
1.   Start by preparing all the ingredients together then combine all the ingredients in your blender then pulse until smooth and well blended.
2.   Pour the smoothies in tall glasses.
3.   Serve and enjoy!

513. Coconut Milk Banana Smoothie

Preparation Time: 5 minutes
Servings: 2
Ingredients:
- 1 banana
- 2 tbsp. almond butter
- ¼ tsp. cinnamon powder
- 2 tbsp. honey
- 1 cup coconut milk

Directions:
1.   Start by preparing all the ingredients together then combine all the ingredients in your blender then pulse until smooth and well blended.
2.   Pour the smoothies in tall glasses.
3.   Serve and enjoy!

514. Mango Pineapple Smoothie

Preparation Time: 5 minutes
Servings: 2
Ingredients:
- ½ cup pineapple
- ½ ripe mango, cut in cubes
- 1 ripe banana, quartered
- 1/3 cup orange juice
- 3-4 ice cubes

Directions:

1.   Start by preparing all the ingredients together then combine all the ingredients in your blender then pulse until smooth and well blended.
2.   Pour the smoothies in tall glasses.
3.   Serve and enjoy!

515. Raspberry Green Smoothie

Preparation Time: 5 minutes
Servings: 2
Ingredients:
- ½ cup chopped kale
- 2 leaves kale
- ½ ripe banana
- 1 cup sliced cucumber
- 3-4 ice cubes

Directions:
1.   Start by preparing all the ingredients together then combine all the ingredients in your blender then pulse until smooth and well blended.
2.   Pour the smoothies in tall glasses.
3.   Serve and enjoy!

516. Loaded Berries Smoothie

Preparation Time: 5 minutes
Servings: 2
Ingredients:
- 1 ripe banana
- ½ cup chopped strawberries
- ½ cup blueberries
- ½ cup blackberries
- 1/2 cup unsweetened soy milk

Directions:
1.   Start by preparing all the ingredients together then combine all the ingredients in your blender then pulse until smooth and well blended.
2.   Pour the smoothies in tall glasses.
3.   Serve and enjoy!

517. Papaya Banana and Kale Smoothie

Preparation Time: 5 minutes
Servings: 2
Ingredients:
- 3 ice cubes
- 1 cup papaya, chopped
- ½ cup fresh orange juice
- 2 pcs ripe bananas
- 3 pcs of kale leaves, chopped

Directions:
1.   Start by preparing all the ingredients together then combine all the ingredients in your blender then pulse until smooth and well blended.
2.   Pour the smoothies in tall glasses.
3.   Serve and enjoy!

518. Green Orange Smoothie

Preparation Time: 5 minutes
Servings: 2
Ingredients:
- 2 cups of chopped kale
- 1 cup of chopped carrots
- 1 cup fresh orange juice
- 3 ice cubes

Directions:
1.   Start by preparing all the ingredients together then combine all the ingredients in your blender then pulse until smooth and well blended.
2.   Pour the smoothies in tall glasses.
3.   Serve and enjoy!

519. Double Berries Smoothie

Preparation Time: 5 minutes
Servings: 2
Ingredients:
- ½ cup fresh cranberries
- ½ chopped cucumber
- ½ cup fresh raspberries
- ½ cup of water
- 5 pcs ice cubes

Directions:
1.   Start by preparing all the ingredients together then combine all the ingredients in your blender then pulse until smooth and well blended.
2.   Pour the smoothies in tall glasses.
3.   Serve and enjoy!

520. Energizing Protein Bars

Preparation Time: 20 minutes
Servings: 4
Ingredients:
- 1 cup pumpkin purée
- 2 eggs
- 1/2 cup almond butter
- 4 oz. vanilla flavoured protein powder
- 1/2 cup maple syrup
- 1 tsp. pure vanilla extract
- 1 cup whole wheat flour
- 1 tsp. baking soda
- 1 tsp. ground cinnamon
- 1/4 tsp. nutmeg
- 1/8 tsp. ground cloves
- 1 cup rolled oats
- 2 tbsp. chocolate chips

Directions:
1.   Start by preparing all the ingredients together then preheat your oven to 350 degrees F then spray a pan with cooking spray.
2.   In a medium-sized bowl, use an electric mixer to combine pumpkin puree, almond butter, protein powder, maple syrup, and vanilla and then beat in the eggs.
3.   Add in the flour, baking soda, and spices until a smooth batter forms then add in the rolled oats.
4.   Spread batter equally into the prepared pan and sprinkle with chocolate chips.
5.   Bake for 15 minutes.
6.   Check the protein bards by inserting toothpick and when the toothpick comes out clean, and then they are done.

7.   Serve and enjoy!

521. Peanut Butter and Fruit Sandwich

Preparation Time: 20 minutes
Servings: 4
Ingredients:
- 1 cup rolled oats
- 4 regular sized apples
- 2 tbsp. ground flaxseeds
- 1 tsp. ground cinnamon
- 2 tbsp. orange juice
- 2 tbsp. honey
- 1 tbsp. packed brown sugar
- 1 tsp. vegetable oil
- 1/2 tsp. vanilla extract
- 1/4 cup raisins
- 1/3 cup creamy peanut butter
- Salt

Directions:
1.   Start by preparing all the ingredients together then preheat your oven to 300° F.
2.   Combine the rolled oats, flaxseeds, ground cinnamon in a medium bowl.
3.   In a sauce pan, add in the orange juice, honey and brown sugar on medium heat until the sugar dissolves while stirring continuously.
4.   Remove from the heat then add in oil and vanilla.
5.   Pour honey mixture over oat mixture, stirring to combine well. Spread mixture in a thin layer onto a roll pan coated with a bit of olive oil.
6.   Bake for about 20 minutes or until golden brown while stirring well halfway through.
7.   Add in raisins and let cool completely.
8.   To set the sandwiches, core each apple and cut into ¼-inch slices. Spread two teaspoons of peanut butter on eight apple slices then sprinkle with crushed nuts of your choice.
9.   Top with remaining apple slices, pressing down carefully to make the sandwiches.
10.   Serve and enjoy!

522. Healthy Green Bites

Preparation Time: 5 minutes
Servings: 2
Ingredients:
- 1 cucumber, ends removed and cut into round slices
- ½ Avocado, peeled, seeded and diced
- 1/4 cup red bell pepper, diced
- 1 tbsp.lime juice
- 1 tbsp.cilantro, diced
- 1/2 tsp. cumin
- 1/4 tsp. salt

Directions:
1.   Start by preparing all the ingredients together then get a melon baller then scoop out the centre of the cucumber slices.

2.   In a mixing bowl, pound the avocado, and add diced red bell pepper, lime juice, cilantro, cumin, and salt.
3.   Mix to combine all the added ingredients.
4.   Place avocado mixture in a zip top plastic bag. Cut off one bottom corner of bag and squeeze avocado mixture into hollowed-out cucumber slices.
5.   Serve and enjoy!

523. Kale Salted Chips

Preparation Time: 45 minutes
Servings: 2
Ingredients:
- 1 cup of kale
- 1 tbsp. extra virgin olive oil
- 1/4 tsp. sea salt

Directions:
1.   Start by preparing all the ingredients together then preheat your oven to 250ºF then line two baking sheets with parchment paper.
2.   Break the kale up into bite size pieces removing the stems and ribs.
3.   Rinse the kale in a colander then shake out all excess water.
4.   Place kale into a large bowl and add olive oil and salt.
5.   With the use of your hands, massage the oil and salt onto the kale pieces.
6.   Divide the kale equally onto the two baking sheets and bake for 45 minutes or until the kale becomes crispy.
7.   Serve with your homemade healthy dip and enjoy!

524. Macho Nachos

Preparation Time: 10 minutes
Servings: 2
Ingredients:
- 20 mini sweet peppers, cut in halved and seeded
- 1 pound ground beef, cooked
- 1 tbsp. cumin
- 2 tbsp. Chilli Powder
- 8 oz. Cheddar Cheese, shredded
- 1 Jalapeno sliced
- Salt

For toppings:
- Avocado
- Tomatoes
- Sour cream

Directions:
1.   Start by preparing all the ingredients together then start cooking the beef adding cumin, chilli powder, and salt in a pan.
2.   Prepare the mini sweet pepper halves on a sheet pan.
3.   Sprinkle cooked meat over mini peppers careful not to let the peppers fall through to the pan.
4.   Cover mini peppers with shredded cheese and jalapeno slices.

138

5. Place in oven set to broil for 5 minutes or until cheese is melted.
6. And then add your toppings to complete your nachos.
7. Serve and enjoy!

525. Sweet and Nutty Brownies

Preparation Time: 50 minutes
Servings: 2
Ingredients:
- 2 boxes brownie mix
- 1/2 cup peanut butter
- 11 tablespoons water
- 1/4 cup oil
- 2 organic eggs
- 1 cup muscovado sugar
- 1 cup pure maple syrup
- 1-1/4 cups peanut butter, all natural
- 2 cups dark chocolate chips
- 1/3 cup peanut butter, all natural

Directions:
1. Start by preparing all the ingredients together then preheat your oven to 350 degrees F then grease 13" x 9" pan with non-stick baking spray and set aside.
2. Combine brownie mix in a large bowl, 1/2 cup of peanut butter, water, oil, and eggs; mix until blended, then beat 30 strokes.
3. Pour into prepared pan. Bake for 45 minutes or until brownies are just set; do not over bake. Let cool on wire rack.
4. In medium microwave-safe bowl, combine sugar and maple syrup.
5. Microwave the mixture on high heat for 2 minutes, then remove and stir.
6. Return to microwave and cook on high heat for 1minute longer.
7. Remove from microwave and immediately stir in 1-1/4 cups peanut butter. Mix well with wire whisk and quickly pour over cooled brownies. Spread evenly to cover.
8. Combine dark chocolate chips and 1/3 cup of peanut butter in a small microwave-safe bowl.
9. Microwave on high for 1minute, then remove and stir until chips melt and mixture is smooth.
10. Pour the caramel mixture on and carefully, with the back of a spoon, spread evenly over the caramel mixture.
11. Cut into bars then serve.
12. Enjoy!

526. Peanut Butter Choco Banana Gelato with Mint

Preparation Time: 5 minutes
Servings: 2
Ingredients:
- 2 bananas, peeled and frozen
- 1 tbsp. peanut butter
- 1 tbsp. cocoa powder
- Mint leaves for toppings

Directions:
1. Start by preparing all the ingredients together then cut the bananas into pieces and put them in a food processor or heavy duty blender.
2. Blend until smooth.
3. Add in the peanut butter and cocoa powder and blend until everything is incorporated and smooth.
4. Serve into ice cream cups with mint leaves on top.
5. Enjoy!

527. Cinnamon Peaches and Yogurt

Preparation Time: 5 minutes
Servings: 2
Ingredients:
- 2 large peaches, halved and pitted
- 2 tbsp. raw honey
- ½ tsp. cinnamon powder
- 1 cup low fat plain yogurt
- ¼ cup sliced almonds

Directions:
1. Start by preparing all the ingredients together then drizzle the peach halves with honey and sprinkle with cinnamon powder. Heat a grill pan over medium flame and place the peaches on the grill.
2. Cook until browned then place on serving plates.
3. Top with yogurt and almond slices.
4. Serve and enjoy!

528. Pear Mint Honey Popsicles

Preparation Time: 5 minutes
Servings: 4
Ingredients:
4 cups pears cut into small pieces
- 4 mint leaves
- 1 lime, juiced
- 2 tbsp. raw honey
- 1 tsp. lemon zest

Directions:
1. Start by preparing all the ingredients together then combine all the ingredients in a blender and pulse until smooth.
2. Pour the mixture in a Popsicle mould and freeze at least 3 hours. When done, dip into hot water for a few seconds to unmould them easier.
3. Serve and enjoy!

529. Coconut Spiced Apple Smoothie

Preparation Time: 5 minutes
Servings: 2
Ingredients:
- 1 apple
- 2 tbsp. almond butter
- ¼ tsp. cinnamon powder
- 1 pinch ground ginger
- 2 tbsp. hemp seeds
- 2 tbsp. honey

- 1 cup coconut milk

Directions:
1.   Start by preparing all the ingredients together then combine all the ingredients in your blender then pulse until smooth and well blended.
2.   Pour the smoothies in tall glasses.
3.   Serve and enjoy!

530. Sweet and Nutty Smoothie

Preparation Time: 5 minutes
Servings: 2
Ingredients:
- 1 banana
- ½ cucumbers
- 1 tbsp. peanut butter

Directions:
1.   Start by preparing all the ingredients together then combine all the ingredients in your blender then pulse until smooth and well blended.
2.   Pour the smoothies in tall glasses.
3.   Serve and enjoy!

531. Orange and Peaches Smoothie

Preparation Time: 5 minutes
Servings: 2
Ingredients:
- 2 oranges, cut into segments
- 2 peaches, pitted and sliced
- 1 cup carrot juice
- ¼ tsp. cinnamon powder
- 1 pinch ground ginger
- 2 tbsp. ground flaxseeds
- 1 tbsp. chia seeds

Directions:
1.   Start by preparing all the ingredients together then combine all the ingredients in your blender then pulse until smooth and well blended.
2.   Pour the smoothies in tall glasses.
3.   Serve and enjoy!

532. Ginger Berry Smoothie

Preparation Time: 5 minutes
Servings: 2
Ingredients:
- ½ cup unsweetened almond milk
- 1 cup mix berries
- ½ cup unsweetened plain yogurt
- 1 piece fresh ginger, minced
- 4 or 5 ice cubes

Directions:
1.   Start by preparing all the ingredients together then combine all the ingredients in your blender then pulse until smooth and well blended.
2.   Pour the smoothies in tall glasses.
3.   Serve and enjoy!

533. Vegetarian Friendly Smoothie

Preparation Time: 5 minutes
Servings: 6

Ingredients:
- 950 ml water
- 180 grams romaine lettuce
- 60 grams pineapple, chopped
- 2 tbsp. fresh parsley
- 1 tbsp. minced ginger
- 180 grams cucumber, peeled and finely chopped
- ½ cup kiwi fruit, peeled and sliced
- ½ avocado, sliced
- 1 tbsp. sugar substitute
- Ice cubes for serving

Directions:
1.   Start by preparing all the ingredients together then wash the lettuce leaves properly with water and coarsely chop it using a knife.
2.   Add them in a blender. To this, add chopped pineapple, ginger, cucumber, kiwi, avocado, sugar substitute and water.
3.   Give all the ingredients a whisk. Now add some parsley and blend the mixture into a smooth paste. Make sure there are no lumps. You can also strain this juice if you wish.
4.   Pour the smoothie into a large glass.
5.   Add then the ice cubes and serve chilled.
6.   Enjoy!

534. ChocNut Smoothie

Preparation Time: 5 minutes
Servings: 2
Ingredients:
- 1 large cup coconut milk, full fat
- ½ avocado, ripe
- 30 grams cacao powder
- 180 grams frozen cherries
- ¼ tsp. turmeric powder
- 230 ml cup water
- Ice cubes

Directions:
1.   Start by preparing all the ingredients together then wash the avocado properly with water and coarsely chop it using a knife.
2.   Add it to a blender then stir in the cacao powder, roughly chopped cherries and turmeric powder and give it a whisk.
3.   Add the water, coconut milk and blend all the ingredients until it forms a smooth paste.
4.   Pour it into a large glass and add some ice cubes to serve.
5.   You can also refrigerate the smoothie for about 30 minutes before serving.
6.   Enjoy!

535. Coco Strawberry Smoothie

Preparation Time: 5 minutes
Servings: 2
Ingredients:
- 180 grams frozen strawberries
- 230 ml coconut milk, unsweetened

- 2 tbsp. almond butter
- 1 tbsp. peanut butter
- 2 packets stevia
- 1 tsp. chia seeds
- Crushed ice
- Mint leaves

Directions:

1. Start by preparing all the ingredients together then wash the strawberries properly with water and coarsely chop it using a knife.
2. Add the strawberries to a blender then stir in the almond butter, coconut milk, peanut butter, chia seeds, stevia drops and blend it using a hand blender.
3. Pour in a tall glass and add crushed ice.
4. Garnish with mint leaves and serve.
5. Enjoy!

536. Egg Spinach Berries Smoothie

Preparation Time: 5 minutes
Servings: 2
Ingredients:

- 1 large egg
- 60 ml coconut milk
- 180 grams of berries
- 365 grams baby spinach, thawed
- ¼ avocado, sliced
- Crushed ice

Directions:

1. Start by preparing all the ingredients together then wash the berries properly with water and coarsely chop it using a knife.
2. Wash the baby spinach and chop it up with the knife.
3. Add the chopped spinach, berries and sliced avocado to the blender and whisk.
4. Add the coconut milk, crack an egg and whisk again until smooth.
5. Add crushed ice to this smoothie and serve chilled.
6. Enjoy!

537. Creamy Dessert Smoothie

Preparation Time: 5 minutes
Servings: 2
Ingredients:

- 175 ml cup coconut milk
- 60 ml sour cream
- 2 tbsp. flaxseed meal
- 1 tbsp. macadamia nut oil
- 20 drops of stevia
- ½ tsp. mango essence
- ¼ tsp. banana essence
- Crushed ice

Directions:

1. Start by preparing all the ingredients together then add the flax seed meal to some coconut milk in a bowl and let it soak up for 10 minutes.

2. Stir in the sour cream, macadamia oil, stevia, mango essence, banana essence and mix. Add this to a blender and whisk until smooth.
3. Pour into tall glasses and add crushed ice to them.
4. Serve chilled.
5. Enjoy!

538. Sweet Buns

Preparation Time: 40 minutes
Servings: 8
Ingredients:

- 1/3 cup psyllium husks
- 1/2 cup coconut flour
- 2 tablespoons swerve
- 4 eggs
- 1 teaspoon baking powder
- 1/2 teaspoon cinnamon
- 1/2 teaspoon cloves; ground
- Some chocolate chips; unsweetened
- 1 cup hot water
- A pinch of salt

Directions:

1. In a bowl, mix flour with psyllium husks, swerve, baking powder, salt, cinnamon, cloves and chocolate chips and stir well.
2. Add water and egg; stir well until you obtain a dough, shape 8 buns and arrange them on a lined baking sheet.
3. Introduce in the oven at 350 degrees and bake for 30 minutes
4. Serve these buns with some almond milk and enjoy!

Nutrition Values: Calories: 100; Fat : 3; Fiber : 3; Carbs : 6; Protein : 6

539. EasyMacaroons

Preparation Time: 20 minutes
Servings: 20
Ingredients:

- 2 cup coconut; shredded
- 1 teaspoon vanilla extract
- 4 egg whites
- 2 tablespoons stevia

Directions:

1. In a bowl, mix egg whites with stevia and beat using your mixer.
2. Add coconut and vanilla extract and stir.
3. Roll this mix into small balls and place them on a lined baking sheet.
4. Introduce in the oven at 350 degrees F and bake for 10 minutes
5. Serve your macaroons cold.

Nutrition Values: Calories: 55; Fat : 6; Fiber : 1; Carbs : 2; Protein : 1

540. Delicious Chocolate Truffles

Preparation Time: 16 minutes
Servings: 22
- **Ingredients:**

141

- 1 cup sugar free- chocolate chips
- 2 tablespoons butter
- 2 teaspoons brandy
- 2 tablespoons swerve
- 2/3 cup heavy cream
- 1/4 teaspoon vanilla extract
- Cocoa powder

Directions:

1. Put heavy cream in a heat proof bowl, add swerve, butter and chocolate chips; stir, introduce in your microwave and heat up for 1 minute
2. Leave aside for 5 minutes; stir well and mix with brandy and vanilla.
3. Stir again, leave aside in the fridge for a couple of hours
4. Use a melon baller to shape your truffles, roll them in cocoa powder and serve them.

Nutrition Values: Calories: 60; Fat : 5; Fiber : 4; Carbs : 6; Protein : 1

541. Coconut Pudding

Preparation Time: 20 minutes
Servings: 4
Ingredients:

- 1 2/3 cups coconut milk
- 1/2 teaspoon vanilla extract
- 3 egg yolks
- 1 tablespoon gelatin
- 6 tablespoons swerve

Directions:

1. In a bowl, mix gelatin with 1 tablespoon coconut milk; stir well and leave aside for now.
2. Put the rest of the milk into a pan and heat up over medium heat.
3. Add swerve; stir and cook for 5 minutes
4. In a bowl, mix egg yolks with the hot coconut milk and vanilla extract; stir well and return everything to the pan.
5. Cook for 4 minutes, add gelatin and stir well.
6. Divide this into 4 ramekins and keep your pudding in the fridge until you serve it.

Nutrition Values: Calories: 140; Fat : 2; Fiber : 0; Carbs : 2; Protein : 2

542. Pumpkin Custard

Preparation Time: 15 minutes
Servings: 6
Ingredients:

- 14 ounces canned coconut milk
- 14 ounces canned pumpkin puree
- 2 teaspoons vanilla extract
- 8 scoops stevia
- 3 tablespoons erythritol
- 1 tablespoon gelatin
- 1/4 cup warm water
- A pinch of salt
- 1 teaspoon cinnamon powder
- 1 teaspoon pumpkin pie spice

Directions:

1. In a pot, mix pumpkin puree with coconut milk, a pinch of salt, vanilla extract, cinnamon powder, stevia, erythritol and pumpkin pie spice; stir well and heat up for a couple of minutes
2. In a bowl, mix gelatin and water and stir.
3. Combine the 2 mixtures; stir well, divide custard into ramekins and leave aside to cool down.
4. Keep in the fridge until you serve it.

Nutrition Values: Calories: 200; Fat : 2; Fiber : 1; Carbs : 3; Protein : 5

543. Yummy Orange Cake

Preparation Time: 30 minutes
Servings: 12
Ingredients:

- 1 orange; cut into quarters
- 1 teaspoon vanilla extract
- 1 teaspoon baking powder
- 4 ounces cream cheese
- 4 ounces coconut yogurt
- 9 ounces almond meal
- 2 tablespoons orange zest
- 2 ounces stevia
- 6 eggs
- 4 tablespoons swerve
- A pinch of salt

Directions:

1. In your food processor, pulse orange very well.
2. Add almond meal, swerve, eggs, baking powder, vanilla extract and a pinch of salt and pulse well again.
3. Transfer this into 2 spring form pans, introduce in the oven at 350 degrees F and bake for 20 minutes
4. Meanwhile; in a bowl, mix cream cheese with orange zest, coconut yogurt and stevia and stir well.
5. Place one cake layer on a plate, add half of the cream cheese mix, add the other cake layer and top with the rest of the cream cheese mix.
6. Spread it well, slice and serve

Nutrition Values: Calories: 200; Fat : 13; Fiber : 2; Carbs : 5; Protein : 8

544. Mug Cake

Preparation Time: 5 minutes
Servings: 1
Ingredients:

- 4 tablespoons almond meal
- 1 tablespoon coconut flour
- 2 tablespoon ghee
- 1 teaspoon stevia
- 1/4 teaspoon vanilla extract
- 1/2 teaspoon baking powder
- 1 tablespoon cocoa powder; unsweetened
- 1 egg

Directions:

1.   Put the ghee in a mug and introduce in the microwave for a couple of seconds
2.   Add cocoa powder, stevia, egg, baking powder, vanilla and coconut flour and stir well.
3.   Add almond meal as well; stir again, introduce in the microwave and cook for 2 minutes
4.   Serve your mug cake with berries on top.
Nutrition Values: Calories: 450; Fat : 34; Fiber : 7; Carbs : 10; Protein : 20

545. Marshmallows

Preparation Time: 13 minutes
Servings: 6
Ingredients:
*   12 scoops stevia
*   2 tablespoons gelatin
*   ¾ cup erythritol
*   1/2 cup cold water
*   2 teaspoons vanilla extract
*   1/2 cup hot water
Directions:
1.   In a bowl, mix gelatin with cold water; stir and leave aside for 5 minutes
2.   Put hot water in a pan, add erythritol and stevia and stir well.
3.   Combine this with the gelatin mix, add vanilla extract and stir everything well.
4.   Beat this using a mixer and pour into a baking pan.
5.   Leave aside in the fridge until it sets, then cut into pieces and serve
Nutrition Values: Calories: 140; Fat : 2; Fiber : 1; Carbs : 2; Protein : 4

546. Caramel Custard

Preparation Time: 40 minutes
Servings: 2
Ingredients:
*   1½ teaspoons caramel extract
*   1½ tablespoons swerve
*   2 ounces cream cheese
*   2 eggs
*   1 cup water
*   For the caramel sauce:
*   1/4 teaspoon caramel extract
*   2 tablespoons swerve
*   2 tablespoons ghee
Directions:
1.   In your blender, mix cream cheese with water, 1½ tablespoons swerve, 1½ teaspoons caramel extract and eggs and blend well.
2.   Pour this into 2 greased ramekins, introduce in the oven at 350 degrees F and bake for 30 minutes
3.   Meanwhile; put the ghee in a pot and heat up over medium heat add 1/4 teaspoon caramel extract and 2 tablespoons swerve; stir well and cook until everything melts
4.   Pour this over caramel custard, leave everything to cool down and serve

Nutrition Values: Calories: 254; Fat : 24; Fiber : 1; Carbs : 2; Protein : 8

547. amazing Granola

Preparation Time: 45 minutes
Servings: 4
Ingredients:
*   1 cup coconut; unsweetened and shredded
*   1 cup almonds and pecans; chopped.
*   2 tablespoons coconut oil
*   1 teaspoon nutmeg; ground
*   2 tablespoons stevia
*   1/2 cup pumpkin seeds
*   1/2 cup sunflower seeds
*   1 teaspoon apple pie spice mix
Directions:
1.   In a bowl, mix almonds and pecans with pumpkin seeds, sunflower seeds, coconut, nutmeg and apple pie spice mix and stir well.
2.   Heat up a pan with the coconut oil over medium heat; add stevia and stir until they combine
3.   Pour this over nuts and coconut mix and stir well.
4.   Spread this on a lined baking sheet, introduce in the oven at 300 degrees F and bake for 30 minutes
5.   Leave your granola to cool down, cut and serve it.
Nutrition Values: Calories: 120; Fat : 2; Fiber : 2; Carbs : 4; Protein : 7

548. Chocolate Cookies

Preparation Time: 50 minutes
Servings: 12
Ingredients:
*   1 teaspoon vanilla extract
*   1/2 cup unsweetened chocolate chips
*   1/4 cup swerve
*   1/2 cup ghee
*   1 egg
*   2 tablespoons coconut sugar
*   2 cups almond flour
*   A pinch of salt
Directions:
1.   Heat up a pan with the ghee over medium heat; stir and cook until it browns
2.   Take this off heat and leave aside for 5 minutes
3.   In a bowl, mix egg with vanilla extract, coconut sugar and swerve and stir.
4.   Add melted ghee, flour, salt and half of the chocolate chips and stir everything.
5.   Transfer this to a pan, spread the rest of the chocolate chips on top, introduce in the oven at 350 degrees F and bake for 30 minutes
6.   Slice when it's cold and serve
Nutrition Values: Calories: 230; Fat : 12; Fiber : 2; Carbs : 4; Protein : 5

549. Dessert Smoothie

143

Preparation Time: 5 minutes
Servings: 2
Ingredients:
- 1/2 cup coconut milk
- 1½ cup avocado; pitted and peeled
- 1 mango thinly sliced for serving
- 2 tablespoons green tea powder
- 1 tablespoon coconut sugar
- 2 teaspoons lime zest

Directions:
1. In your smoothie maker, combine milk with avocado, green tea powder and lime zest and pulse well.
2. Add sugar, blend well, divide into 2 glasses and serve with mango slices on top.
Nutrition Values: Calories: 87; Fat : 5; Fiber : 3; Carbs : 6; Protein : 8

550. Peanut Butter And Chia Pudding

Preparation Time: 10 minutes
Servings: 4
Ingredients:
- 1/4 cup peanut butter; unsweetened
- 2 cups almond milk; unsweetened
- 1 teaspoon vanilla extract
- 1/2 cup chia seeds
- 1 teaspoon vanilla stevia
- A pinch of salt

Directions:
1. In a bowl, mix milk with chia seeds, peanut butter, vanilla extract, stevia and pinch of salt and stir well.
2. Leave this pudding aside for 5 minutes, then stir it again, divide into dessert glasses and leave in the fridge for 10 minutes
Nutrition Values: Calories: 120; Fat : 1; Fiber : 2; Carbs : 4; Protein : 2

551. Coconut And Strawberry Desert

Preparation Time: 10 minutes
Servings: 4
Ingredients:
- 1¾ cups coconut cream
- 2 teaspoons granulated stevia
- 1 cup strawberries

Directions:
1. Put coconut cream in a bowl, add stevia and stir very well using an immersion blender.
2. Add strawberries, fold them gently into the mix, divide dessert into glasses and serve them cold.
Nutrition Values: Calories: 245; Fat : 24; Fiber : 1; Carbs : 5; Protein : 4

552. Ricotta Mousse

Preparation Time: 2 hours 10 minutes
Servings: 10
Ingredients:
- 1/2 cup hot coffee
- 2 cups ricotta cheese
- 2½ teaspoons gelatin

- 1 teaspoon espresso powder
- 1 teaspoon vanilla stevia
- 1 teaspoon vanilla extract
- 1 cup whipping cream
- A pinch of salt

Directions:
1. In a bowl, mix coffee with gelatin; stir well and leave aside until coffee is cold.
2. In a bowl, mix espresso, stevia, salt, vanilla extract and ricotta and stir using a mixer.
3. Add coffee mix and stir everything well.
4. Add whipping cream and blend mixture again.
5. Divide into dessert bowls and serve after you've kept it in the fridge for 2 hours
Nutrition Values: Calories: 160; Fat : 13; Fiber : 0; Carbs : 2; Protein : 7

553. Scones

Preparation Time: 20 minutes
Servings: 10
Ingredients:
- 1 cup blueberries
- 1/2 cup coconut flour
- 2 eggs
- 5 tablespoons stevia
- 1/2 cup ghee
- 1/2 cup almond flour
- 2 teaspoons vanilla extract
- 2 teaspoons baking powder
- 1/2 cup heavy cream
- A pinch of salt

Directions:
1. In a bowl, mix almond flour with coconut flour, salt, baking powder and blueberries and stir well.
2. In another bowl, mix heavy cream with ghee, vanilla extract, stevia and eggs and stir well.
3. Combine the 2 mixtures and stir until you obtain your dough.
4. Shape 10 triangles from this mix, place them on a lined baking sheet, introduce in the oven at 350 degrees F and bake for 10 minutes Serve them cold.
Nutrition Values: Calories: 130; Fat : 2; Fiber : 2; Carbs : 4; Protein : 3

554. Delicious Mousse

Preparation Time: 10 minutes
Servings: 12
Ingredients:
- 8 ounces mascarpone cheese
- 1/2 pint blueberries
- 1/2 pint strawberries
- 1 cup whipping cream
- ¾ teaspoon vanilla stevia

Directions:
1. In a bowl, mix whipping cream with stevia and mascarpone and blend well using your mixer.

2.   Arrange a layer of blueberries and strawberries in 12 glasses, then a layer of cream and so on.
3.   Serve this mousse cold!
Nutrition Values: Calories: 143; Fat : 12; Fiber : 1; Carbs : 3; Protein : 2

555. VanillaIce Cream

Preparation Time: 3 hours 10 minutes
Servings: 6
Ingredients:
- 4 eggs; yolks and whites separated
- 1/2 cup swerve
- 1¼ cup heavy whipping cream
- 1 tablespoon vanilla extract
- 1/4 teaspoon cream of tartar

Directions:
1.   In a bowl, mix egg whites with cream of tartar and swerve and stir using your mixer.
2.   In another bowl, whisk cream with vanilla extract and blend very well.
3.   Combine the 2 mixtures and stir gently.
4.   In another bowl, whisk egg yolks very well and then add the two egg whites mix.
5.   Stir gently, pour this into a container and keep in the freezer for 3 hours before serving your ice cream.
Nutrition Values: Calories: 243; Fat : 22; Fiber : 0; Carbs : 2; Protein : 4

556. Jello Dessert

Preparation Time: 2 hours 15 minutes
Servings: 12
Ingredients:
- 2 ounces packets sugar free jello
- 1 teaspoon vanilla extract
- 3 tablespoons erythritol
- 1 cup cold water
- 1 cup hot water
- 1 cup heavy cream
- 1 cup boiling water
- 2 tablespoons gelatin powder

Directions:
- Put jello packets in a bowl, add 1 cup hot water; stir until it dissolves and then mix with 1 cup cold water.
- Pour this into a lined square dish and keep in the fridge for 1 hour.
- Cut into cubes and leave aside for now.
- Meanwhile; in a bowl, mix erythritol with vanilla extract, 1 cup boiling water, gelatin and heavy cream and stir very well.
- Pour half of this mix into a silicon round mold, spread jello cubes, then top with the rest of the gelatin.
- Keep in the fridge for 1 more hour and then serve
Nutrition Values: Calories: 70; Fat : 1; Fiber : 0; Carbs : 1; Protein : 2

557. Nutella

Preparation Time: 10 minutes
Servings: 6
Ingredients:
- 2 ounces coconut oil
- 4 tablespoons cocoa powder
- 1 cup walnuts; halved
- 4 tablespoons stevia
- 1 teaspoon vanilla extract

Directions:
1.   In your food processor, mix cocoa powder with oil, vanilla, walnuts and stevia and blend very well.
2.   Keep in the fridge for a couple of hours and then serve
Nutrition Values: Calories: 100; Fat : 10; Fiber : 1; Carbs : 3; Protein : 2

558. Avocado Pudding

Preparation Time: 10 minutes
Servings: 4
Ingredients:
- 2 avocados; pitted, peeled and chopped.
- 1 tablespoon lime juice
- 2 teaspoons vanilla extract
- 14 ounces canned coconut milk
- 80 drops stevia

Directions:
1.   In your blender, mix avocado with coconut milk, vanilla extract, stevia and lime juice, blend well, spoon into dessert bowls and keep in the fridge until you serve it.
Nutrition Values: Calories: 150; Fat : 3; Fiber : 3; Carbs : 5; Protein : 6

559. Cookie Dough Balls

Preparation Time: 10 minutes
Servings: 10
Ingredients:
- 1/2 cup almond butter
- 1/2 teaspoon vanilla extract
- 3 tablespoons coconut sugar
- 1 teaspoon cinnamon; powder
- 3 tablespoons coconut flour
- 3 tablespoons coconut milk
- 15 drops vanilla stevia
- A pinch of salt

For the topping:
- 3 tablespoons granulated swerve
- 1½ teaspoon cinnamon powder

Directions:
2.   In a bowl, mix almond butter with 1 teaspoon cinnamon, coconut flour, coconut milk, coconut sugar, vanilla extract, vanilla stevia and a pinch of salt and stir well.
3.   Shape balls out of this mix.
4.   In another bowl mix 1½ teaspoon cinnamon powder with swerve and stir well.

5. Roll balls in cinnamon mix and keep them in the fridge until you serve
Nutrition Values: Calories: 89; Fat : 1; Fiber : 2; Carbs : 4; Protein : 2

560. Chocolate Biscotti

Preparation Time: 22 minutes
Servings: 8
Ingredients:
- 2 cups almonds
- 1/4 cup cocoa powder
- 1/4 cup coconut oil
- 2 tablespoons chia seeds
- 1 egg
- 2 tablespoons stevia
- 1 teaspoon baking soda
- 1/4 cup coconut; shredded
- A pinch of salt

Directions:
1. In your food processor, mix chia seeds with almonds and blend well.
2. Add coconut, egg, coconut oil, cocoa powder, a pinch of salt, baking soda and stevia and blend well.
3. Shape 8 biscotti pieces out of this dough, place on a lined baking sheet, introduce in the oven at 350 degrees and bake for 12 minutes
4. Serve them warm or cold.
Nutrition Values: Calories: 200; Fat : 2; Fiber : 1; Carbs : 3; Protein : 4

561. Lime Cheesecake

Preparation Time: 12 minutes
Servings: 10
Ingredients:
- 4 ounces almond meal
- 2 tablespoons ghee; melted
- 2 teaspoons granulated stevia
- 1/4 cup coconut; unsweetened and shredded
- For the filling:
- 1 pound cream cheese
- 2 cup hot water
- 2 sachets sugar free lime jelly
- Zest from 1 lime
- Juice from 1 lime

Directions:
1. Heat up a small pan over medium heat; add ghee and stir until it melts
2. In a bowl, mix coconut with almond meal, ghee and stevia and stir well.
3. Press this on the bottom of a round pan and keep in the fridge for now.
4. Meanwhile; put hot water in a bowl, add jelly sachets and stir until it dissolves
5. Put cream cheese in a bowl, add jelly and stir very well.
6. Add lime juice and zest and blend using your mixer.
7. Pour this over base, spread and keep the cheesecake in the fridge until you serve it.
Nutrition Values: Calories: 300; Fat : 23; Fiber : 2; Carbs : 5; Protein : 7

562. Cherry And Chia Jam

Preparation Time: 27 minutes
Servings: 22
Ingredients:
- 2 ½ cups cherries; pitted
- 10 drops stevia
- 1 cup water
- 3 tablespoons chia seeds
- Peel from 1/2 lemon; grated
- 1/4 cup erythritol
- 1/2 teaspoon vanilla powder

Directions:
1. Put cherries and the water in a pot, add stevia, erythritol, vanilla powder, chia seeds and lemon peel; stir, bring to a simmer and cook for 12 minutes
2. Take off heat and then leave your jam aside for 15 minutes at least.
3. Serve cold.
Nutrition Values: Calories: 60; Fat : 1; Fiber : 1; Carbs : 2; Protein : 0.5

365-DAY MEAL PLAN

DAY	BREAKFAST	LUNCH/DINNER	DESSERT
1	Shrimp Skillet	Spinach Rolls	Matcha Crepe Cake
2	Coconut Yogurt with Chia Seeds	Goat Cheese Fold-Overs	Pumpkin Spices Mini Pies
3	Chia Pudding	Crepe Pie	Nut Bars
4	Egg Fat Bombs	Coconut Soup	Pound Cake
5	Morning "Grits"	Fish Tacos	Tortilla Chips with Cinnamon Recipe
6	Scotch Eggs	Cobb Salad	Granola Yogurt with Berries
7	Bacon Sandwich	Cheese Soup	Berry Sorbet
8	Noatmeal	Tuna Tartare	Coconut Berry Smoothie
9	Breakfast Bake with Meat	Clam Chowder	Coconut Milk Banana Smoothie
10	Breakfast Bagel	Asian Beef Salad	Mango Pineapple Smoothie
11	Egg and Vegetable Hash	Keto Carbonara	Raspberry Green Smoothie
12	Cowboy Skillet	Cauliflower Soup with Seeds	Loaded Berries Smoothie
13	Feta Quiche	Prosciutto-Wrapped Asparagus	Papaya Banana and Kale Smoothie
14	Bacon Pancakes	Stuffed Bell Peppers	Green Orange Smoothie
15	Waffles	Stuffed Eggplants with Goat Cheese	Double Berries Smoothie
16	Chocolate Shake	Korma Curry	Energizing Protein Bars
17	Eggs in Portobello Mushroom Hats	Zucchini Bars	Sweet and Nutty Brownies
18	Matcha Fat Bombs	Mushroom Soup	Keto Macho Nachos
19	Keto Smoothie Bowl	Stuffed Portobello Mushrooms	Peanut Butter Choco Banana Gelato with Mint
20	Salmon Omelet	Lettuce Salad	Cinnamon Peaches and Yogurt
21	Hash Brown	Onion Soup	Pear Mint Honey Popsicles
22	Black's Bangin' Casserole	Asparagus Salad	Orange and Peaches Smoothie
23	Bacon Cups	Cauliflower Tabbouleh	Coconut Spiced Apple Smoothie
24	Spinach Eggs and Cheese	Beef Salpicao	Sweet and Nutty Smoothie
25	Taco Wraps	Stuffed Artichoke	Ginger Berry Smoothie
26	Coffee Donuts	Spinach Rolls	Vegetarian Friendly Smoothie
27	Egg Baked Omelet	Goat Cheese Fold-Overs	ChocNut Smoothie
28	Ranch Risotto	Crepe Pie	Coco Strawberry Smoothie
29	Scotch Eggs	Coconut Soup	Egg Spinach Berries Smoothie
30	Fried Eggs	Fish Tacos	Creamy Dessert Smoothie
31	Shrimp Skillet	Spinach Rolls	Matcha Crepe Cake
32	Coconut Yogurt with Chia Seeds	Goat Cheese Fold-Overs	Pumpkin Spices Mini Pies
33	Chia Pudding	Crepe Pie	Nut Bars
34	Egg Fat Bombs	Coconut Soup	Pound Cake
35	Morning "Grits"	Fish Tacos	Tortilla Chips with Cinnamon Recipe
36	Scotch Eggs	Cobb Salad	Granola Yogurt with Berries
37	Bacon Sandwich	Cheese Soup	Berry Sorbet
38	Noatmeal	Tuna Tartare	Coconut Berry Smoothie
39	Breakfast Bake with Meat	Clam Chowder	Coconut Milk Banana Smoothie
40	Breakfast Bagel	Asian Beef Salad	Mango Pineapple Smoothie
41	Egg and Vegetable Hash	Keto Carbonara	Raspberry Green Smoothie
42	Cowboy Skillet	Cauliflower Soup with Seeds	Loaded Berries Smoothie
43	Feta Quiche	Prosciutto-Wrapped Asparagus	Papaya Banana and Kale Smoothie
44	Bacon Pancakes	Stuffed Bell Peppers	Green Orange Smoothie
45	Waffles	Stuffed Eggplants with Goat	Double Berries Smoothie

		Cheese	
46	Chocolate Shake	Korma Curry	Energizing Protein Bars
47	Eggs in Portobello Mushroom Hats	Zucchini Bars	Sweet and Nutty Brownies
48	Matcha Fat Bombs	Mushroom Soup	Keto Macho Nachos
49	Keto Smoothie Bowl	Stuffed Portobello Mushrooms	Peanut Butter Choco Banana Gelato with Mint
50	Salmon Omelet	Lettuce Salad	Cinnamon Peaches and Yogurt
51	Hash Brown	Onion Soup	Pear Mint Honey Popsicles
52	Black's Bangin' Casserole	Asparagus Salad	Orange and Peaches Smoothie
53	Bacon Cups	Cauliflower Tabbouleh	Coconut Spiced Apple Smoothie
54	Spinach Eggs and Cheese	Beef Salpicao	Sweet and Nutty Smoothie
55	Taco Wraps	Stuffed Artichoke	Ginger Berry Smoothie
56	Coffee Donuts	Spinach Rolls	Vegetarian Friendly Smoothie
57	Egg Baked Omelet	Goat Cheese Fold-Overs	ChocNut Smoothie
58	Ranch Risotto	Crepe Pie	Coco Strawberry Smoothie
59	Scotch Eggs	Coconut Soup	Egg Spinach Berries Smoothie
60	Fried Eggs	Fish Tacos	Creamy Dessert Smoothie
61	Shrimp Skillet	Spinach Rolls	Matcha Crepe Cake
62	Coconut Yogurt with Chia Seeds	Goat Cheese Fold-Overs	Pumpkin Spices Mini Pies
63	Chia Pudding	Crepe Pie	Nut Bars
64	Egg Fat Bombs	Coconut Soup	Pound Cake
65	Morning "Grits"	Fish Tacos	Tortilla Chips with Cinnamon Recipe
66	Scotch Eggs	Cobb Salad	Granola Yogurt with Berries
67	Bacon Sandwich	Cheese Soup	Berry Sorbet
68	Noatmeal	Tuna Tartare	Coconut Berry Smoothie
69	Breakfast Bake with Meat	Clam Chowder	Coconut Milk Banana Smoothie
70	Breakfast Bagel	Asian Beef Salad	Mango Pineapple Smoothie
71	Egg and Vegetable Hash	Keto Carbonara	Raspberry Green Smoothie
72	Cowboy Skillet	Cauliflower Soup with Seeds	Loaded Berries Smoothie
73	Feta Quiche	Prosciutto-Wrapped Asparagus	Papaya Banana and Kale Smoothie
74	Bacon Pancakes	Stuffed Bell Peppers	Green Orange Smoothie
75	Waffles	Stuffed Eggplants with Goat Cheese	Double Berries Smoothie
76	Chocolate Shake	Korma Curry	Energizing Protein Bars
77	Eggs in Portobello Mushroom Hats	Zucchini Bars	Sweet and Nutty Brownies
78	Matcha Fat Bombs	Mushroom Soup	Keto Macho Nachos
79	Keto Smoothie Bowl	Stuffed Portobello Mushrooms	Peanut Butter Choco Banana Gelato with Mint
80	Salmon Omelet	Lettuce Salad	Cinnamon Peaches and Yogurt
81	Hash Brown	Onion Soup	Pear Mint Honey Popsicles
82	Black's Bangin' Casserole	Asparagus Salad	Orange and Peaches Smoothie
83	Bacon Cups	Cauliflower Tabbouleh	Coconut Spiced Apple Smoothie
84	Spinach Eggs and Cheese	Beef Salpicao	Sweet and Nutty Smoothie
85	Taco Wraps	Stuffed Artichoke	Ginger Berry Smoothie
86	Coffee Donuts	Spinach Rolls	Vegetarian Friendly Smoothie
87	Egg Baked Omelet	Goat Cheese Fold-Overs	ChocNut Smoothie
88	Ranch Risotto	Crepe Pie	Coco Strawberry Smoothie
89	Scotch Eggs	Coconut Soup	Egg Spinach Berries Smoothie
90	Fried Eggs	Fish Tacos	Creamy Dessert Smoothie
91	Shrimp Skillet	Spinach Rolls	Matcha Crepe Cake
92	Coconut Yogurt with Chia	Goat Cheese Fold-Overs	Pumpkin Spices Mini Pies

	Seeds		
93	Chia Pudding	Crepe Pie	Nut Bars
94	Egg Fat Bombs	Coconut Soup	Pound Cake
95	Morning "Grits"	Fish Tacos	Tortilla Chips with Cinnamon Recipe
96	Scotch Eggs	Cobb Salad	Granola Yogurt with Berries
97	Bacon Sandwich	Cheese Soup	Berry Sorbet
98	Noatmeal	Tuna Tartare	Coconut Berry Smoothie
99	Breakfast Bake with Meat	Clam Chowder	Coconut Milk Banana Smoothie
100	Breakfast Bagel	Asian Beef Salad	Mango Pineapple Smoothie
101	Egg and Vegetable Hash	Keto Carbonara	Raspberry Green Smoothie
102	Cowboy Skillet	Cauliflower Soup with Seeds	Loaded Berries Smoothie
103	Feta Quiche	Prosciutto-Wrapped Asparagus	Papaya Banana and Kale Smoothie
104	Bacon Pancakes	Stuffed Bell Peppers	Green Orange Smoothie
105	Waffles	Stuffed Eggplants with Goat Cheese	Double Berries Smoothie
106	Chocolate Shake	Korma Curry	Energizing Protein Bars
107	Eggs in Portobello Mushroom Hats	Zucchini Bars	Sweet and Nutty Brownies
108	Matcha Fat Bombs	Mushroom Soup	Keto Macho Nachos
109	Keto Smoothie Bowl	Stuffed Portobello Mushrooms	Peanut Butter Choco Banana Gelato with Mint
110	Salmon Omelet	Lettuce Salad	Cinnamon Peaches and Yogurt
111	Hash Brown	Onion Soup	Pear Mint Honey Popsicles
112	Black's Bangin' Casserole	Asparagus Salad	Orange and Peaches Smoothie
113	Bacon Cups	Cauliflower Tabbouleh	Coconut Spiced Apple Smoothie
114	Spinach Eggs and Cheese	Beef Salpicao	Sweet and Nutty Smoothie
115	Taco Wraps	Stuffed Artichoke	Ginger Berry Smoothie
116	Coffee Donuts	Spinach Rolls	Vegetarian Friendly Smoothie
117	Egg Baked Omelet	Goat Cheese Fold-Overs	ChocNut Smoothie
118	Ranch Risotto	Crepe Pie	Coco Strawberry Smoothie
119	Scotch Eggs	Coconut Soup	Egg Spinach Berries Smoothie
120	Fried Eggs	Fish Tacos	Creamy Dessert Smoothie
121	Shrimp Skillet	Spinach Rolls	Matcha Crepe Cake
122	Coconut Yogurt with Chia Seeds	Goat Cheese Fold-Overs	Pumpkin Spices Mini Pies
123	Chia Pudding	Crepe Pie	Nut Bars
124	Egg Fat Bombs	Coconut Soup	Pound Cake
125	Morning "Grits"	Fish Tacos	Tortilla Chips with Cinnamon Recipe
126	Scotch Eggs	Cobb Salad	Granola Yogurt with Berries
127	Bacon Sandwich	Cheese Soup	Berry Sorbet
128	Noatmeal	Tuna Tartare	Coconut Berry Smoothie
129	Breakfast Bake with Meat	Clam Chowder	Coconut Milk Banana Smoothie
130	Breakfast Bagel	Asian Beef Salad	Mango Pineapple Smoothie
131	Egg and Vegetable Hash	Keto Carbonara	Raspberry Green Smoothie
132	Cowboy Skillet	Cauliflower Soup with Seeds	Loaded Berries Smoothie
133	Feta Quiche	Prosciutto-Wrapped Asparagus	Papaya Banana and Kale Smoothie
134	Bacon Pancakes	Stuffed Bell Peppers	Green Orange Smoothie
135	Waffles	Stuffed Eggplants with Goat Cheese	Double Berries Smoothie
136	Chocolate Shake	Korma Curry	Energizing Protein Bars
137	Eggs in Portobello Mushroom Hats	Zucchini Bars	Sweet and Nutty Brownies

138	Matcha Fat Bombs	Mushroom Soup	Keto Macho Nachos
139	Keto Smoothie Bowl	Stuffed Portobello Mushrooms	Peanut Butter Choco Banana Gelato with Mint
140	Salmon Omelet	Lettuce Salad	Cinnamon Peaches and Yogurt
141	Hash Brown	Onion Soup	Pear Mint Honey Popsicles
142	Black's Bangin' Casserole	Asparagus Salad	Orange and Peaches Smoothie
143	Bacon Cups	Cauliflower Tabbouleh	Coconut Spiced Apple Smoothie
144	Spinach Eggs and Cheese	Beef Salpicao	Sweet and Nutty Smoothie
145	Taco Wraps	Stuffed Artichoke	Ginger Berry Smoothie
146	Coffee Donuts	Spinach Rolls	Vegetarian Friendly Smoothie
147	Egg Baked Omelet	Goat Cheese Fold-Overs	ChocNut Smoothie
148	Ranch Risotto	Crepe Pie	Coco Strawberry Smoothie
149	Scotch Eggs	Coconut Soup	Egg Spinach Berries Smoothie
150	Fried Eggs	Fish Tacos	Creamy Dessert Smoothie
151	Shrimp Skillet	Spinach Rolls	Matcha Crepe Cake
152	Coconut Yogurt with Chia Seeds	Goat Cheese Fold-Overs	Pumpkin Spices Mini Pies
153	Chia Pudding	Crepe Pie	Nut Bars
154	Egg Fat Bombs	Coconut Soup	Pound Cake
155	Morning "Grits"	Fish Tacos	Tortilla Chips with Cinnamon Recipe
156	Scotch Eggs	Cobb Salad	Granola Yogurt with Berries
157	Bacon Sandwich	Cheese Soup	Berry Sorbet
158	Noatmeal	Tuna Tartare	Coconut Berry Smoothie
159	Breakfast Bake with Meat	Clam Chowder	Coconut Milk Banana Smoothie
160	Breakfast Bagel	Asian Beef Salad	Mango Pineapple Smoothie
161	Egg and Vegetable Hash	Keto Carbonara	Raspberry Green Smoothie
162	Cowboy Skillet	Cauliflower Soup with Seeds	Loaded Berries Smoothie
163	Feta Quiche	Prosciutto-Wrapped Asparagus	Papaya Banana and Kale Smoothie
164	Bacon Pancakes	Stuffed Bell Peppers	Green Orange Smoothie
165	Waffles	Stuffed Eggplants with Goat Cheese	Double Berries Smoothie
166	Chocolate Shake	Korma Curry	Energizing Protein Bars
167	Eggs in Portobello Mushroom Hats	Zucchini Bars	Sweet and Nutty Brownies
168	Matcha Fat Bombs	Mushroom Soup	Keto Macho Nachos
169	Keto Smoothie Bowl	Stuffed Portobello Mushrooms	Peanut Butter Choco Banana Gelato with Mint
170	Salmon Omelet	Lettuce Salad	Cinnamon Peaches and Yogurt
171	Hash Brown	Onion Soup	Pear Mint Honey Popsicles
172	Black's Bangin' Casserole	Asparagus Salad	Orange and Peaches Smoothie
173	Bacon Cups	Cauliflower Tabbouleh	Coconut Spiced Apple Smoothie
174	Spinach Eggs and Cheese	Beef Salpicao	Sweet and Nutty Smoothie
175	Taco Wraps	Stuffed Artichoke	Ginger Berry Smoothie
176	Coffee Donuts	Spinach Rolls	Vegetarian Friendly Smoothie
177	Egg Baked Omelet	Goat Cheese Fold-Overs	ChocNut Smoothie
178	Ranch Risotto	Crepe Pie	Coco Strawberry Smoothie
179	Scotch Eggs	Coconut Soup	Egg Spinach Berries Smoothie
180	Fried Eggs	Fish Tacos	Creamy Dessert Smoothie
181	Shrimp Skillet	Spinach Rolls	Matcha Crepe Cake
182	Coconut Yogurt with Chia Seeds	Goat Cheese Fold-Overs	Pumpkin Spices Mini Pies
183	Chia Pudding	Crepe Pie	Nut Bars
184	Egg Fat Bombs	Coconut Soup	Pound Cake
185	Morning "Grits"	Fish Tacos	Tortilla Chips with Cinnamon

			Recipe
186	Scotch Eggs	Cobb Salad	Granola Yogurt with Berries
187	Bacon Sandwich	Cheese Soup	Berry Sorbet
188	Noatmeal	Tuna Tartare	Coconut Berry Smoothie
189	Breakfast Bake with Meat	Clam Chowder	Coconut Milk Banana Smoothie
190	Breakfast Bagel	Asian Beef Salad	Mango Pineapple Smoothie
191	Egg and Vegetable Hash	Keto Carbonara	Raspberry Green Smoothie
192	Cowboy Skillet	Cauliflower Soup with Seeds	Loaded Berries Smoothie
193	Feta Quiche	Prosciutto-Wrapped Asparagus	Papaya Banana and Kale Smoothie
194	Bacon Pancakes	Stuffed Bell Peppers	Green Orange Smoothie
195	Waffles	Stuffed Eggplants with Goat Cheese	Double Berries Smoothie
196	Chocolate Shake	Korma Curry	Energizing Protein Bars
197	Eggs in Portobello Mushroom Hats	Zucchini Bars	Sweet and Nutty Brownies
198	Matcha Fat Bombs	Mushroom Soup	Keto Macho Nachos
199	Keto Smoothie Bowl	Stuffed Portobello Mushrooms	Peanut Butter Choco Banana Gelato with Mint
200	Salmon Omelet	Lettuce Salad	Cinnamon Peaches and Yogurt
201	Hash Brown	Onion Soup	Pear Mint Honey Popsicles
202	Black's Bangin' Casserole	Asparagus Salad	Orange and Peaches Smoothie
203	Bacon Cups	Cauliflower Tabbouleh	Coconut Spiced Apple Smoothie
204	Spinach Eggs and Cheese	Beef Salpicao	Sweet and Nutty Smoothie
205	Taco Wraps	Stuffed Artichoke	Ginger Berry Smoothie
206	Coffee Donuts	Spinach Rolls	Vegetarian Friendly Smoothie
207	Egg Baked Omelet	Goat Cheese Fold-Overs	ChocNut Smoothie
208	Ranch Risotto	Crepe Pie	Coco Strawberry Smoothie
209	Scotch Eggs	Coconut Soup	Egg Spinach Berries Smoothie
210	Fried Eggs	Fish Tacos	Creamy Dessert Smoothie
211	Shrimp Skillet	Spinach Rolls	Matcha Crepe Cake
212	Coconut Yogurt with Chia Seeds	Goat Cheese Fold-Overs	Pumpkin Spices Mini Pies
213	Chia Pudding	Crepe Pie	Nut Bars
214	Egg Fat Bombs	Coconut Soup	Pound Cake
215	Morning "Grits"	Fish Tacos	Tortilla Chips with Cinnamon Recipe
216	Scotch Eggs	Cobb Salad	Granola Yogurt with Berries
217	Bacon Sandwich	Cheese Soup	Berry Sorbet
218	Noatmeal	Tuna Tartare	Coconut Berry Smoothie
219	Breakfast Bake with Meat	Clam Chowder	Coconut Milk Banana Smoothie
220	Breakfast Bagel	Asian Beef Salad	Mango Pineapple Smoothie
221	Egg and Vegetable Hash	Keto Carbonara	Raspberry Green Smoothie
222	Cowboy Skillet	Cauliflower Soup with Seeds	Loaded Berries Smoothie
223	Feta Quiche	Prosciutto-Wrapped Asparagus	Papaya Banana and Kale Smoothie
224	Bacon Pancakes	Stuffed Bell Peppers	Green Orange Smoothie
225	Waffles	Stuffed Eggplants with Goat Cheese	Double Berries Smoothie
226	Chocolate Shake	Korma Curry	Energizing Protein Bars
227	Eggs in Portobello Mushroom Hats	Zucchini Bars	Sweet and Nutty Brownies
228	Matcha Fat Bombs	Mushroom Soup	Keto Macho Nachos
229	Keto Smoothie Bowl	Stuffed Portobello Mushrooms	Peanut Butter Choco Banana Gelato with Mint
230	Salmon Omelet	Lettuce Salad	Cinnamon Peaches and Yogurt

231	Hash Brown	Onion Soup	Pear Mint Honey Popsicles
232	Black's Bangin' Casserole	Asparagus Salad	Orange and Peaches Smoothie
233	Bacon Cups	Cauliflower Tabbouleh	Coconut Spiced Apple Smoothie
234	Spinach Eggs and Cheese	Beef Salpicao	Sweet and Nutty Smoothie
235	Taco Wraps	Stuffed Artichoke	Ginger Berry Smoothie
236	Coffee Donuts	Spinach Rolls	Vegetarian Friendly Smoothie
237	Egg Baked Omelet	Goat Cheese Fold-Overs	ChocNut Smoothie
238	Ranch Risotto	Crepe Pie	Coco Strawberry Smoothie
239	Scotch Eggs	Coconut Soup	Egg Spinach Berries Smoothie
240	Fried Eggs	Fish Tacos	Creamy Dessert Smoothie
241	Shrimp Skillet	Spinach Rolls	Matcha Crepe Cake
242	Coconut Yogurt with Chia Seeds	Goat Cheese Fold-Overs	Pumpkin Spices Mini Pies
243	Chia Pudding	Crepe Pie	Nut Bars
244	Egg Fat Bombs	Coconut Soup	Pound Cake
245	Morning "Grits"	Fish Tacos	Tortilla Chips with Cinnamon Recipe
246	Scotch Eggs	Cobb Salad	Granola Yogurt with Berries
247	Bacon Sandwich	Cheese Soup	Berry Sorbet
248	Noatmeal	Tuna Tartare	Coconut Berry Smoothie
249	Breakfast Bake with Meat	Clam Chowder	Coconut Milk Banana Smoothie
250	Breakfast Bagel	Asian Beef Salad	Mango Pineapple Smoothie
251	Egg and Vegetable Hash	Keto Carbonara	Raspberry Green Smoothie
252	Cowboy Skillet	Cauliflower Soup with Seeds	Loaded Berries Smoothie
253	Feta Quiche	Prosciutto-Wrapped Asparagus	Papaya Banana and Kale Smoothie
254	Bacon Pancakes	Stuffed Bell Peppers	Green Orange Smoothie
255	Waffles	Stuffed Eggplants with Goat Cheese	Double Berries Smoothie
256	Chocolate Shake	Korma Curry	Energizing Protein Bars
257	Eggs in Portobello Mushroom Hats	Zucchini Bars	Sweet and Nutty Brownies
258	Matcha Fat Bombs	Mushroom Soup	Keto Macho Nachos
259	Keto Smoothie Bowl	Stuffed Portobello Mushrooms	Peanut Butter Choco Banana Gelato with Mint
260	Salmon Omelet	Lettuce Salad	Cinnamon Peaches and Yogurt
261	Hash Brown	Onion Soup	Pear Mint Honey Popsicles
262	Black's Bangin' Casserole	Asparagus Salad	Orange and Peaches Smoothie
263	Bacon Cups	Cauliflower Tabbouleh	Coconut Spiced Apple Smoothie
264	Spinach Eggs and Cheese	Beef Salpicao	Sweet and Nutty Smoothie
265	Taco Wraps	Stuffed Artichoke	Ginger Berry Smoothie
266	Coffee Donuts	Spinach Rolls	Vegetarian Friendly Smoothie
267	Egg Baked Omelet	Goat Cheese Fold-Overs	ChocNut Smoothie
268	Ranch Risotto	Crepe Pie	Coco Strawberry Smoothie
269	Scotch Eggs	Coconut Soup	Egg Spinach Berries Smoothie
270	Fried Eggs	Fish Tacos	Creamy Dessert Smoothie
271	Shrimp Skillet	Spinach Rolls	Matcha Crepe Cake
272	Coconut Yogurt with Chia Seeds	Goat Cheese Fold-Overs	Pumpkin Spices Mini Pies
273	Chia Pudding	Crepe Pie	Nut Bars
274	Egg Fat Bombs	Coconut Soup	Pound Cake
275	Morning "Grits"	Fish Tacos	Tortilla Chips with Cinnamon Recipe
276	Scotch Eggs	Cobb Salad	Granola Yogurt with Berries
277	Bacon Sandwich	Cheese Soup	Berry Sorbet
278	Noatmeal	Tuna Tartare	Coconut Berry Smoothie

279	Breakfast Bake with Meat	Clam Chowder	Coconut Milk Banana Smoothie
280	Breakfast Bagel	Asian Beef Salad	Mango Pineapple Smoothie
281	Egg and Vegetable Hash	Keto Carbonara	Raspberry Green Smoothie
282	Cowboy Skillet	Cauliflower Soup with Seeds	Loaded Berries Smoothie
283	Feta Quiche	Prosciutto-Wrapped Asparagus	Papaya Banana and Kale Smoothie
284	Bacon Pancakes	Stuffed Bell Peppers	Green Orange Smoothie
285	Waffles	Stuffed Eggplants with Goat Cheese	Double Berries Smoothie
286	Chocolate Shake	Korma Curry	Energizing Protein Bars
287	Eggs in Portobello Mushroom Hats	Zucchini Bars	Sweet and Nutty Brownies
288	Matcha Fat Bombs	Mushroom Soup	Keto Macho Nachos
289	Keto Smoothie Bowl	Stuffed Portobello Mushrooms	Peanut Butter Choco Banana Gelato with Mint
290	Salmon Omelet	Lettuce Salad	Cinnamon Peaches and Yogurt
291	Hash Brown	Onion Soup	Pear Mint Honey Popsicles
292	Black's Bangin' Casserole	Asparagus Salad	Orange and Peaches Smoothie
293	Bacon Cups	Cauliflower Tabbouleh	Coconut Spiced Apple Smoothie
294	Spinach Eggs and Cheese	Beef Salpicao	Sweet and Nutty Smoothie
295	Taco Wraps	Stuffed Artichoke	Ginger Berry Smoothie
296	Coffee Donuts	Spinach Rolls	Vegetarian Friendly Smoothie
297	Egg Baked Omelet	Goat Cheese Fold-Overs	ChocNut Smoothie
298	Ranch Risotto	Crepe Pie	Coco Strawberry Smoothie
299	Scotch Eggs	Coconut Soup	Egg Spinach Berries Smoothie
300	Fried Eggs	Fish Tacos	Creamy Dessert Smoothie
301	Shrimp Skillet	Spinach Rolls	Matcha Crepe Cake
302	Coconut Yogurt with Chia Seeds	Goat Cheese Fold-Overs	Pumpkin Spices Mini Pies
303	Chia Pudding	Crepe Pie	Nut Bars
304	Egg Fat Bombs	Coconut Soup	Pound Cake
305	Morning "Grits"	Fish Tacos	Tortilla Chips with Cinnamon Recipe
306	Scotch Eggs	Cobb Salad	Granola Yogurt with Berries
307	Bacon Sandwich	Cheese Soup	Berry Sorbet
308	Noatmeal	Tuna Tartare	Coconut Berry Smoothie
309	Breakfast Bake with Meat	Clam Chowder	Coconut Milk Banana Smoothie
310	Breakfast Bagel	Asian Beef Salad	Mango Pineapple Smoothie
311	Egg and Vegetable Hash	Keto Carbonara	Raspberry Green Smoothie
312	Cowboy Skillet	Cauliflower Soup with Seeds	Loaded Berries Smoothie
313	Feta Quiche	Prosciutto-Wrapped Asparagus	Papaya Banana and Kale Smoothie
314	Bacon Pancakes	Stuffed Bell Peppers	Green Orange Smoothie
315	Waffles	Stuffed Eggplants with Goat Cheese	Double Berries Smoothie
316	Chocolate Shake	Korma Curry	Energizing Protein Bars
317	Eggs in Portobello Mushroom Hats	Zucchini Bars	Sweet and Nutty Brownies
318	Matcha Fat Bombs	Mushroom Soup	Keto Macho Nachos
319	Keto Smoothie Bowl	Stuffed Portobello Mushrooms	Peanut Butter Choco Banana Gelato with Mint
320	Salmon Omelet	Lettuce Salad	Cinnamon Peaches and Yogurt
321	Hash Brown	Onion Soup	Pear Mint Honey Popsicles
322	Black's Bangin' Casserole	Asparagus Salad	Orange and Peaches Smoothie
323	Bacon Cups	Cauliflower Tabbouleh	Coconut Spiced Apple Smoothie
324	Spinach Eggs and Cheese	Beef Salpicao	Sweet and Nutty Smoothie

325	Taco Wraps	Stuffed Artichoke	Ginger Berry Smoothie
326	Coffee Donuts	Spinach Rolls	Vegetarian Friendly Smoothie
327	Egg Baked Omelet	Goat Cheese Fold-Overs	ChocNut Smoothie
328	Ranch Risotto	Crepe Pie	Coco Strawberry Smoothie
329	Scotch Eggs	Coconut Soup	Egg Spinach Berries Smoothie
330	Fried Eggs	Fish Tacos	Creamy Dessert Smoothie
331	Shrimp Skillet	Spinach Rolls	Matcha Crepe Cake
332	Coconut Yogurt with Chia Seeds	Goat Cheese Fold-Overs	Pumpkin Spices Mini Pies
333	Chia Pudding	Crepe Pie	Nut Bars
334	Egg Fat Bombs	Coconut Soup	Pound Cake
335	Morning "Grits"	Fish Tacos	Tortilla Chips with Cinnamon Recipe
336	Scotch Eggs	Cobb Salad	Granola Yogurt with Berries
337	Bacon Sandwich	Cheese Soup	Berry Sorbet
338	Noatmeal	Tuna Tartare	Coconut Berry Smoothie
339	Breakfast Bake with Meat	Clam Chowder	Coconut Milk Banana Smoothie
340	Breakfast Bagel	Asian Beef Salad	Mango Pineapple Smoothie
341	Egg and Vegetable Hash	Keto Carbonara	Raspberry Green Smoothie
342	Cowboy Skillet	Cauliflower Soup with Seeds	Loaded Berries Smoothie
343	Feta Quiche	Prosciutto-Wrapped Asparagus	Papaya Banana and Kale Smoothie
344	Bacon Pancakes	Stuffed Bell Peppers	Green Orange Smoothie
345	Waffles	Stuffed Eggplants with Goat Cheese	Double Berries Smoothie
346	Chocolate Shake	Korma Curry	Energizing Protein Bars
347	Eggs in Portobello Mushroom Hats	Zucchini Bars	Sweet and Nutty Brownies
348	Matcha Fat Bombs	Mushroom Soup	Keto Macho Nachos
349	Keto Smoothie Bowl	Stuffed Portobello Mushrooms	Peanut Butter Choco Banana Gelato with Mint
350	Salmon Omelet	Lettuce Salad	Cinnamon Peaches and Yogurt
351	Hash Brown	Onion Soup	Pear Mint Honey Popsicles
352	Black's Bangin' Casserole	Asparagus Salad	Orange and Peaches Smoothie
353	Bacon Cups	Cauliflower Tabbouleh	Coconut Spiced Apple Smoothie
354	Spinach Eggs and Cheese	Beef Salpicao	Sweet and Nutty Smoothie
355	Taco Wraps	Stuffed Artichoke	Ginger Berry Smoothie
356	Coffee Donuts	Spinach Rolls	Vegetarian Friendly Smoothie
357	Egg Baked Omelet	Goat Cheese Fold-Overs	ChocNut Smoothie
358	Ranch Risotto	Crepe Pie	Coco Strawberry Smoothie
359	Scotch Eggs	Coconut Soup	Egg Spinach Berries Smoothie
360	Fried Eggs	Fish Tacos	Creamy Dessert Smoothie
361	Shrimp Skillet	Spinach Rolls	Matcha Crepe Cake
362	Coconut Yogurt with Chia Seeds	Goat Cheese Fold-Overs	Pumpkin Spices Mini Pies
363	Chia Pudding	Crepe Pie	Nut Bars
364	Egg Fat Bombs	Coconut Soup	Pound Cake
365	Morning "Grits"	Fish Tacos	Tortilla Chips with Cinnamon Recipe

CPSIA information can be obtained
at www.ICGtesting.com
Printed in the USA
LVHW051115091222
734879LV00050B/920

9 781649 848901